Antibody-Mediated Delivery Systems

Targeted Diagnosis and Therapy

Editor

John D. Rodwell
Vice President, Discovery Research
CYTOGEN Corporation
Princeton, New Jersey

1. Antibody-Mediated Delivery Systems, *edited by John D. Rodwell*

Antibody-Mediated Delivery Systems

edited by

John D. Rodwell

CYTOGEN Corporation
Princeton, New Jersey

Marcel Dekker, Inc. **New York • Basel**

Library of Congress Cataloging-in-Publication Data

Antibody-mediated delivery systems.

(Targeted diagnosis and therapy series ; 1)
Includes index.
1. Antibody-drug conjugates. I. Rodwell, John D.
II. Series.
RS201.A56A67 1988 615'.37 88-3715
ISBN 0-8247-7960-6

MARCEL DEKKER, INC.
270 Madison Avenue, New York, New York, 10016

Current printing (last digit):
10 9 8 7 6 5 4 3 2 1

PRINTED IN THE UNITED STATES OF AMERICA

Introduction to the Series

Targeted Diagnosis and Therapy is a series intended to collect new knowledge generated in the research and development of self-directed diagnostic and therapeutic agents. The powerful tools of recombinant DNA and monoclonal antibody technologies have contributed immensely to our understanding of the concept of molecular recognition as well as protein structure-function relationships. This has yielded a view of the future that includes the use of a variety of new pharmaceutical products. These products will have the property of localizing to a predetermined site, with a consequent diagnostic or therapeutic effect. The clinical use of these products will include the treatment in vivo of malignant organs or tissues as well as elimination of specific cell types in ex vivo bone marrow-purging procedures. Each volume will focus on one product or strategy, and contain the relevant preclinical and/or clinical experience. The list of near-term subjects includes a variety of antibody conjugates, the interferons, the interleukins, tissue plasminogen activator, and gene therapy. Other volumes will deal with the next generation of agents, such as genetically engineered toxins and fusion proteins. It is expected that the series will be useful for basic researchers and clinicians alike.

New frontiers lie ahead. The opportunities for research and development of important new pharmaceutical products are considerable. It is hoped that Targeted Diagnosis and Therapy will assist in the efforts to achieve this goal.

John D. Rodwell
Editor

Preface

The development of monoclonal antibody technology in 1975 by George Köhler and Caesar Milstein caused a rebirth of interest in the use of antibodies to target substances for diagnosis and treatment of human diseases. This rebirth was accompanied by a great deal of optimism by members of the biomedical, business, and financial communities. Medical researchers were faced with an array of promising antibodies and a long list of substances (toxins, isotopes, drugs) that were candidates for chemical coupling. A great deal of effort followed, in which a variety of antibody conjugates were prepared and evaluated. Now, more than a decade later, the high hopes are as yet unrealized. This is true despite hard work and the expenditure of millions of dollars in public and private money. There are a number of reasons for this, some of which are described below.

First, it is now apparent that more careful specificity analyses are needed in choosing antibodies for in vivo use. For example, many antibodies originally thought to be specific for antigens unique to tumor cells were found in practice to cross-react to varying degrees with normal tissue. To the extent that this occurred, antibody conjugates were diverted from their intended target to normal tissue.

Second, the importance of the properties intrinsic to substances being attached to antibodies has become recognized. For example, toxins, due to their potency, were considered highly attractive candidates for conjugation, despite the fact that they had targeting properties of their own. When immunotoxins were prepared, these targeting properties competed with antibody specificity and caused conjugates to localize in normal tissue, sometimes with disastrous results. The use of toxin fragments, which lacked the tissue receptor portion, did not circumvent the nontarget localization problems of immunoconjugates. Upon injection, these rapidly localized to elements of the reticuloendothelial system. Nevertheless, because of their potency, toxins are still viewed as appealing candidates, and a variety of genetic engineering approaches to modified molecules are being explored in an effort to make them useful.

In another example of the importance of intrinsic properties, conjugates prepared with hydrophobic chemotherapeutic agents (e.g., doxorubicin) may seem to carry a large number of covalently attached drugs when in fact many molecules are merely adsorbed. After injection, the loss of adsorbed drugs to serum proteins and other receptors made experiments with such "conjugates" difficult to interpret or reproduce.

Third, there evolved a more refined appreciation for the potential effect of the chemistry of conjugation on antibody reactivity. Specifically, scientists realized that there were practical limits to the degree of chemical treatment or covalent modification of antibodies which, when exceeded, compromised immunoreactivity.

Recognition of the above and other points has led to more careful experimentation which provides both a sound foundation for future work and a reason for sustained optimism. The purpose of this volume is to collect the most current methodologies for preparing a variety of antibody conjugates useful for targeted diagnosis and therapy. These methodologies take into account the latter two issues identified above and represent the best efforts of each contributor. A number of books already exist that collect the expertise of scientists who are pursuing monoclonal antibodies of more appropriate specificity (the first issue above), so this aspect is not treated here. The contributors to this volume were requested to write a detailed review of their experience with a particular type of conjugate, highlighting both the rationale for its preparation and the conjugation chemistry used. These include antibodies coupled to biological response modifiers, photosensitizers, several diagnostic and therapeutic radiometal chelates, and a variety of chemotherapeutic agents. An appendix to each chapter on a subject conjugate details the specifics of preparation and analysis. It is hoped that readers interested in targeted diagnosis or therapy with antibody conjugates will be encouraged to prepare and evaluate one or another of those described in this volume, benefiting in the process from the contributors' experiences.

No one succeeds in an undertaking such as this without assistance. First, my humble thanks go to the authors who contributed extremely interesting and instructive manuscripts. Next, I thank Drs. Vernon Alvarez and Daniel Coughlin, two of my colleagues at CYTOGEN Corporation, who helped me review some of the chemistry described herein. I am also grateful to the staff of the publisher, Marcel Dekker, Inc. Their encouragement and enthusiasm for this project never wavered. Last, but far from least, I would like to thank my editorial assistant and secretary Ms. Carol Peevey. As many of the authors can attest, her cheerful determination to encourage them to submit manuscripts on time was a great help, as was her ability to keep me organized.

John D. Rodwell

Contents

Contributors

Vernon L. Alvarez, Ph.D. Director, Chemical Research, CYTOGEN Corporation, Princeton, New Jersey

Eric L. Andrews, B.S. Laboratory Technician, Department of Immunology, Lilly Research Laboratories, Indianapolis, Indiana

Lynn D. Apelgren, M.S. Assistant Senior Immunologist, Department of Immunology, Lilly Research Laboratories, Indianapolis, Indiana

A. Leroy Baker, Ph.D. Senior Research Scientist, Department of Chemical, Cancer, and Virology Research, Lilly Research Laboratories, Indianapolis, Indiana

A. Huntley Blair, Ph.D. Professor of Biochemistry and Associate Professor of Pathology, Departments of Biochemistry and Pathology, Dalhousie University, Halifax, Nova Scotia, Canada

Stephen L. Briggs, B.S. Assistant Organic Chemist, Department of Chemical, Cancer, and Virology Research, Lilly Research Laboratories, Indianapolis, Indiana

Thomas F. Bumol, Ph.D. Research Scientist, Department of Immunology Research, Lilly Research Laboratories, Indianapolis, Indiana

Rei K. Chiou, Ph.D.* Professor, Department of Urologic Surgery, University of Minnesota and Veterans Administration Medical Center, Minneapolis, Minnesota

Daniel J. Coughlin, Ph.D. Group Leader, Organic Synthesis, CYTOGEN Corporation, Princeton, New Jersey

Heather Deal, B.A. Graduate Student, Department of Microbiology, University of British Columbia, Vancouver, British Columbia, Canada

Sonja V. DeHerdt, B.S. Associate Immunologist, Department of Immunology Research, Lilly Research Laboratories, Indianapolis, Indiana

Erwin Diener, Ph.D. Professor and Chairman, Department of Immunology, University of Alberta, Edmonton, Alberta, Canada

Michael K. Elson, Ph.D. Research Scientist, Department of Nuclear Medicine, Veterans Administration Medical Center, Minneapolis, Minnesota

A. A. Epenetos, Ph.D. Senior Lecturer and Consultant, Department of Clinical Oncology, Hammersmith Hospital, London, England

Steve D. Figard, Ph.D.† Post-doctoral Staff Member, Medical Radioisotopes Research Program, Los Alamos National Laboratory, Los Alamos, New Mexico

Arthur E. Frankel, M.D. Associate Professor of Medicine, Department of Medicine, Duke University Medical Center, Durham, North Carolina

Tarunendu Ghose, Ph.D. Professor of Pathology and Associate Professor of Microbiology, Dalhousie University and Associate Pathologist, Victoria General Hospital, Halifax, Nova Scotia, Canada

D. J. Hnatowich, Ph.D. Research Scientist, Department of Nuclear Medicine, University of Massachusetts Medical Center, Worcester, Massachusetts

Jaroslav Kralovec, Ph.D. Research Associate, Departments of Biochemistry and Pathology, Dalhousie University, Halifax, Nova Scotia, Canada

Paul H. Lange, M.D. Professor and Vice-Chairman, Department of Urologic Surgery, Veterans Administration Medical Center and University of Minnesota, Minneapolis, Minnesota

David K. Lavallee, Ph.D. Professor, Department of Chemistry, Hunter College of the City University of New York, New York, New York.

**Current Affiliation*: Associate Professor, Department of Urology, George Washington University, Washington, D.C.

†*Current Affiliation*: Research Biochemist, OB/GYN Research and Development 1/M Physiological Diagnostics, Abbot Laboratories, Abbot Park, Illinois

Chyi Lee, Ph.D. Senior Scientist, Organic Synthesis, CYTOGEN Corporation, Princeton, New Jersey

Julia Levy, Ph.D. Professor, Department of Microbiology, University of British Columbia, Vancouver, British Columbia, Canada

Daniel Liu, Ph.D. Research Scientist, Department of Research and Development, Quadralogic Technologies, Inc., Vancouver, British Columbia, Canada

B. Michael Longenecker, Ph.D. Professor, Department of Immunology, University of Alberta, Edmonton, Alberta, Canada

A. Dwight Lopes, Ph.D. Group Leader, Antibody Evaluations, CYTOGEN Corporation, Princeton, New Jersey

Molly Mammen, B.S. Senior Technologist, Department of Pathology, Dalhousie University, Halifax, Nova Scotia, Canada

Thomas J. McKearn, Ph.D. Senior Vice President, Scientific Affairs, CYTOGEN Corporation, Princeton, New Jersey

Ian Farquhar Campbell McKenzie, Ph.D. Professor, Research Centre for Cancer and Transplantation, Department of Pathology, University of Melbourne, Parkville, Victoria, Australia

Janet A. Mercer-Smith, Ph.D. Principal Investigator, Medical Radioisotopes Research Program, Los Alamos National Laboratory, Los Alamos, New Mexico

Donald F. Palme II, M.S. Research Assistant and Graduate Student, Department of Microbiology, University of Minnesota, Minneapolis, Minnesota

Geoffrey A. Pietersz, Ph.D. Senior Research Fellow, Research Centre for Cancer and Transplantation, Department of Pathology, University of Melbourne, Parkville, Victoria, Australia

Jeanette C. Roberts, Ph.D. J. Robert Oppenheimer Fellow, Medical Radioisotopes Research Program, Los Alamos National Laboratory, Los Alamos, New Mexico

John D. Rodwell, Ph.D. Vice President, Discovery Research, CYTOGEN Corporation, Princeton, New Jersey

G. Rowlinson, Ph.D. Research Scientist, Department of Clinical Oncology, Hammersmith Hospital, London, England

David M. Schlossman, Ph.D. Assistant Professor, Department of Medicine, Duke University Medical Center, Durham, North Carolina

A. A. Sinha, Ph.D. Professor, Department of Immunology, University of Alberta, Edmonton, Alberta, Canada

Mark J. Smyth, B.S. Doctorial Student, Research Centre for Cancer and Transplantation, Department of Pathology, University of Melbourne, Parkville, Victoria, Australia

D. Snook, Ph.D. Research Scientist, Department of Clinical Oncology, Hammersmith Hospital, London, England

Marshall E. Spearman, Ph.D. Senior Pharmacologist, Department of Drug Disposition, Lilly Research Laboratories, Indianapolis, Indiana

Anthea Tench Stammers, M.S. Research Scientist, Department of Microbiology, University of British Columbia, Vancouver, British Columbia, Canada

J. Kevin Steele, B.S.* Graduate Student, Department of Microbiology, University of British Columbia, Vancouver, British Columbia, Canada

S. Stewart, Ph.D. Research Scientist, Department of Clinical Oncology, Hammersmith Hospital, London, England

P. O. Uadia, Ph.D. Professor, Department of Biochemistry, University of Port Harcourt, Port Harcourt, Nigeria

Robert L. Vessella, Ph.D. Assistant Professor, Department of Urologic Surgery, Veterans Administration Medical Center and University of Minnesota, Minneapolis, Minnesota

Carl-Wilhelm Vogel, Ph.D. Associate Professor, Department of Biochemistry and Medicine, Vincent T. Lombardi Cancer Center, and International Center of Interdisciplinary Studies of Immunology, Georgetown University School of Medicine, Washington, D.C.

Philip C. Welsh, M.S. Research Analyst, Department of Medicine, Duke University Medical Center, Durham, North Carolina

Barry W. Wessels, Ph.D. Associate Professor, Department of Radiology, The George Washington University Medical Center, Washington, D.C.

Stephen Whitney, B.S.† Professor, Department of Microbiology, University of British Columbia, Vancouver, British Columbia, Canada

David Ian Withers, B.S. Research Technician, Department of Medicine, Duke University Medical Center, Durham, North Carolina

Shusheng Xie, M.D. Visiting Scientist, Department of Immunology, University of Alberta, Edmonton, Alberta, Canada

Lizhang Yu, M.D. Visiting Scientist, Department of Immunology, University of Alberta, Edmonton, Alberta, Canada

---

**Current Affiliation*: Research Fellow, Department of Pathology, Harvard Medical School, Boston, Massachusetts.

†*Current Affiliation*: Research Scientist, Research and Development, Quadralogic Technologies, Inc., Vancouver, British Columbia, Canada

1

Experimental Application of Target-Specific Immunoconjugates Containing Daunomycin as the Cytocidal Component

ERWIN DIENER, SHUSHENG XIE, LIZHANG YU, B. MICHAEL LONGENECKER, and A. A. SINHA
University of Alberta, Edmonton, Alberta, Canada

I. INTRODUCTION

The use of toxic proteins, such as ricin, a disulfide-linked heterodimer, as the conjugand with cell-specific targeting carriers raises the serious problem of nonspecific toxicity due to the presence on the toxin's B chain of binding sites for oligosaccharides present on all cells of the body (1,2, reviewed in Ref. 3). Although it is possible to reveal the target specificity of a ricin- or abrin-containing immunotoxin in vitro by blocking these receptors with lactose or galactose (4,5), such a procedure is not feasible in vivo (6). The separate, potentially toxic A chain of ricin, whose entry into the target cell depends on endocytosis, may fail to exert cytotoxicity if endosomes fuse with lysosomes before the peptide is translocated from endocytic vesicles to the cytosol. Thus, delayed fusion of endosomes with lysosomes favorably affects the efficacy of these immunotoxins whose cytocidal conjugand consists of a peptide. The importance of this concept has been impressively documented in a recent study showing that the degree of resistance of target cells to a ricin A chain-containing immunotoxin correlates with the rapidity at which it enters the lysosomal compartment (7). A survey of the literature reveals the following criteria as being important in the choice of an immunotoxin's cytocidal component:

1. Its pharmacological property must resist the acidic intralysosomal environment.
2. When part of an immunotoxin, it must be reversibly conjugated with the target-specific carrier so as to be cleaved from the latter inside the cell without loss of the toxic potential.
3. Its physicochemical properties must allow it to exit from the endolysosomal compartment into the cytosol.
4. It must have no binding affinity for cell surface structures.

For peptide immunotoxins to come close in meeting these criteria, their application in vitro, and more so in vivo, requires manipulative procedures whose complexity calls in question their practicability, particularly for use in vivo. In contrast, cytocidal drugs, such as anthracyclines, after having been delivered to cells by an appropriate antibody, resist the intralysosomal environment and, once freed from the carrier, may readily enter the cytosol. One of the major problems with drugs as conjugands has been their dependence on proteolysis for release from the protein carrier. This process has proven difficult due to steric hindrance preventing access of intralysosomal peptidases to the peptide linkage between the drug and the carrier, and to the amino bond not being adjacent to an asymmetric carbon (8). The introduction of a *cis*-aconityl (CA) group as acid-sensitive spacer between a cytocidal drug, for example, daunomycin (DM), and the target-specific carrier (Fig. 1) alleviates this problem by providing a reversible linkage; the drug is released from the spacer group unaltered and, hence, without loss of its cytotoxic potency, only within the acidic environment of the lysosome (9). At the intravascular physiologic pH, however, DM remains co-

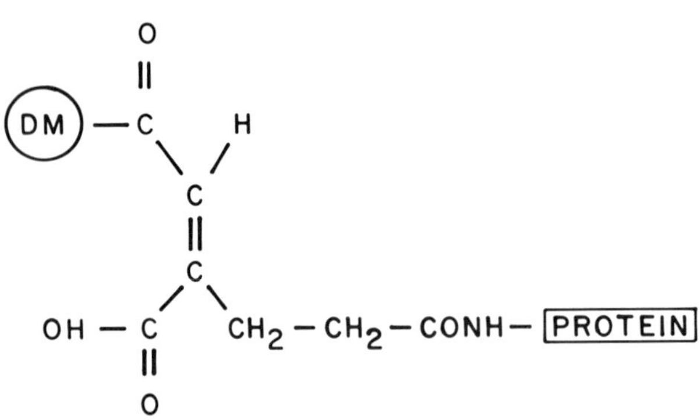

Figure 1 Chemical structure of the *cis*-aconityl spacer between the protein carrier (PROTEIN) and daunomycin (DM).

valently attached to the CA-carrier complex. Once released inside the target cell, DM is a molecule small enough to exit through the lysosomal membrane into the cytosol. Following penetration of the nuclear membrane, it renders template DNA unavailable to DNA and RNA polymerases through intercalation (10,11). In th following section, we describe the successful application of DM-CA-containing immunoconjugates directed at various kinds of target cells in a variety of experimental models.

II. RESULTS

A. Daunomycin Conjugated via an Acid-sensitive Spacer Group to Antigen as the Target-specific Carrier Causes Antigen-specific Unresponsiveness in B Lymphocytes

Immunocompetent bone marrow-derived (B) lymphocyte populations are clonally diverse with respect to the recognition specificities that are expressed by surface immunoglobulin receptors for antigen. Antigen selectively binds to those clones of B cells whose antigen receptors bear stereospecificity for a particular antigenic determinant. It follows that if one constructed a conjugate whose target-seeking carrier of the cytotoxic drug is an antigen, one would be able to selectively eliminate the B-lymphocyte clone that recognizes it.

Following these premises, we constructed a drug conjugate prototype in which the target-specific carrier was a trinitrophenol (TNP) hapten derivative of ovalbumin (OVA). As predicted, in vitro exposure of murine spleen cells to (TNP-OVA)-(CA-DM) at 4°C for 2 to 3 hr followed by thorough washing caused TNP-specific B lymphocytes to become deleted. Thus, splenocytes that had been treated with the DM conjugate failed to generate a TNP-specific antibody response in vitro to the strongly immunogenic hapten TNP-substituted microorganism *Brucella abortus* (TNP-Ba). Importantly, the conjugate did not affect immunocompetence of the spleen cells to haptens other than TNP, i.e., nitrophenylacetic acid (NIP) or fluorescein isothiocyanate (FLU). Conversely, (NIP-OVA)-(CA-DM) caused the deletion of NIP-specific B cells without affecting B cells recognizing TNP (Fig. 2). Presumably the hapten TNP on the conjugate was recognized by TNP-specific immunoglobulin surface receptors on B cells, whereupon the entire complex became endocytosed. Appropriate control experiments showed that the specific immunosuppressive effect was critically dependent on the presence of DM, since butacaine (BC), a compound of similar molecular weight as that of the anthracyclin but without cytotoxic activity, was ineffective as conjugand. Furthermore, DM, when directly linked to the target-specific carrier, failed to exert cytotoxicity (12) (Fig. 3).

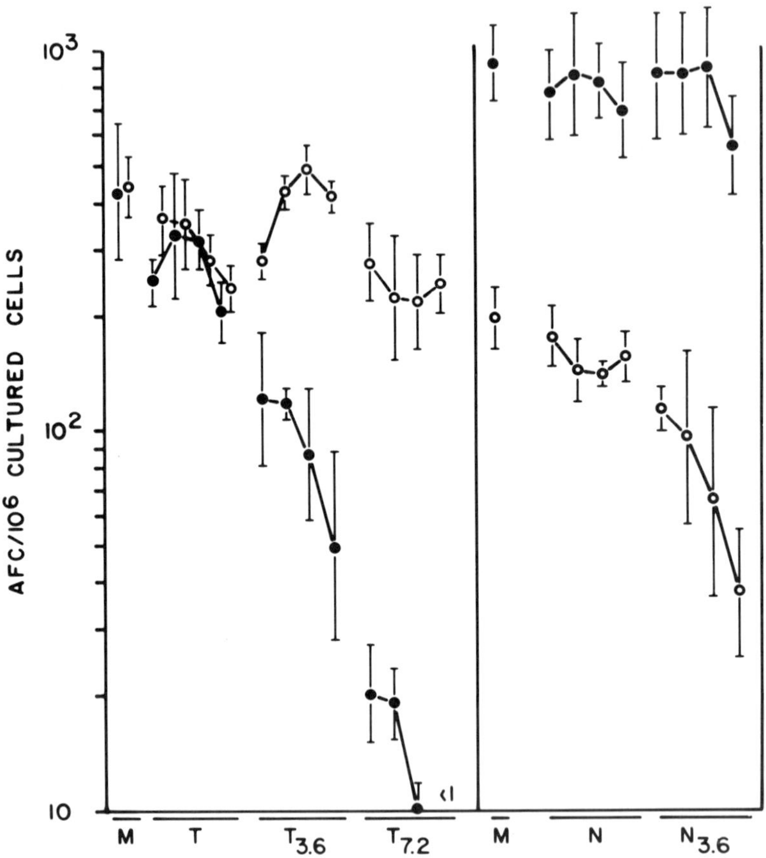

Figure 2 TNP- or NIP-specific immunosuppression induced in vitro with (TNP-OVA)-(CA-DM) or (NIP-OVA)-(CA-DM). In each group, interconnected symbols represent treatment of splenocytes (4×10^6 cells/ml) for 2 hr at 4°C with the indicated conjugate at 50, 100, 250, and 500 μg/ml. M, medium alone; T, TNP_7-OVA; $T_{3.6}$, $(TNP_7\text{-OVA})\text{-}(CA\text{-}DM)_{3.6}$; $T_{7.2}$, $(TNP\text{-OVA})\text{-}(CA\text{-}DM)_{7.2}$; N, NIP_3-OVA; $N_{3.6}$, $(NIP_3\text{-OVA})\text{-}(CA\text{-}DM)_{3.6}$. The treated cells were washed and challenged with TNP-Ba (closed circles) or NIP-Ficoll (open circles) in vitro for 4 days. Mean numbers of antibody-forming cells (AFC) ± standard deviation are indicated on the ordinate. Reproduced with the permission of *Science*, Diener et al. (1986), *Science 231*:148-150.

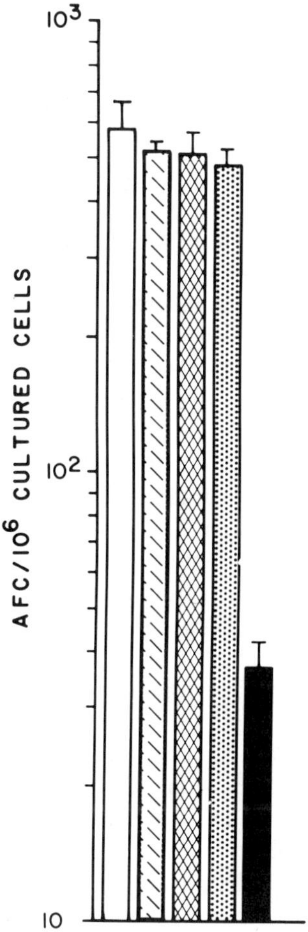

Figure 3 Effectiveness of (TNP-OVA)-(CA-DM) depends on the attachment of DM to the protein carrier by the acid-sensitive spacer molecule CA. Treatment of splenocytes as described in Figure 1 with medium alone (open bar), TNP_3-OVA-CA (hatched bar), TNP_3-OVA-DM (cross-hatched bar), (TNP_3-OVA)-$(CA\text{-}BC)_{54}$ (dotted bar), or (TNP_3-OVA)-$(CA\text{-}DM)_{54}$ (solid bar; final concentration of conjugate was 500 μg/ml. The mean numbers of cells forming IgM antibodies (AFC) to TNP ± standard deviation are shown. Reproduced with the permission of *Science*, Diener et al. (1986), *Science 231*:148-150.

B. A Cytotoxic Immunoconjugate Whose Targeting Moiety Is an Antibody Specifically Eliminates Lymphocyte Subpopulations

B lymphocytes, by virtue of displaying surface immunoglobulin receptors, should also be susceptible to killing by an immunoconjugate whose targeting moiety is an anti-immunoglobulin antibody. Unlike the antigen-containing immunoconjugate used in the above experiment, an Ig-specific cytotoxic immunoconjugate is expected to eliminate all Ig receptor-bearing B lymphocytes, regardless of antigen recognition specificity. This we have tested using an IgG goat anti-mouse immunoglobulin conjugated to CA-DM. The wide recognition spectrum of this immunoconjugate, covering all B-lymphocyte clones, required us to challenge purged spleen cells with the B-cell polyclonal mitogen lipopolysaccharide (LPS) in order to determine the extent to which (anti-Ig)-(CA-DM) had been effective. To provide for specificity control, purged cells were challenged with the T-cell polyclonal mitogen Concanavalin A (Con A). This experiment showed that our Ig-specific immunoconjugate was, indeed, able to eliminate a sufficiently large portion of the B-lymphocyte population so as to render the LPS response deficient, without affecting the T-cell response to Con A (Table 1).

Bone marrow transplantation between individuals whose antigens encoded by the major histocompatibility complex (MHC) are different from each other inevitably leads to failure due to immunological reactivity between host and donor lymphocytes. If the lymphocytes of an allogeneic bone marrow receipient have been destroyed by irradiation prior to grafting, the lymphocytes contained in the bone marrow inoculum will, within a few days, kill the host by so-called graft-versus-host disease (GVHD). Such GVHD has been shown to be due to T cells (13-18). Because of the clinical importance of bone marrow transplantation, efforts to prevent GVHD from occurring have aimed at the elimination of mature and, hence, immunocompetent T lymphocytes contaminating the bone marrow. Among other less effective methods, this has included the purging in vitro of T cells from donor bone marrow by means of immunotoxins selectively directed at T-cell surface markers (18,19). To assess the spectrum of potential applications of a DM-containing immunoconjugate, it was thus important to test its effectiveness when directed at murine T cells by a monoclonal, Thy-1.2-specific IgM antibody. Applying the same in vitro treatment protocol as was used to purge B lymphocytes (anti-Thy-1)-(CA-DM) was shown to delete the proliferative response of mouse splenocytes in a dose-dependent fashion to a challenge with the T-cell polyclonal activator Con A (Fig. 4). However, the same immunoconjugate had no effect on B lymphocytes; the proliferative response to the B cell mitogen LPS by spleen cells from which T cells had been purged was no different from that of untreated controls (12).

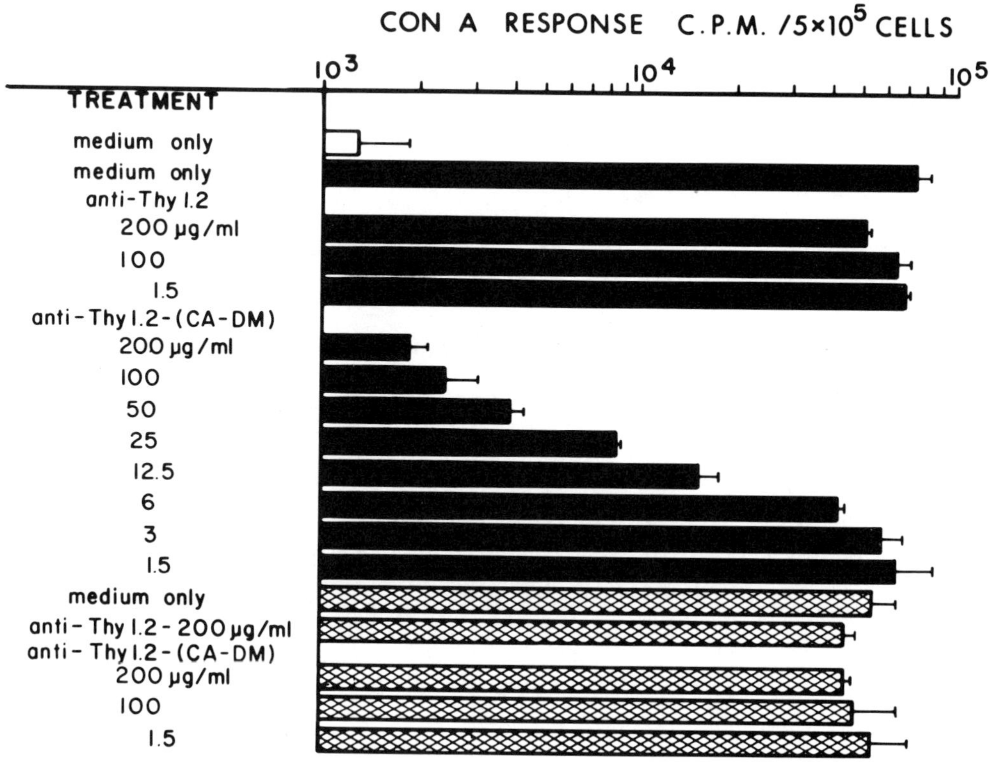

Figure 4 Immunosuppression of T-cell response to Con A by treatment of spleen cells in vitro with (anti-Thy-1.2)-(CA-DM). The antibody used in these experiments was of the IgM class. Uptake of [^{3}H]-thymidine is expressed ± standard deviation for the responses by unstimulated cells (open bar), by cells stimulated with Con A (solid bars), or by cells stimulated with LPS (cross-hatched bars). Numbers at the top of the bars represent concentrations in µg/ml. The amount of DM contained in anti-Thy-1.2 at 200 µg of protein/ml was 10 µg. The concentraiton of conjugated DM required to suppress the Con A response 50% was 0.3 µg/ml. Free DM at 0.1 µg/ml suppressed the Con A response 50%. Reproduced with the premission of *Science*, Diener et al. (1986), *Science 231*:148-150.

Table 1 Immunosuppression of the Murine B-Cell Response by (anti-Ig)-(CA–DM) in Vitro

CBA/CaJ spleen cells (5×10^5/well) Incubated with	Stimulated with	$[^3H]$–Thymidine incorporation mean ± SD (cpm)
medium	–	2,384 ± 824
anti-Ig (20 μg/ml)[a]	LPS	65,842 ± 4,284
(anti-Ig)-(CA–DM)[b]	LPS	
2.0 μg/ml		8,581 ± 725
1.0 μg/ml		12,452 ± 1,280
0.5 μg/ml		28,458 ± 3,258
0.25 μg/ml		39,876 ± 2,894
0.125 μg/ml		54,209 ± 3,785
anti-Ig (20 μg/ml)[a]	Con A	148,092 ± 8,562
(anti-Ig)-(CA–DM)[b]	Con A	
2.0 μg/ml		159,728 ± 4,648
1.0 μg/ml		140,780 ± 6,452
0.5 μg/ml		130,898 ± 9,805
0.25 μg/ml		143,210 ± 5,878
0.125 μg/ml		160,872 ± 9,280

Following treatment of cells with the immunoconjugate, they were washed and cultured for 3 days, at which time they were pulsed for $[^3H]$–thymidine uptake

[a]Concentration refers to the content of antibody at the highest dose of immunoconjugate used.

[b]Concentrations refer to the content of DM in amounts/ml of immunoconjugate used to treat the cells. The conjugation ratio between DM and the carrier remained the same at all concentrations of immunoconjugate used.

C. CA-DM-Containing Immunoconjugates Directed at Neoplastic Cells

Encouraged by the above results, we undertook to further explore the versatility of DM-containing immunoconjugates by directing them at neoplastic cells of different tissue origins. The LoVo tumor cell line grown from a human colorectal adenocarcinoma (20) was incubated in vitro for 2.5 hr at 4°C with different concentrations of CA-DM coupled to the murine monoclonal IgG antibody 50H.19. This antibody was shown to detect a 24,000 MW glycoprotein, which is associated with protein kinase activity (21). Following incubation, the cells were washed free of unbound immunoconjugate, cultured for 3 days, and tested for DNA replication as measured by [^{3}H]-thymidine uptake. The rate of growth inhibition directly depended on the concentration of (50H.19)-(CA-DM) with which the LoVo cells were treated. The antibody alone, when added to a concentration equivalent to that contained in the highest dose of the immunoconjugate used, had no inhibitory effect on cell growth. Most important, even at the highest concentration, the growth inhibitory effect of (50H.19)-(CA-DM) was entirely specific for LoVo cells and did not affect the K562 human chronic myelogenous leukemia (Fig. 5). Finally, in another experiment, a Thy-1.2-specific immunoconjugate was shown to specifically kill cells of a murine Thy-1.2-bearing thymoma (EL-4) but not a Thy-1.1-bearing thymoma (BW5147.3) or a mouse lymphoma (P388D_1) (Table 2).

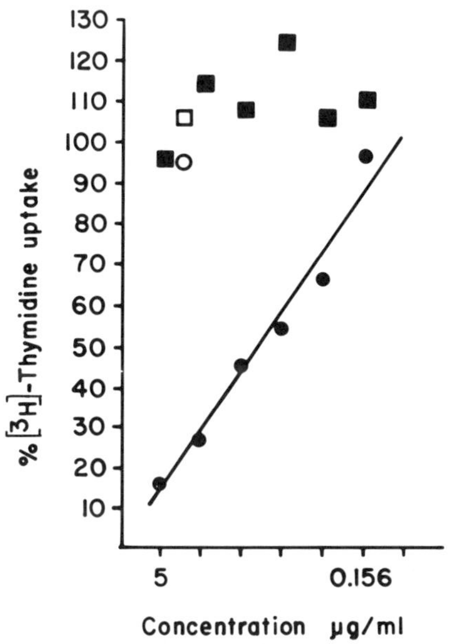

Figure 5 Selective killing in vitro of human colorectal carcinoma cells (LoVo) by (50H.19)-(CA-DM) (filled circles). Note that the viability of the human chronic myelogenous leukemia cell line K562 (filled square) is not affected by the immunoconjugate. LoVo cells treated with 50H.19 antibody only (open circle) or K562 cells treated with 50H.19 antibody only (open square) remained unaffected. The concentrations on the abscissa refer to the amounts of DM contained in each ml of immunoconjugate-containing medium with which the cells were treated before culture.

D. A CA-DM-Containing Immunoconjugate is Effective In Vivo

We have pointed out the clinical relevance of immunoconjugates that are specifically cytotoxic in vivo. CA-DM coupled to an appropriate carrier meets this requirement. Mice injected intravenously with (TNP-OVA)-(CA-DM) underwent a marked reduction in their TNP-specific antibody response when challenged with TNP-Ba as compared to untreated controls. Upon challenge with fluorescein isothiocyanate (FLU), a hapten unrelated to TNP, attached to the immunogenic carrier Ba, these same mice generated a normal FLU-specific immune response (Fig. 6). Importantly, our immunoconjugate was specifically immuno-

Table 2 Inhibition of Growth of Murine EL-4 Thymoma Cells by (anti-Thy-1.2)-(CA–DM)

Treatment with	EL-4	BW5147.3	$P388D_1$
(anti-Thy-1.2)-(CA–DM)			
10.00 μg/ml	8,920 ± 230	103,287 ± 13,286	65,968 ± 8,976
5.00 μg/ml	10,321 ± 4,578	138,653 ± 19,895	74,321 ± 9,625
2.50 μg/ml	13,208 ± 1,252	123,956 ± 1,489	86,581 ± 6,578
1.25 μg/ml	73,542 ± 4,896	142,396 ± 15,698	74,896 ± 3,241
0.60 μg/ml	107,981 ± 10,381	110,837 ± 13,286	97,884 ± 7,685
0.30 μg/ml	145,926 ± 8,956	138,678 ± 19,764	79,868 ± 5,679
cells alone	158,432 ± 10,982	129,685 ± 12,860	89,685 ± 6,423
anti-Thy-1.2			
50 μg/ml	165,726± 46,792	112,939 ± 35,674	93,768 ± 4,321
anti-Thy-1.2 (50 μg/ml) + DM (10 μg/ml)	5,642 ± 256	6,541 ± 193	5,786 ± 327
DM			
10 μg/ml	5,876 ± 142	7,932 ± 186	5,321 ± 489

Cells were treated with either the immunoconjugate, antibody, DM, or a mixture of antibody and DM, washed, and cultured for 24 hr, at which time they were pulsed for [^{3}H]–thymidine uptake. The concentrations of DM and of anti-Thy-1.2 correspond to the content of each ligand in amounts/ml of immunoconjugate used to treat the cells. The conjugation ratio between DM and the carrier remained the same at all concentrations of immunoconjugate used. Values represent counts per minute expressed as mean + standard deviation from the groups of 5 cultures individually tested.
EL-4 is a thymoma expressing Thy-1.2.
BW5147.3 is a thymoma expressing Thy-1.1.
$P388D_1$ is a mouse lymphoma.

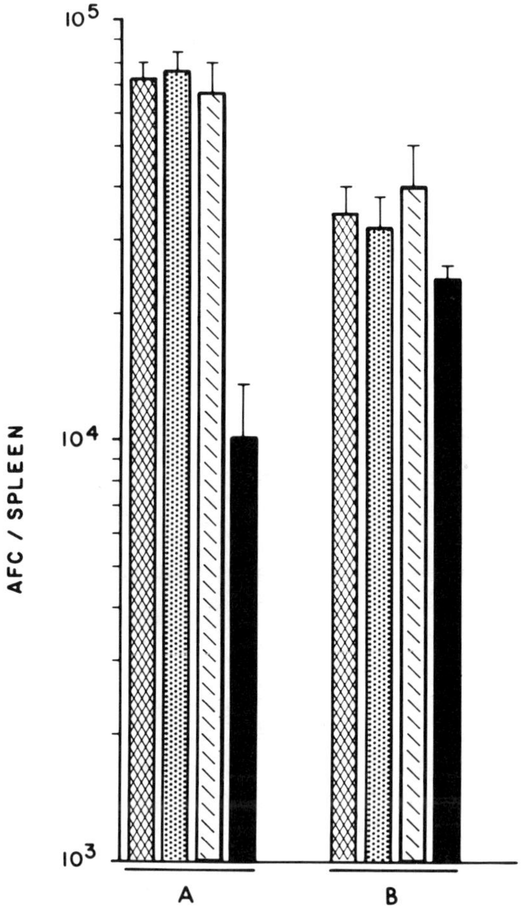

Figure 6 TNP-specific immunosuppression induced in vivo with (TNP-OVA)-(CA-DM). Mice in groups of five were each injected intravenously with saline (cross-hatched bars), 600 μg of TNP_3-OVA-CA (dotted bars), (TNP_3-OVA)-$(CA\text{-}BC)_{72}$ (hatched bars), or (TNP_3-OVA)-$(CA\text{-}DM)_{72}$ (solid bars). The mice were simultaneously challenged with TNP-Ba and FLU-Ba 24 hr later. Mean numbers ± standard deviations of spleen cells forming IgM antibodies (AFC) to TNP are shown in (A) and to FLU in (B). Reproduced with the permission of *Science*, Diener et al. (1986), *Science 231*:148-150.

suppressive without visibly affecting the health of the animals during the course of the experiment (12).

E. The Application of a CA-DM-Containing Immunoconjugate to Allogeneic Bone Marrow Transplantation

The clinical application of specifically cytotoxic immunoconjugates promises to be successful in the therapy of bone marrow malignancies, notably leukemia. A therapeutic protocol may include the autologous hematopoietic reconstitution of a patient's bone marrow following whole-body irradiation and/or chemotherapy. Bone marrow, secured from the patient prior to irradiation, is purged of leukemic cells in vitro with a tumor-specific immunoconjugate that spares pluripotent hematopoietic stem cells. Autologous bone marrow transplantation is not always feasible, in which case the grafting of allogeneic hematopoietic tissue is necessary. In such cases, GVHD generated by T lymphocytes is expected to ensue unless the potentially alloreactive T lymphocytes are purged from the donor bone marrow prior to inoculation into the immunocompromised recipient. Our success in specifically eliminating T cells from murine spleen with (anti-Thy-1.2)-(CA-DM) prompted experiments to see if we could construct fully allogeneic irradiation chimeras with purged bone marrow. In this respect, it was important to know whether the immunoconjugate would spare hematopoietic stem cells from being affected by the purging procedure, since these cells are the source of hematopoietic reconstitution once inside the irradiated recipient. Thus, murine bone marrow was treated with (anti-Thy-1.2)-(CA-DM) as described and tested in vitro for content of hematopoietic stem cells and of the more mature committed progenitor cells of the granulocyte macrophage line.

Hematopoietic stem cells acting as colony-forming units in vitro may be enumerated using the multilineage mixed-colony assay (CFU-ML) (22). Similarly available is an assay for colony-forming units in culture (CFU-C), which is representative of committed progenitor cells (23). These tests showed that, at a concentration of immunoconjugate deemed optimal for the purging of T lymphocytes, neither hematopoietic stem cells nor progenitor cells were affected (Table 3). The preservation of these cells is noteworthy in view of reports that Thy-1.2 appears to represent a differentiation antigen characteristic of murine erythroid and myeloid hematopoietic stem cells (24). Possibly, in our experiment, the pluripotent stem cells giving rise to the mixed colonies in vitro displayed Thy-1.2 antigen in amounts too low to bring about the intracellular accumulation of lethal doses of DM. Having thus confirmed that bone marrow stem cells are spared destruction by the T-cell-specific immunoconjugate, we set out to construct fully allogeneic chimeras by repopulating lethally irradiated BALB/cCr male mice with a T-cell-depleted mixture of 25×10^6 bone marrow cells and 25×10^6 spleen cells administered intravenously. Due to the addi-

Table 3 Effect of (Thy-1.2)-(CA–DM) on the Viability of Murine Hematopoietic Progenitor and Pluripotent Stem Cells and on Con A Response by Spleen Cell

Treatment with	Number of CFU–C/ 5 X 10^5 bone marrow cells ± SD[a]	Number of CFU–ML/ 5 X 10^5 bone marrow cells ± SD[a]	Con A response by spleen cells (cpm ± SD)[b]
anti-Thy-1.2-CA–DM (10 μg/ml)	250 ± 25	40 ± 5	1,256 ± 289
anti-Thy-1.2 (50 μg/ml)	280 ± 38	42 ± 4	171,564 ± 7,551
DM (10 μg/ml)	<1	<1	1,758 ± 519
DM + anti-Thy-1.2 (10 μg/ml + 50 μg/ml)	<1	<1	n.d.
untreated control	240 ± 23	50 ± 5	191,875 ± 4,207

Bone marrow and spleen cells were separately treated with either the immunoconjugate, antibody, DM, or a mixture of antibody and DM, washed, and cultured. The concentrations of DM and of anti-Thy-1.2 correspond to the content of each ligand in amounts/ml of immunoconjugate used to treat the cells. The conjugation ratio between DM and the carrier remained the same at all concentrations of immunoconjugate used.

[a]Mean and standard deviation (SD) of numbers of colonies generated by 6 independent cultures.

[b]Incorporation of [^{3}H]-thymidine; mean counts per minute (cpm) ± standard deviation.

Reproduced with the permission of *Transplantation*, Xie et al. (1987), *Transplantation* (in press).

tional contribution of large numbers of potentially alloreactive T lymphocytes by the spleen cells added to the bone marrow inoculum, allogeneic recipients of unpurged donor cell mixtures died from severe GVHD within 50 days. Treatment of the inoculum with anti-Thy-1.2 antibody alone, although it prolonged the allogeneic bone marrow/spleen recipient's lifespan significantly beyond that of mice repopulated with untreated donor cells, eventually failed to prevent their death within 125 days. In contrast, in this experiment 49 out of 50 BALB/cCr mice repopulated with the allogeneic bone marrow/spleen mixture from which T cells had been purged were still alive at time of killing >200 days after reconstitution (25) (Fig. 7). The mouse of this group that died did so shortly after inoculation for unknown reasons other than GVHD. Autopsy of five

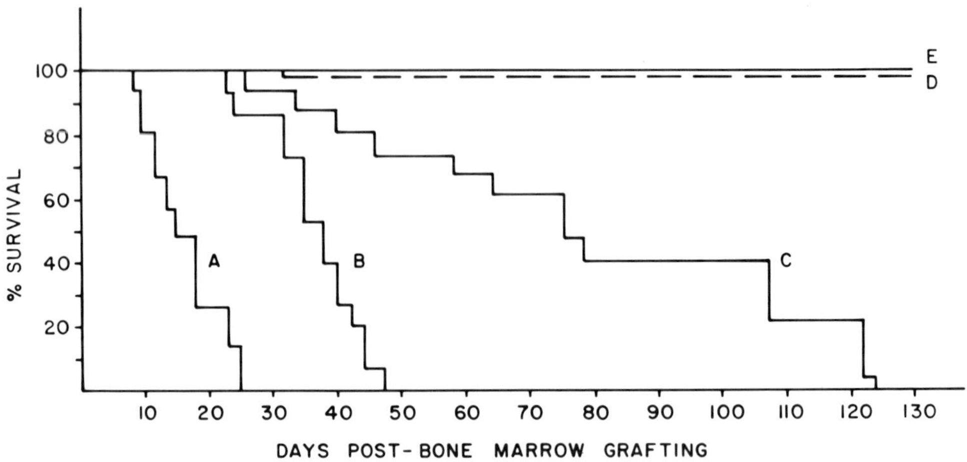

Figure 7 Long-term survival of irradiated BALB/c mice injected with a mixture of 25 × 10^6 bone marrow and 25 × 10^6 C57BL/6J spleen cells from which T cells have been purged. (A) Irradiated BABL/c mice (950 rad). (B) Irradiated BALB/c mice grafted with untreated C57BL/6J cells. (C) Irradiated BABL/c mice grafted with C57BL/6J cells treated with anti-Thy-1.2 antibody only. (D) Irradiated BABL/c mice grafted with C57BL/6J cells purged of T cells with (anti-Thy-1.2)–(CA-DM) as described in text to Figure 3. (E) Irradiated BABL/c mice grafted with syngeneic bone marrow. Reproduced with the permission of *Transplantation*, Xie et al. (1987), *Transplantation* (in press).

immunoconjugate-facilitated allogeneic chimeras 90 days after transplantation showed no sign of subclinical GVHD as judged by size and weight of secondary lymphoid organs (i.e., spleen and lymph nodes).

Besides concerns over GVHD when dealing with clinical allogeneic bone marrow transplantation, the degree to which donor stem cells achieve engraftment in the MHC-incompatible environment of the recipient represents one of the most crucial parameters reflecting therapeutic success or failure. To determine the degree of hematopoietic chimerism in our immunoconjugate-facilitated allogeneically reconstituted mice, we made use of the polymorphic glucose phosphate isomerase (GPI) marker (26). BALB/cCr and C57BL/6J mice used in our experiments differ for the Gpi gene, whose alleles are designated Gpi-1^a and Gpi-1^b, respectively. Their enzyme products from chimeric cell lysates were separated from each other by gel electrophoresis and quantitatively assessed by densitometry (27). Twelve weeks following transplantation, the blood of immunoconjugate-facilitated, allogeneically reconstituted mice was 100% donor type in 8 out of 10 BALB/cCr recipients of C57BL/6J bone marrow (25). The GPI test applied to lymphocytes of chimeric mice 250 days following reconstitution yielded similar results indicating that their hematopoietic system was predominantly of donor origin (Table 4).

It is of paramount importance that allogeneic chimeras, in order to remain physiologically viable, display full immunocompetence to extrinsic antigens while being tolerant to self, which includes mutual tolerance between donor and host lymphocytes. A state of immunocompetence to extrinsic antigens is not a self-evident expectation in allogeneic chimeras in view of early reports that the acquisition of a normal antigen recognition repertoire by thymocyte precursors in the environment of an MHC-incompatible thymic epithelium is severely curtailed (28). This notion is particularly valid in view of recently published data showing that, contrary to earlier claims (29,30), intrathymic MHC restriction is controlled by the thymic epithelium rather than by bone marrow-derived cells of the reticuloendothelial system (31). For these reasons, we tested both T-cell- and B-cell-mediated immunocompetence in immunoconjugate-

Table 4 Hematopoietic Reconstitution with Donor Cells in Irradiated Recipients of Immunoconjugate-treated Allogeneic Bone Marrow

4 weeks		8 weeks		12 weeks	
BALB/c	C57BL/6J	BALB/c	C57BL/6J	BALB/c	C57BL/6J
40	59	13	86	<1	100
37	62	<1	100	4	95
35	64	2	98	<1	100
42	57	<1	100	<1	100
39	68	<1	100	<1	100
43	56	<1	100	<1	100
39	60	20	79	<1	100
32	67	7	92	<1	100
<1	100	<1	100	14	85
<1	100	<1	100	<1	100

Percentage of peripheral red blood cells bearing the GPI-A or GPI-B isozyme marker of BALB/c receipient or of C57BL/6J donor origin, respectively, at 4, 8, and 12 weeks post-transplantation. Each of the 10 mice was individually monitored for chimerism. Reproduced with the permission of *Transplantation*, Xie et al (1987), *Transplantation* (in press).

facilitated allogeneic bone marrow chimeras. The proliferative response in vitro by splenic T lymphocytes from these mice was assessed in the presence of irradiated BALB/cCr (H-2[d]), C57BL/6J (H-2[b]), or CBA/CaJ (H-2[k]) stimulator splenocytes. Likewise, mixed-lymphocyte reactions and MHC-specific tytotoxic T cells generated from chimeric spleen cells in vitro in the presence of irradiated BABL/cCr, C57BL/6J, or CBA/CaJ stimulator cells were determined in a standard cytotoxicity test (25). To measure immunocompetence with respect to antibody responses, chimeric mice were injected with sheep erythrocytes as a foreign immunogen and their spleens assayed for content of IgM- and IgG-forming cells (25). These tests showed that the chimeric T-lymphocyte populations, while fully tolerant of each other's MHC haplotype, were immunocompetent towards third-party MHC antigens to the same extent as T lymphocytes from syngeneically reconstituted mice (Tables 5,6). Similarly, allogeneic chimeras were equally immunocompetent with respect to the SRBC-specific antibody response, as were syngeneically reconstituted mice (25) (Table 7). Finally, five out of five immunoconjugate-facilitated chimeras, while tolerant of allogeneic skin grafts derived from the bone marrow donor, rejected third-party allografts as promptly as did mice reconstituted with syngeneic bone marrow.

Table 5 MLR by Spleen Cells from Immunoconjugate-facilitated Allogeneically C57BL/6J → BABL/c or Syngeneically BALB/c → BALB/c Reconstituted Mice

	Responders: [^{3}H]–thymidine incorporation[a]		
Stimulators[b]	BALB/c	BALB/c → BALB/c	C57BL/6J → BALB/c
–	6,203 ± 782	3,850 ± 258	4,366 ± 835
BALB/c	7,082 ± 625	4,029 ± 486	4,799 ± 1.088
C57BL/6J	34,808 ± 2,402	28,972 ± 3,214	6,159 ± 1,133
CBA	45,864 ± 4,871	36,412 ± 8,670	35,452 ± 8,119

[a]Values represent counts per minute expressed as mean ± standard deviation from groups of 5 mice individually tested.

[b]4×10^5 irradiated stimulator spleen cells were mixed with 4×10^5 responder spleen cells, cultured for 4 days, and pulsed with [^{3}H]–thymidine. [^{3}H]–Thymidine incorporation is taken as a measure of MLR reactivity.

Reproduced with the permission of *Transplantation*, Xie et al. (1987). *Transplantation* (in press).

Table 6 Reactivity by Spleen Cells from Immunoconjugate-facilitated Allogeneically C57BL/6J → BALB/c or Syngeneically BALB/c → BALB/c Reconstituted Mice[a]

	Responders: % specific lysis ± SEM[b]		
Stimulators	BALB/c	BALB/c → BALB/c	C57BL/6J → BALB/c
BALB/c	1.5 ± 1.8	0.8 ± 2.0	0.5 ± 0.5
C56BL/6J	49.0 ± 1.4	43.0 ± 1.5	1.8 ± 0.9
CBA	51.0 ± 3.5	48.0 ± 2.0	40.6 ± 6.0

[a]5 × 10^5 responder spleen cells were cultured with 5 × 10^5 irradiated stimulator spleen cells for 5 days. The target effector cell ratio was 10:1.
[b]Mean and standard error of the mean (SEM) from groups of 5 mice each individually tested. Specific lysis is reflected in the amount of ^{51}Cr released from target cell.
Reproduced with the permission of *Transplantation*, Xie et al. (1987), *Transplantation* (in press).

Table 7 In vivo IgM and IgG Antibody-forming Cell Response by Spleen Cells from Immunoconjugate-facilitated Allogeneic C57BL/6J → BALB/c Chimeras

Groups of mice	AFC/spleen ± SD IgM	AFC/spleen ± SD IgG
(1) Normal BALB/c	179,311 ± 13,231	35,460 ± 5,422
(2) Syngeneically reconstituted BALB/c → BALB/c	127,950 ± 8,584	35,550 ± 5,727
(3) Allogeneically reconstituted C57BL/6 → BALB/c	116,596 ± 12,062	32,625 ± 8,062

Mean and standard deviation (SD) of numbers of antibody-forming cells (AFC) per spleen generated by 10 mice in groups (2) and (3), and 5 mice in group (1). IgM AFC measured 4 days after immunization. IgG AFC measured 10 days after immunization. Reproduced with the permission of *Transplantation*, Xie et al (1986), *Transplantation* (in press).

F. Concluding Remarks

Historically, research on the design of cytotoxic drug-immunoconjugates has met with little success mainly because drugs tend to irreversibly lose toxicity when directly conjugated to a carrier. The description by Shen and Ryser (9) of an acid-sensitive spacer between drug and carrier enabled us to demonstrate, in a variety of biological models, the use of specifically effective cytotoxic drug-immunoconjugates. For reasons described in this chapter, such immunoconjugates offer distinct advantages over immunotoxins: They suffer little variability in specific activity when applied to different types of target cells, remain specifically active within a wide range of concentrations, and may be administered in vivo. Of practical relevance is the ease with which drug immunoconjugates may be constructed in the laboratory in quantities limited only by the supply of target-specific carriers.

The clinical use of target cell-specific cytotoxic agents is currently of immediate relevance to bone marrow transplantation. We consider our experimental data on this subject sufficiently convincing to encourage the use in clinical trials of drug immunoconjugates of the type described in this chapter.

G. Methodology

1. Comments Regarding the Exposure of Cell Suspensions to Immunoconjugate

It is presumed that cell surface marker-immunoconjugate complexes become endocytosed at a rate proportional to the degree to which the markers are cross-linked by the ligand. Cells maintained at 37°C undergo ligand-induced antigen modulation within minutes, thereby reducing the density of residual surface markers to levels at which cross-linking by the immunoconjugate and hence endocytosis become less efficient. For these reasons, we have chosen to expose target-cell suspensions to the immunoconjugates on ice at a temperature at which cells are metabolically inactive and endocytosis does not occur. In our experience, this allows for maximal accumulation of cell-surface-bound immunoconjugate to levels which may not be obtained when ligand binding is to occur at 37°C. Thus, intracellular accumulation of immunoconjugate is optimal when cells are incubated with a ligand at 4°C, washed, and subsequently warmed to 37°C to facilitate endocytosis. This must be taken into consideration when one quantitatively compares cellular uptake of free DM with that of conjugated DM. In the case of conjugated DM, only amounts of drug actually bound to the cell surface will be internalized by the cell.

2. Preparation of Cytotoxic Immunoconjugates Following the Method of Shen and Ryser (9).

a. Preparation of CA-DM A solution containing 5 mg of DM in 1 ml of double-distilled water is kept on ice and the pH adjusted to 8.5 with 0.1 N NaOH. An equal quantity of solid *cis*-aconityl anhydride (CA) is added slowly while the pH is maintained at 8.5-9.0. This step may be facilitated by dissolving CA in 1 ml of dioxane, which, when added dropwise to the ice-cold solution of DM, allows for more accurate control of the pH. After the solution has been kept on ice for 10 min, 0.1 N HCl is added slowly, which results in the formation of a precipitate that is collected by centrifugation at 500 *g* for 2 min. The pellet is then resuspended in 1 ml of double-distilled water and the pH increased by addition of 0.1 N NaOH until a clear solution is obtained. The precipitation procedure is repeated, and the final precipitate is redissolved in 1 ml of phosphate-buffered saline (PBS) and adjusted to pH 7.2.

b. Coupling of CA-DM to the Target-Specific Protein 0.2 ml of the CA-DM solution containing 5 mg of DM per ml and 60 μl of 1-ethyl-3-(3-dimethylaminopropyl) carbodiimide (10 mg/ml in PBS) are added to 1 ml of target-specific protein (2 mg/ml in PBS) while being stirred at room temperature. After 20 hr, the mixture is centrifuged and the supernatant applied to a medium or coarse Sephadex G25 column that has previously been equilibrated with PBS. The conjugate is collected as the excluded fraction from the column, concentrated, and filtered.

3. Cell Cultures

Mice were killed by cervical dislocation and their spleens removed into PBS containing 5% fetal calf serum (FCS) (Grand Island Biological Co., Grand Island, NY). Spleens were cut with fine scissors and the cells were gently pressed through a stainless steel sieve. Cell suspensions were left standing for 15 min in order to permit clumps of cellular debris to settle out. After washing by centrifugation at 500 *g* for 7 min, the cells were resuspended in RPMI 1640 medium (Gibco Canada, Ltd., Calgary, Canada), supplemented with 10% FCS, 50 nM 2-mercaptoethanol and 0.5% penicillin-streptomycin (Gibco). Following adjustment of cell density, numbers of cells as required in 200 μl/well were cultured in flat-bottomed, 96-well plates (Linbro Scientific Co., Hamden, CT). For B-cell stimulation, LPS from *E coli*, serotype 0.5S.B5 (Sigma Chemical Co., St. Louis, MO), and for T-cell stimulation, Concanavalin A (Con A) (Sigma) were used at concentrations of 10 μl/ml and 2 μg/ml, respectively. Tumor cell lines were grown in RPMI 1640 as described above. Cultures were incubated at 37°C in a humidified atmosphere of 7% CO_2 in air.

4. Measurement of $[^3H]$-Thymidine Incorporation

Cell cultures were pulsed with 2 μCi/well of $[^3H]$-thymidine (NEN, 2 μCi/mM) for 4-6 hr and harvested. Radioactivity was measured by scintillation counting.

5. Enumeration of Antibody-Forming Cells

Spleens from mice immunized by intraperitoneal injection of 0.4 ml sheep red blood cells (5% v/v) were dissociated into cell suspensions and assayed for content of IgM and IgG plaque-forming cells (32). For assessment of IgG responses, rabbit anti-mouse gamma globulin (Cappel Laboratories, Cochraneville, PA) was used at a concentration previously determined to be optimal. Numbers of cells secreting IgG immunoglobulin were reported as the difference between assays done in the presence or absence of anti-immunoglobulin antibody.

6. Chimeras

Mice were irradiated with 950 rad from a 137 Cs source (Atomic Energy of Canada Ltd., Ottawa, Canada) and reconstituted intravenously within 24 hr with a mixture of 25×10^6 bone marrow and 25×10^6 spleen cells (hereafter referred to as bone marrow) from an allogeneic or syngeneic donor. Purging of bone marrow was by a 2-hr incubation on ice of the cell suspension in RPMI 1640 tissue culture medium containing 10% FCS, with appropriate concentrations of immunoconjugate equivalent to 10 μg/ml of DM. Thereafter, the cells were washed three times and injected intravenously into recipient mice. Degrees of hematopoietic chimerism were assessed in bone marrow-reconstituted mice using the polymorphic glucose phosphate isomerase enzyme (GPI) marker (26). BALB/c and C57BL/6J mice used in the experiments differ for the Gpi gene, whose alleles are designated Gpi-1^a and Gpi-1^b, respectively. Their products were separated from each other by gel electrophoresis and quantitatively assessed by densitometry (27).

7. Mixed Lymphocyte Reaction

4×10^5/well irradiated (2,000 rad) splenic stimulator cells were cultured with 4×10^5/well splenic responder cells in 200 μl/well of RPMI 1640 tissue culture medium supplemented with 10% FCS. Cultures were at 37°C in 6-mm flat-bottomed microtitre wells placed in a humidified incubator containing a mixture of 7% CO_2 in air. On the fourth day of culture, each well was separately assayed for $[^3H]$-thymidine (pulsed for 8 hr) with 1 μCi/well incorporation using a liquid scintillation counter.

8. Cell-Mediated Cytotoxicity

5×10^5/well irradiated (2,000 rad) splenic stimulator cells were cultured with 5×10^5/well responder cells in 200 μl/well of RPMI 1640 tissue culture medium supplemented with 10% FCS. Cultures were at 37°C in 6-mm flat-bottomed microtitre wells. On the fifth day of culture, each well was separately assayed for the presence of cytotoxic lymphocytes using ^{51}Cr-labeled Con A blasts as targets. The effector-to-target cell ratio in this 4-hr assay was 10:1. Cytotoxicity was expressed as percent of specific lysis.

9. Colony Assay for Hematopoietic Progenitor Cells and Multilineage Stem Cells

Hematopoietic progenitor cells giving rise to macrophage-granulocytic colonies in vitro (CFU-C) were assayed by standard methods (23). Multilineage colony-forming cells (CFU-ML) giving rise to mixed colonies were assayed according to published methods (22) modified as follows: Spleen cells were plated out in 35 X 10-mm dishes in 1 ml of Iscove's Modified Dulbeco's Medium (Gibco, Grand Island, NY) supplemented with 0.8% methylcellulose, 20% heat-inactivated FCS and 0.05 mM 2-mercaptoethanol. Pokeweed mitogen-stimulated spleen-condition medium at a concentration of 10% was used as a source of colony-stimulating factor. For optimal growth of mixed colonies, 10% WEHI-3-conditioned medium and 1 unit/ml of erythropoietin (Step I) (Terry Fox Cancer Research Lab, Vancouver, Canada) were added to cultures. After 10-14 days of incubation at 37°C in a mixture of 7% CO_2 in air, mixed colonies composed of more than 50 cells were counted and analyzed.

10. Skin Grafting

Full-thickness skin grafting on the animal's back was performed eight weeks after bone marrow reconstitution, following the method of Billingham (33).

REFERENCES

1. Thorpe, P. E. (1985). Antibody carriers of cytotoxic agents in cancer therapy: A review. *Monoclonal Antibodies: Biological and Clinical Applications* (Pinchera, A., Dora, G., Dammacco, F., and Bargellesi, A., Eds.). Editrice Kurtis, Milan, p. 475.
2. Olsnes, S. (1981). Directing toxins to cancer cells *Nature 290*:84.
3. Neville, D. M., Youle, R. J. (1982). Monoclonal antibody-ricin or ricin A chain hybrids: Kinetic analysis of cell killing for tumor therapy. *Immunol. Rev. 62*:75–91.
4. Youle, R. J., and Neville, D. M. (1980). Anti-Thy-1.2 monoclonal antibody linked to ricin as a potent cell-type specific toxin. *Proc. Natl. Acad. Sci. USA 77*:5483-5486.
5. Thorpe, P. E., Cumber, A. J., Williams, N., Edwards, D. C., Ross, W. C. J., and Davies, A. J. S. (1981). Abrogation of the non-specific toxicity of abrain conjugated to anti-lymphocyte globulin. *Clin. Exp. Immunol. 43*: 195-200.
6. Blakey, D. C., and Thorpe, P. E. (1986). Immunotoxins. *Bio. Assays 4*:292.

7. Press, O. W., Vitetta, E. S., Farr, A. G., Hansen, J. A., and Martin, P. J. (1986). Evaluation of ricin A-chain immunotoxins directed against human T cells. *Cell. Immunol. 102*:10-20.
8. Truet, A., Baurain, R., Masomelier, M., and Deprez-De Campeneere, D. (1982). Covalent and reversible linkage of daunorubicin to proteins. Lysosomal hydrolysis and antitumoral activity of conjugates prepared with oligopeptidic spacer arms. *EORTC Symposium*: "*Promising New Anti-Cancer Agents in Clinical Trials*" (Mathe, G., Ed.). Masson, Paris.
9. Shen, W. C., and Ryser, H. J. P. (1981). *Cis*-aconityl spacer between daunomycin and macromolecular carriers: A model of pH-sensitive linkage releasing drug from a liposomotrophic conjugate. *Biochem. Biophys. Res. Comm. 102*:1048-1054.
10. Calendi, E., Di Marco, A., Reggiani, M., Scarpinato, B., and Valentini, L. (1965). On physico-chemical interactions between daunomycin and nucleic acids. *Biophys. Acta 103*:25-49.
11. Di Marco, A. (1975). Adriamycin (NSC-123127): Mode and mechanism of action. *Cancer Chemother. Rep. 6*:91-106.
12. Diener, E., Diner, U. E., Sinha, A., Xie, S., and Vergidis, R. (1986). Specific immunosuppression by immunotoxins containing daunomycin. *Science 231*:148-150.
13. Tyan, M. E. (1973). Modification of severe graft-versus-host disease with antisera to the theta antigen or to whole serum. *Transplantation 15*:601-604.
14. Rodt, H., Thierfelder, S., and Eulitz, M. (1974). Anti-lymphocyte antibodies and marrow transplantation. III. Effect of heterologous anti-brain antibodies on acute secondary disease in mice. *Eur. J. Immunol. 4*:25-29.
15. Von Boehmer, H., and Sprent, J. (1976). T cell function in bone marrow chimeras: Absence of host-reactive T cells and cooperation of helper T cells across allogeneic barriers. *Transplant. Rev. 29*:3-23.
16. Korngold, R., and Sprent, J. (1978). Lethal graft-versus-host disease after bone marrow transplantation across major histocompatibility barriers in mice. *J. Exp. Med. 148*:1687-1698.
17. Onoe, K., Fernandes, G., and Good, R. A. (1980). Humoral and cell-mediated immune responses in full allogeneic bone marrow chimeras in mice. *J. Exp. Med. 151*:115-132.
18. Vallera, D. A., Soderling, C. C. B., Carlson, G. J., and Kersey, J. H. (1981). Bone marrow transplantation across major histocompatibility barriers in mice: Effect of elimination of T cells from donor grafts by treatment with monoclonal Thy-1.2 plus complement or antibody alone. *Transplantation 31*:218-222.
19. Vallera, D. A., Youle, R. J. Neville, D. M., and Kersey J. H. (1982). Bone marrow transplantation across major histocompatibility barriers. V. Protection of mice from lethal graft-versus-host disease by pretreatment of donor cells with monoclonal anti-1.2 coupled to the toxin ricin. *J. Exp. Med. 155*:949-954.

20. Drewinko, B., Yang, L. Y., and Barlogie, B. (1978). Further biologic characterization of a human carcinoembryonic antigen-producing colon carcinoma cell line. *JNCI 61*:75-83.
21. Seehafer, J., Longenecker, B. M., and Shaw, A. R. E. (1984). Biochemical characterization of human carcinoma surface antigen associated with protein kinase activity. *Int. J. Cancer 34*:815-819.
22. Keller, G., Paige, C., Gilboa, E., and Wagner, E. F. (1985). Expression of a foreign gene in myeloid and lymphoid cells derived from multipotent hematopoietic precursors. *Nature 318*:149-154.
23. Bradley, T. R., and Metcalf, D. (1966). The growth of mouse bone marrow cells in vitro. *Aust. J. Exp. Biol. Med. Sci. 44*:287-300.
24. Miller, B. A., Lipton, J. M., Linch, D. C. Burakoff, S. J., and Nathan, D. G. (1985). Thy-1 is a differentiation antigen that characterizes immature erythroid and myeloid hematopoietic progenitors. *J. Cell. Physiol. 123*: 25-32.
25. Xie, S., Inazawa, M., Sinha, N., Sawada, S., Vergidis, R., and Diener, E. Facilitation of allogeneic bone marrow transplantation by a T cell-specific immunotoxin containing daunomycin. *Transplantation* (in press).
26. Peterson, A. C., Frair, P. M., and Wong, G. G. (1978). A technique for detection and relative quantitative analysis of glucose phosphate isomerase from nanogram tissue samples. *Biochem. Genet. 16*:681.
27. Frauncescutti, L. H., Gambel, P., and Wegmann, T. G. (1985). Characterization of hematopoietic stem cell chimerism in antibody facilitated bone marrow chimeras. *Transplantation 40*:7-11.
28. Rayfield, L. S., and Brent, L. (1983). Tolerance, immunocompetence, and secondary disease in fully allogeneic radiation chimeras. *Transplantation 36*:183.
29. Longo, D. L., and Davis, M. L. (1983). Early appearance of donor-type antigen-presenting cells in the thymuses of 1200 r radiation-induced bone marrow chimeras correlates with self recognition of donor I region gene products. *J. Immunol. 130*:2525-2527.
30. Longo, D. L., Kruisbeek, A. M., Davis, M. L., and Matis, L. A. (1985). Bone marrow-derived thymic antigen-presenting cells determine self recognition of Ia-restricted T lymphocytes. *Proc. Natl. Acad. Sci. USA 82*: 5900-5904.
31. Ron, Y., Lo, D., and Sprent J. (1986). T cell specificity in twice-irradiated F_1-parent bone marrow chimeras: Failure to detect a role for immigrant marrow-derived cells in imprinting intrathymic H-2 recognition. *J. Immunol. 137*:1764-1771.
32. Cunningham, A., and Szenberg, A. (1968). Further improvement in the plaque technique for detecting antibody-forming cells. *Immunology 4*:599.
33. Billingham, R. E. (1961). Free skin grafting in mammals. *Transplantation of Tissues and Cells* (Billingham, R. E., and Silvers, W. K., Eds.). The Wistar Institute Press, Philadelphia, p. 1.

2

The Use of Anthracycline-Antibody Complexes for Specific Antitumor Activity

GEOFFREY A. PIETERSZ, MARK J. SMYTH, and IAN FARQUHAR CAMPBELL McKENZIE

Research Centre for Cancer and Transplantation, University of Melbourne, Parkville, Victoria, Australia

I. INTRODUCTION

The advent of monoclonal antibodies has reawakened the "magic bullet" concept of Ehrlich, whereby antibodies can be used to specifically target materials toxic to tumors (1,2). This concept has been studied for years, but the major problem has been the production of high titer, specific antitumor antibodies. The production of monoclonal antibodies with high tumor reactivity (even if not completely tumor specific) has led to a new appraisal of the concept using isotopes, drugs, and toxins such as ricin, abrin, and diptheria toxin (3-5). Relatively few studies have been reported with drug-antibody complexes in comparison to toxin-antibody complexes, probably because most drugs are complex organic molecules which can only be coupled to antibodies with difficulty.

The anthracyclines, which include daunomycin and adriamycin (Ad), are an important group of antitumor agents in current use (6). Due to their potency against solid tumors they are used extensively, but their use is accompanied by the occasional case of cardiotoxicity, in addition to systemic effects on bone marrow seen with all cytotoxic drugs. If these compounds could be coupled to antibodies with retention of the antitumor effects but with reduced nonspecific toxic effects, it would be of great benefit. Most attempts on the coupling of anthracyclines to antibody have used daunomycin. Early studies involved the coupling of daunomycin via the daunosamine sugar moiety; periodate oxidation of the sugar and subsequent reaction with antibody to form Schiff bases, subsequently reduced with borohydride, gave conjugates that were cytotoxic to tumor cells (7). Using this method conjugates of daunomycin to antitumor antibody led to loss of drug and antibody activity (8), nevertheless, daunomycin was coupled to yield an active conjugate of melanotropin (9), concanavalin A (10), and thyrotropin (11). In addition, coupling daunomycin and antibody using glutaraldehyde gave conjugates with moderate activity, whereas using carbodiimide yielded inactive conjugates (7). An alternative means of binding the two moieties is via a dextran bridge which serves as an inert carrier, and such conjugates have been able to eradicate tumors growing in the peritoneum (12). Very few studies have been performed with adriamycin, probably because of its lower solubility and stability in comparison to daunomycin. However, there have been two reports on the conjugation of adriamycin to antibodies, using polyaldehyde dextran (13) or by the oxidation of the daunosamine sugar moiety (7); in the former case there was no in vitro activity (although in vivo activity could be demonstrated), in the latter case the conjugate had low activity. It was noted that the use of borohydride for the stabilization of the Schiff bases caused a loss of activity when adriamycin is used (14).

After a number of unsuccessful attempts to couple adriamycin to antibodies using these procedures (7,13), we made suitably functionalized analogs and then coupled these to antibodies. The amino group of adriamycin is known to be involved in the binding of DNA (15) and should, preferably, not be disturbed by the coupling procedure, however, a number of analogs that do not bind DNA have been shown to be active (16). As an alternative approach, the C14 of anthracyclines was evaluated as being a possible site of attachment to antibody. Such a coupling procedure has been described with the use of the analog bromodaunomycin (17). The bromo group of bromodaunomycin can be displaced by either carboxy, amino, or sulfhydryl groups, to form covalent complexes with proteins. Gallego et al. have coupled daunomycin to antibodies using this procedure (18) to yield conjugates active in vitro. We have used a more potent anthracycline analog 4-demethoxydaunomycin (Idarubicin, Ida), to produce conjugates of extremely high in vitro and in vivo activity. These will also be described below.

II. RESULTS

A. Coupling of Adriamycin to Monoclonal Antibodies

Prior to attempting to establish new ways of coupling adriamycin to monoclonal antibodies, existing methods reported in the literature as being successful were tried (7,13). The first method used to synthesize an adriamycin-antibody conjugate involved periodate oxidation of the anthracycline amino sugar moiety (7);

this led to a drug-antibody conjugate devoid of drug activity, although the antibody activity was retained (unpublished data). We next used glutaraldehyde or carbodiimide to couple adriamycin to antibody using the amino group; both methods led to the complete loss of either drug or antibody activity. The failure of these coupling techniques, attempted many times with the same results, prompted us to investigate alternative methods of conjugation, involving the synthesis of chemically defined adriamycin intermediates, which were prepared by reaction with various heterobifunctional cross-linking agents with the amino group of adriamycin such that they can be specifically linked to reactive groups of monoclonal antibodies (either introduced or inherent).

1. Preparation and Biological Activity of Adriamycin Analogs

Adriamycin was coupled to monoclonal antibodies using three different intermediates prepared by modifying the amino group of the sugar moiety of adriamycin (Fig. 1A). Adriamycin hydrochloride was first converted to its free base with silver carbonate; the reaction of this with succinimidyl maleimidophenylbutyrate (SMPB) gave the derivative maleimidophenylbutyryl adriamycin (MPB-Ad) (yield = 78%) (Fig. 1B); this derivative had a maleimide residue capable of reacting with free sulfhydryl groups of antibody (Fig. 2). A similar reaction with succinic anhydride gave the derivative succinyl adriamycin (Succ-Ad) (yield = 66%) (Fig. 1C); Succ-Ad has a carboxylic acid group which on activation will react with free amino groups of antibody (Fig. 3). Adriamycin was also reacted with succinimidyl iodoacetate to yield iodoacetyl adriamycin (IA-Ad) (Fig. 1D) (yield = 75%), which can react with free sulfhydryl groups of antibody (Fig. 4). Thin layer chromatography analysis demonstrated that these compounds were considered to be pure and, prior to coupling to antibody, were tested for retention of activity by their ability to inhibit DNA synthesis in vitro.

Cytotoxicity studies of each of the three intermediates on the colon carcinoma cell line (HT29) were performed (Fig. 5), where inhibition of [^{3}H]-methylthymidine incorporation (relative to a dimethyl sulfoxide control) at different concentrations of the adriamycin analog were examined. It should be noted that with the exception of Succ-Ad, all the analogs were insoluble in water but soluble in dimethyl sulfoxide (DMSO), so that cytotoxicity studies had to be performed in dilute DMSO and the results compared with those obtained on control samples containing a similar amount of DMSO (5% DMSO at the highest concentration). It was clear that all three intermediates showed a *reduced* toxicity compared with free adriamycin (Fig. 5). DMSO itself had some inhibitory activity, but inhibition obtained by the analogs, in the presence of DMSO, were clearly different from that obtained with DMSO alone. MPB-Ad was almost totally without activity; however the IA-Ad derivative gave inhibition which was not greatly different from free Ad—indeed at levels > 4 μg/ml the two were indistinguishable. Succ-Ad had reduced toxicity (50% reduction at 3.4 μg/ml)

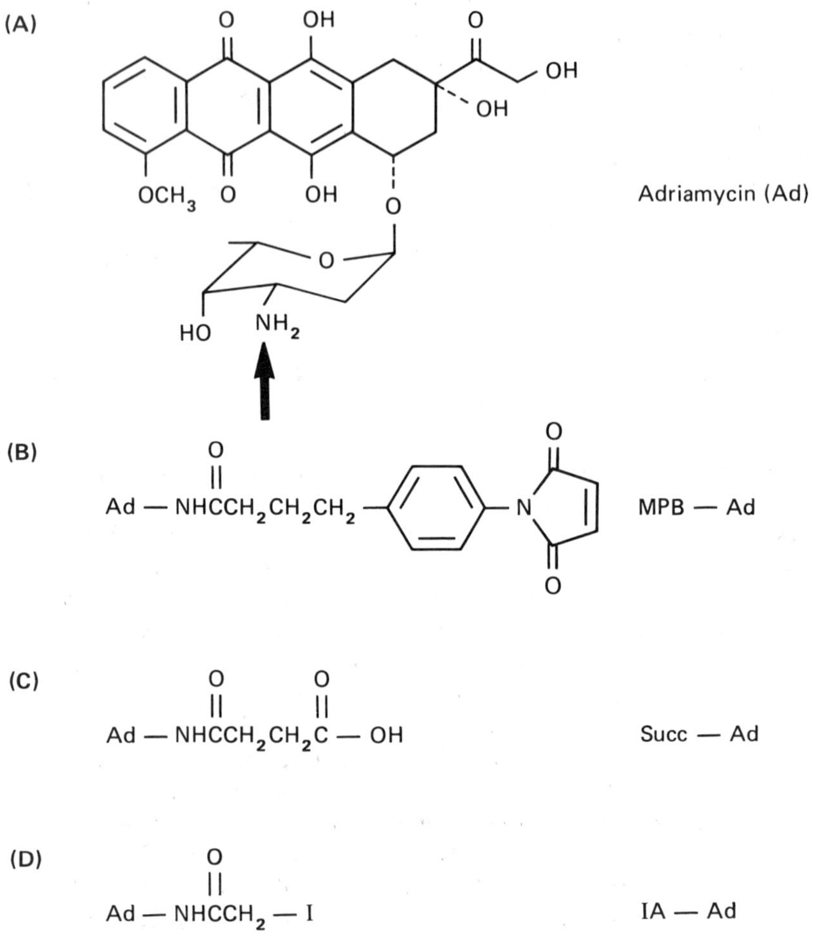

Figure 1 Chemical structure of adriamycin (A), and analogs; (B) maleimidophenylbutyryl adriamycin; (C) succinyl adriamycin; (D) iodoacetyl adriamycin. The analogs were made using the amino groups of the sugar (arrow).

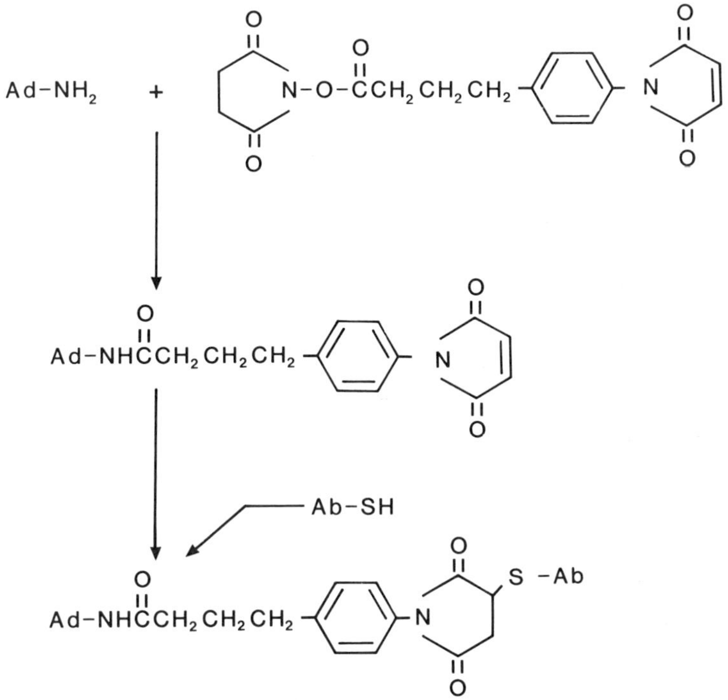

Figure 2 Reaction scheme showing the prepration of maleimidophenylbutyryl adriamycin (MPB-Ad) and conjugation to antibody.

compared to free Ad and was less active than the IA-Ad derivative. Clearly the activity of Ad was less effected by modification to form IA-Ad than with the formation of the other derivatives, nonetheless all three analogs were coupled to antibodies for further study.

2. Preparation and Activity of an Adriamycin-Antibody Conjugate Using the MPB-Ad Analog (Method A)

Conjugation of MPB-Ad to antibody required the modification of antibody using succinimidyl pyridyldithiopropionate (SPDP) to introduce new sulfhydryl groups (Fig. 2). The number of sulfhydryl groups incorporated into antibody was measured as a function of the molar excess of SPDP(Table 1), and it was apparent that the thiolation of antibody led to a dramatic loss of activity. For instance, with the addition of eight thiol groups, the activity of monoclonal antibody 250-30.6 fell from 1/16,384 to 1/4096 (a loss of >75% of activity); with further increases in the number of -SH groups, the antibody activity pro-

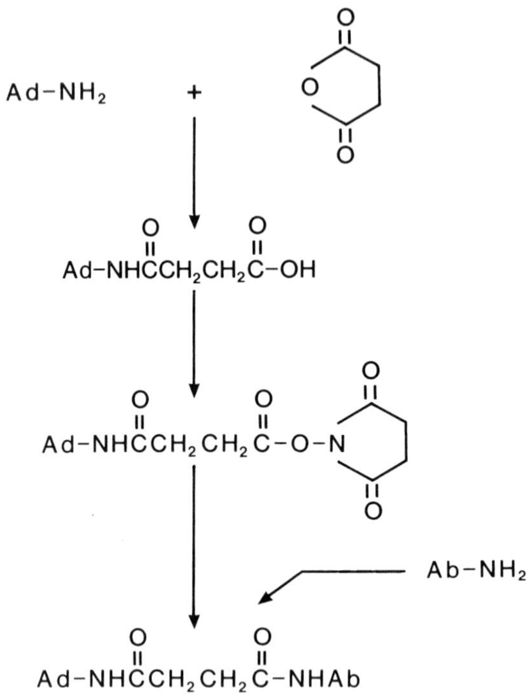

Figure 3 Reaction scheme showing the preparation of succinyl adriamycin (Succ-Ad) and conjugation to antibody via the active ester.

gressively fell and there was virtually no activity in the presence of 24 sulfhydryl groups. The loss of antibody activity appeared to be due to loss of protein due to precipitation resulting from the neutralization of charged lysyl residues by chemical modification and to modification of the antibody. On the basis of these results, 8-10 sulfhydryl groups per antibody molecule (88% recovery) were regularly used, and reasonable retention of antibody activity occurred. For conjugation of MPB-Ad to antibody, a solution containing excess MPB-Ad was added to the thiolated antibody, to yield, after purification, an adriamycin-antibody conjugate in which adriamycin and antibody were linked via a thioether bond. When this conjugate was tested, most of the antibody activity had been lost, and it was found (Table 2) that most of the loss occurred in the final step after the addition of MPB-Ad (Table 2). Drug activity was tested on the HT29 cell line and, like antibody activity, was also lost. As this coupling procedure resulted in the loss of both drug and antibody activity, it was considered to be unsuitable for further study, particularly as studies using other antibodies gave similar results.

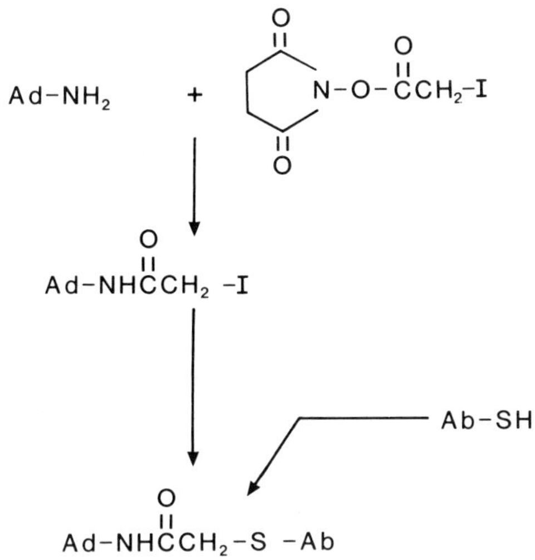

Figure 4 Reaction scheme showing the prepration of iodoacetyl adriamycin (IA-Ad) and conjugation to antibody.

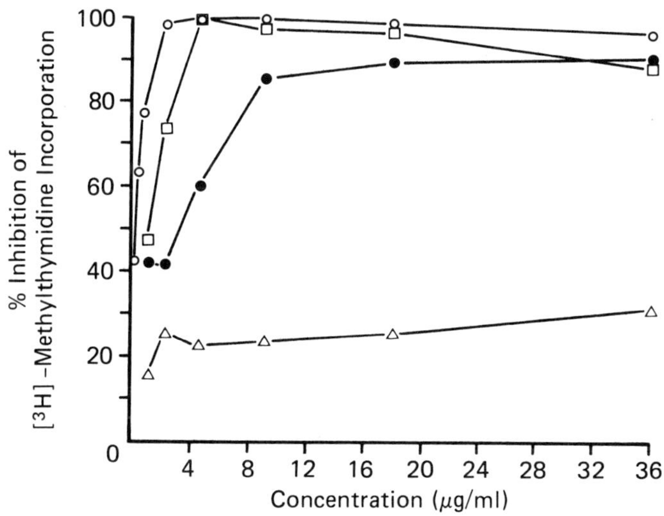

Figure 5 Cytotoxicity of adriamycin analogs on the human colon carcinoma, HT 29, showing the concentration of drug (horizontal axis) and the percentage of incorporation of [^{3}H]-methylthymidine (vertical axis); ○, adriamycin; □, iodoacetyl adriamycin; ●, succinyl adriamycin; △, maleimidophenylbutyryl adriamycin.

Table 1 The Use of SPDP to Introduce Thiol Groups into Immunoglobulin

Molar excess of SPDP	Number of thiol groups introduced	Protein recovery (%)	Antibody titer^{-1}
0	0	100	16384
10	8	88	4096
30	11	88	4096
50	14	80	128
100	24	16	4

See text for further details; antibody 250-30.6 used; titer measured by the rosetting assay.

3. Preparation and Biological Activity of Adriamycin-Antibody Conjugate Prepared Using Succ-Ad Analog (Method B)

Conjugation of Succ-Ad to either 250-30.6 or anti-Ly-2.1 antibodies required activation of the carboxylic acid group of Succ-Ad by treating it with N-hydroxysuccinimide and dicyclohexylcarbodiimide in dimethylformamide (DMF), to produce the intermediate active ester which was used in solution (Fig. 3). The resulting conjugate containe 8-10 molecules of adriamycin per antibody molecule and had an antibody titer of 1/256, compared with 1/4096 for the unmodified antibody. The cytotoxicity of the conjugate was then tested on HT29 cells and showed only a 15-20% inhibition of incorporation of isotope at

Table 2 Effect of Chemical Manipulations on the Titer of Monoclonal Antibody 250-30.6 Conjugated to MPB-Adriamycin

Antibody	Titer
Pure antibody (0.8 mg/ml)	500,000
Thiolated antibody in DTT (0.4 mg/ml)	250,000
Thiolated antibody after removal of reducing agent (0.4 mg/ml)	250,000
Thiolated antibody at room temperature overnight (0.4 mg/ml)	250,000
Thiolated antibody in 10% DMSO (0.4 mg/ml)	250,000
Antibody conjugated to Adriamycin (0.2 mg/ml)	16

The antibody concentration is shown in parentheses; the titer was measured in the rosetting assay.

a concentration of 5.6 μg/ml, while free adriamycin showed 85% inhibition (data not shown). Due to poor drug and antibody activity, these conjugates were not further studied.

4. Preparation and Testing of an Adriamycin-Antibody Conjugate Using the IA-Ad Analog (Method C)

Iodoacetyl adriamycin has the capacity to react with sulfhydryl groups of antibody to yield a thioether bond (Fig. 4). Monoclonal antibody anti-Ly-2.1 was treated with dithiothreitol (DTT) such that selective cleavage of intrachain disulphide bonds occurred without further chemical modification; this partially reduced antibody was then reacted with IA-Ad. Conjugates made in this way showed an antibody titer of 1/32,000 compared to 1/128,000 for unmodified antibody, i.e., there was a reasonable retention of antibody activity. The cytotoxicity of the conjugate was tested (Fig. 6) and showed an inhibition of 50% DNA synthesis ($I.D._{50}$) at a concentration of 2.6×10^{-6} M (with respect to adriamycin). The conjugate showed a comparable toxicity to the free IA-Ad analog ($I.D._{50}$ 8×10^{-6} M) but a reduced toxicity when compared with free adriamycin ($I.D._{50}$ 2.3×10^{-7} M, Fig. 7). There were two important points to note in this study: (a) free Ad was approximately 40 times more potent than IA-Ad, and (b) IA-Ad and IA-Ad-MAb were of comparable potency. This latter finding is of interest, as it clearly demonstrates that covalently binding IA-Ad to antibody did not drastically affect Ad activity—a significant finding in that IA-Ad can freely diffuse or be transported into the cell compared with the IA-Ad antibody conjugate (see below).

As the conjugate was active in vitro it was important to demonstrate that the binding and cytotoxicity was specific, i.e., that antibody was truly "targeting" the drug to the tumor. In the previous cytotoxicity assay, the conjugate was exposed to the target cell throughout the whole period of the assay, whereas in the 30-min inhibition assay the conjugate was exposed to the target cell line for 30 min at room temperature and washed. During this time, antibody would be expected to bind to the tumor cell and selectively convey adriamycin to the target. For specificity testing another adriamycin conjugate was made using the 17.1 antibody which did not react with the $Ly\text{-}2^+$ E3 tumor; this conjugate had the same number of adriamycin residues as the IA-Ad-anti-Ly-2.1 conjugate. E3 cells were exposed to various concentrations of the two conjugates and assayed for their cytotoxic effects (Fig. 8). Only the Ly-2.1 antibody conjugate was cytotoxic to the $Ly\text{-}2.1^+$ target cells, as shown by a 50% inhibition at 1×10^{-6} M while 17.1 antibody conjugate showed only a 5% inhibition on 17.1^- E3 cells at this concentration, i.e., the reactive antibody conjugate was many times more toxic than the nonreactive antibody conjugate.

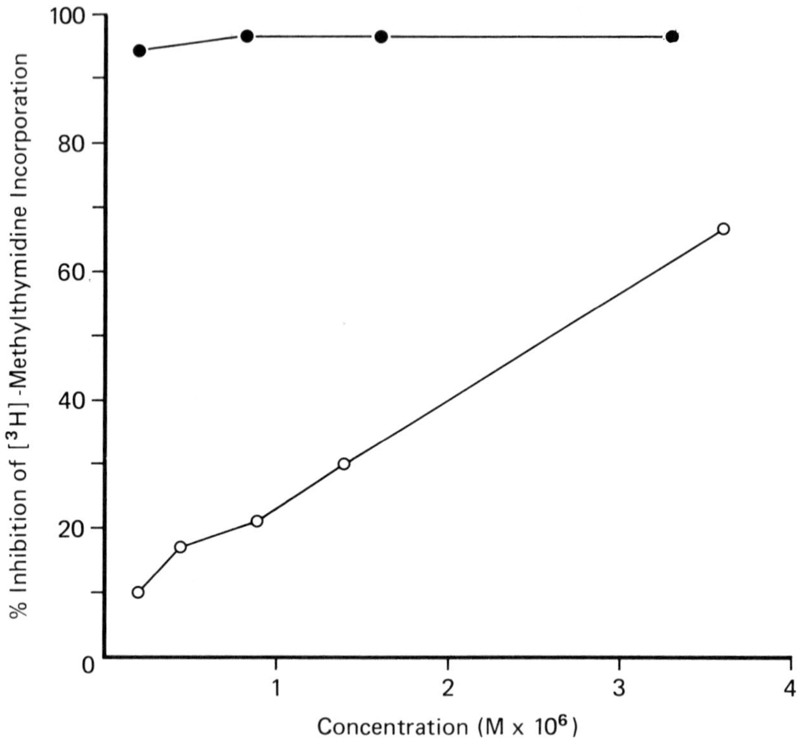

Figure 6 Cytotoxicity of adriamycin (●) and adriamycin-antibody (anti-Ly-2.1) conjugate prepared using IA-Ad analog (○) on the mouse thymoma ITT(1)75NS E3. The horizontal axis shows the concentration of the drug, the vertical axis the % inhibition of uptake of [^{3}H]-methylthymidine.

5. In Vivo Efficacy of Iodoacetyl-Adriamycin-Anti-Ly-2.1 Conjugate

The antitumor activity was tested in (C57BL/6 × BALB/c)F_1 (BCF_1) mice with intraperitoneal thymomas. Groups of mice were injected intraperitoneally on day 1, 3, 5, and 7 with (1) PBS, (2) a mixture of adriamycin and anti-Ly-2.1, and (3) IA-Ad-anti-Ly-2.1 conjugate receiving a total of 4 μg adriamycin and 50 μg antibody either free or in conjugate form. Mice that received PBS were all dead by day 28 due to ascites, whereas 30% of those receiving conjugate survived indefinitely (Fig. 9); a mixture of adriamycin and antibody led to a survival until day 32. In addition, the anti-Ly-2.1 antibody has a slight antitumor effect. These studies were also performed on mice with subcutaneous tumors (Fig. 10) with similar results. However, while it was clear that these conjugates had *some* therapeutic effect, it was not impressive and so derivatives with a greater potency were sought.

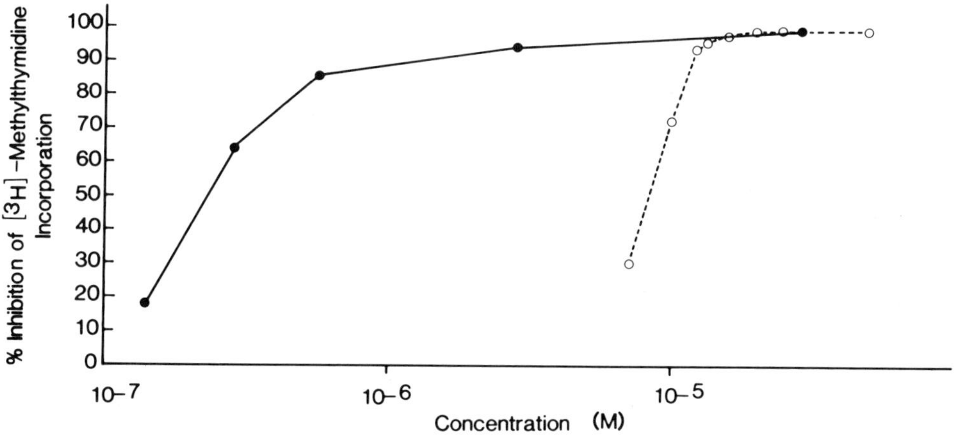

Figure 7 Cytotoxicity of adriamycin (●) and iodoacetyl adriamycin (○) on the mouse thymoma ITT(1)75NS E3. Axes as for Figure 6.

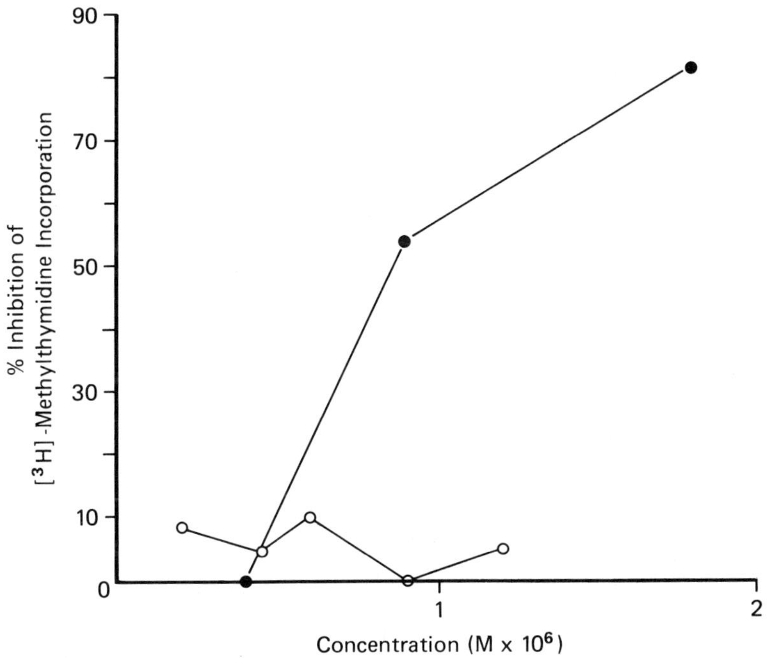

Figure 8 Specific cytotoxicity of adriamycin-antibody conjugate prepared using IA-Ad on the mouse thymoma ITT(1)75NS E3. (●) IA-Ad-anti-Ly-2.1; (○) IA-Ad-17.1 antibody. Axes as for Figure 6.

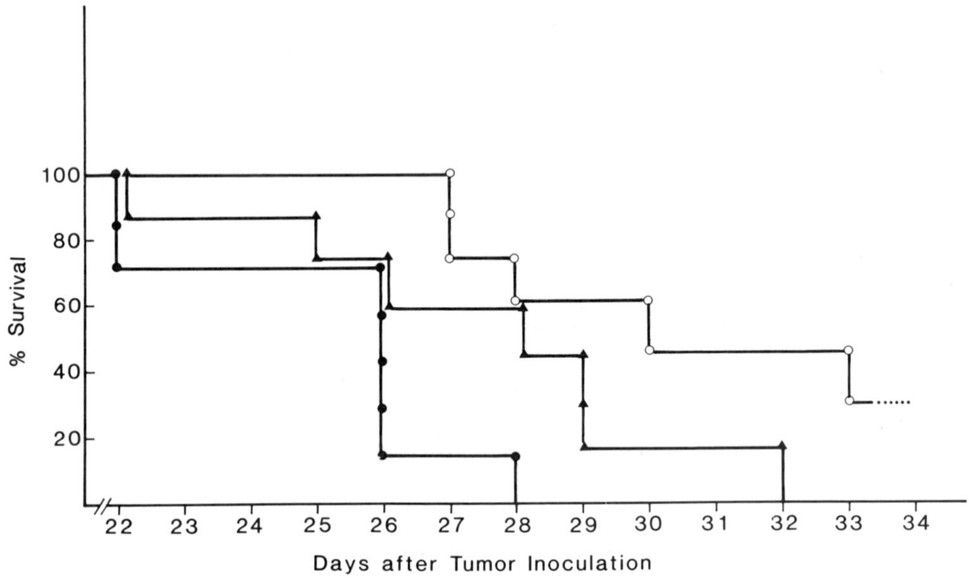

Figure 9 Survival of CBF_1 mice bearing the ITT(1)75NS E3 thymoma. Groups of 7 mice were inoculated i.p. with 10^5 cells per mouse; 24 hours later, mice received i.p. PBS (●), a mixture of anti-Ly-2.1 and adriamycin (▲), and IA-Ad-anti-Ly-2.1 (○).

B. Coupling of Idarubicin to Monoclonal Antibodies

1.Preparation of Idarubicin-Antibody Conjugates

A derivative of idarubicin-bromoidarubicin (BrIda) was used, as it is capable of reacting with the amino and carboxyl groups of antibodies (Fig. 11). To establish optimum coupling conditions, reactions were performed with excess amounts of BrIda and a constant amount of anti-colon carcinoma antibody 250-30.6 (Fig. 12). A 20-fold excess of BrIda gave a conjugate with six residues of Ida/mol antibody with 60% protein recovery; adding increasing amounts of BrIda led to poor protein recovery. The stability of the conjugate was tested in alkaline (pH 9.0) and acid (pH 4.5) conditions and resulted in the loss of 50% of drug under the former conditions, suggesting that at least 50% of the drug is coupled to the antibody via an ester linkage.

2. Antibody Activity

The antibody activity of the conjugates were tested and it was found that the coupling of 2-6 residues gave rise to conjugates with acceptable antibody activity (Fig. 13) (titers of 1:16000 and 1:11000 cf neat 250-30.6 titer of 1:33000 on the target cell COLO 205).

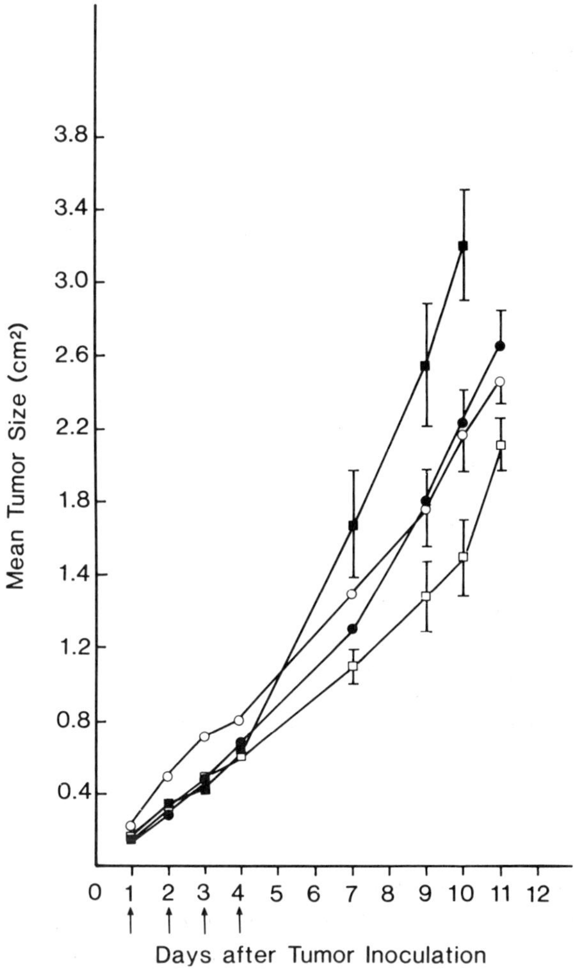

Figure 10 Growth of the thymoma ITT(1)75NS E3 in CBF_1 mice injected s.c. with 3×10^6 cells. Groups of 10 mice were given treatments i.p., denoted (↑); PBS (■), adriamycin (○), a mixture of adriamycin and anti-Ly-2.1 (●), and IA-Ad-anti-Ly-2.1 conjugate (□). Error bars represent ± standard error of the mean tumor size.

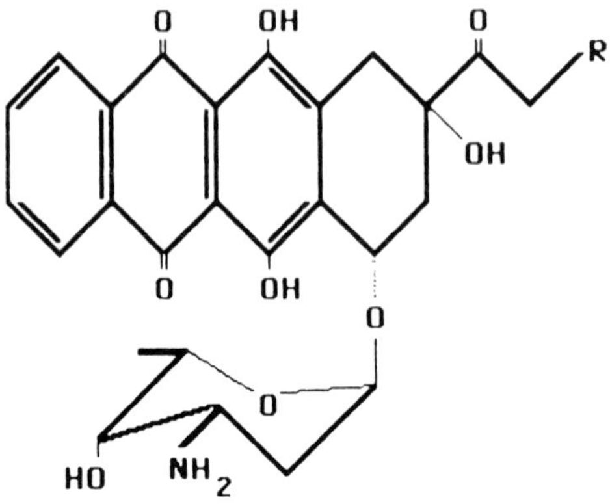

IDARUBICIN	R = H
BROMOIDARUBICIN	R = Br
AMINE LINK	R = NH–MAb
ESTER LINK	R = O–C(=O)–MAb

Figure 11 Structure of bromoidarubicin and its reaction with antibody.

3. In Vitro Activity of Idarubicin-Antibody Conjugates

Free drug and conjugates were tested by their ability to inhibit the incorporation of [^{3}H]-thymidine using conjugates with up to six residues of idarubicin/mol of antibody. The 250-30.6-Id conjugates were slightly less active than free idarubicin (Fig. 14a); free idarubicin had an I.D.$_{50}$ at 6×10^{-8} M, while the conjugate had an I.D.$_{50}$ of 3.5×10^{-7} M on the target cell line COLO 205. Similar activities were demonstrated by other antibody conjugates (anti-Ly-2.1 and antitransferrin receptor) prepared in a similar manner (19). The specificity of these conjugates was tested on COLO 205 (250-30.6 +ve) and E3 (250-30.6 -ve) cell lines. Both cell lines showed a similar dose response to free drug, i.e., 9.2×10^{-7} M for COLO 205 and 9.8×10^{-7} M for E3, however, the 250-30.6-Id conjugate was four times more toxic to COLO 205 than the antibody nonreactive E3 cell line (Fig. 14b). In addition free antibody could inhibit the killing of antigen-reactive cells with the conjugate (not shown).

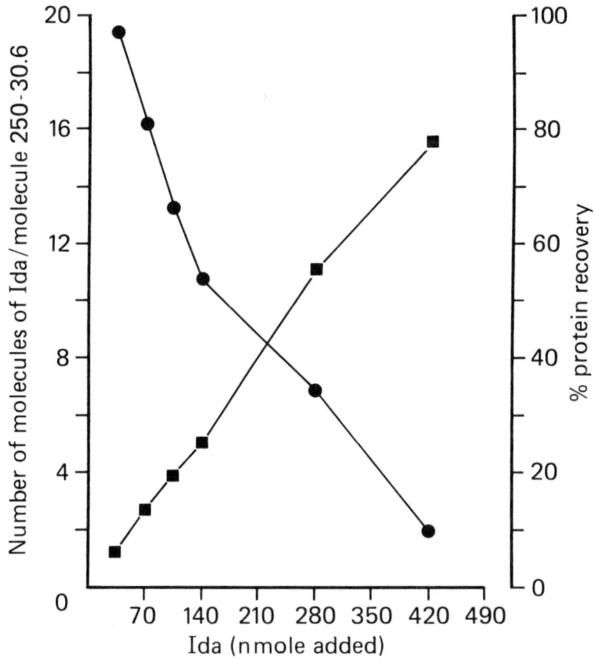

Figure 12 Coupling of Ida to 250-30.6 (0.5 mg). Moles of Ida incorporated per molecule 250-30.6 (■) and protein recovery (●) are shown as a function of the number of nanomoles of BrIda in the reaction mixture.

4. In Vivo Efficacy of Idarubicin-Antibody Conjugates

The in vivo antitumor activity of the 250-30.6-Id conjugate was tested in nude mice bearing COLO 205 palpable human tumor xenografts. Mice were then treated on days 4, 5, 6, 10, and 12 after tumor innoculation with (1) PBS, (2) 250-30.6 antibody, (3) idarubicin and 250-30.6 (nonconjugated), (4) idarubicin, and (5) Ida-250-30.6 conjugate. A total of 275 μg of Ida was given intravenously. No therapeutic effect was apparent in the groups of mice treated with PBS and unconjugated 250-30.6 (Fig. 15a); with Ida, 20% of the mice survived while all the mice in the nonconjugated Id and 250-30.6 groups were dead by day 7 with symptoms of toxicity, such as previous weight loss. However, mice treated with the Ida-antibody conjugate showed a dramatic reduction of mean tumor size (Fig. 15a) and tumor growth curves for individual mice (Fig. 15b) showed that 5/10 mice had tumors that had regressed by day 7; these tumors then proceeded to grow, leaving 2/10 mice without tumors, and the mice did not show any effects due to toxicity. To determine whether there had been

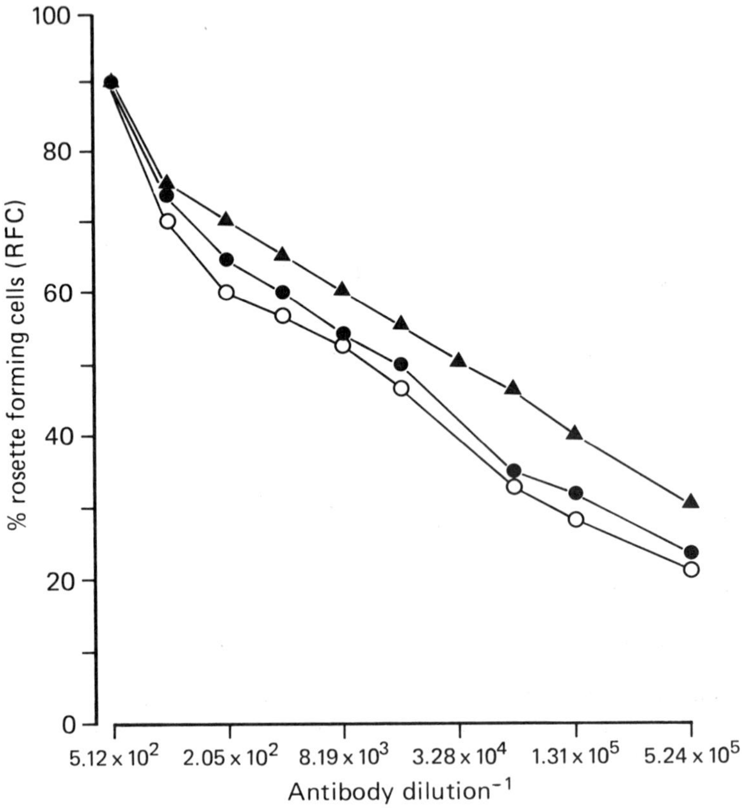

Figure 13 Percentage of rosette-forming cells vs. antibody dilution of different 250-30.6 conjugates on COLO 205 target cells. Unconjugated 250-30.6 (▲) and 6 (○) and 2 (●) molecules of Ida/molecule conjugates.

some selection for antigen-negative variants, the tumors that reappeared were tested for 250-30.6 antigen density by rosetting or flow cytometry, but no differences were seen from the tumors obtained from mice treated with PBS (data not shown). The anti-Ly-2.1-Ida conjugates were also tested in CBF_1 mice with subcutaneously growing thymomas (Fig. 16). A total of 10 μg of idarubicin in the form of conjugate inhibited the growth by up to 75% on day 7 and 60% by day 11, some of the most impressive results we have seen with this form of therapy.

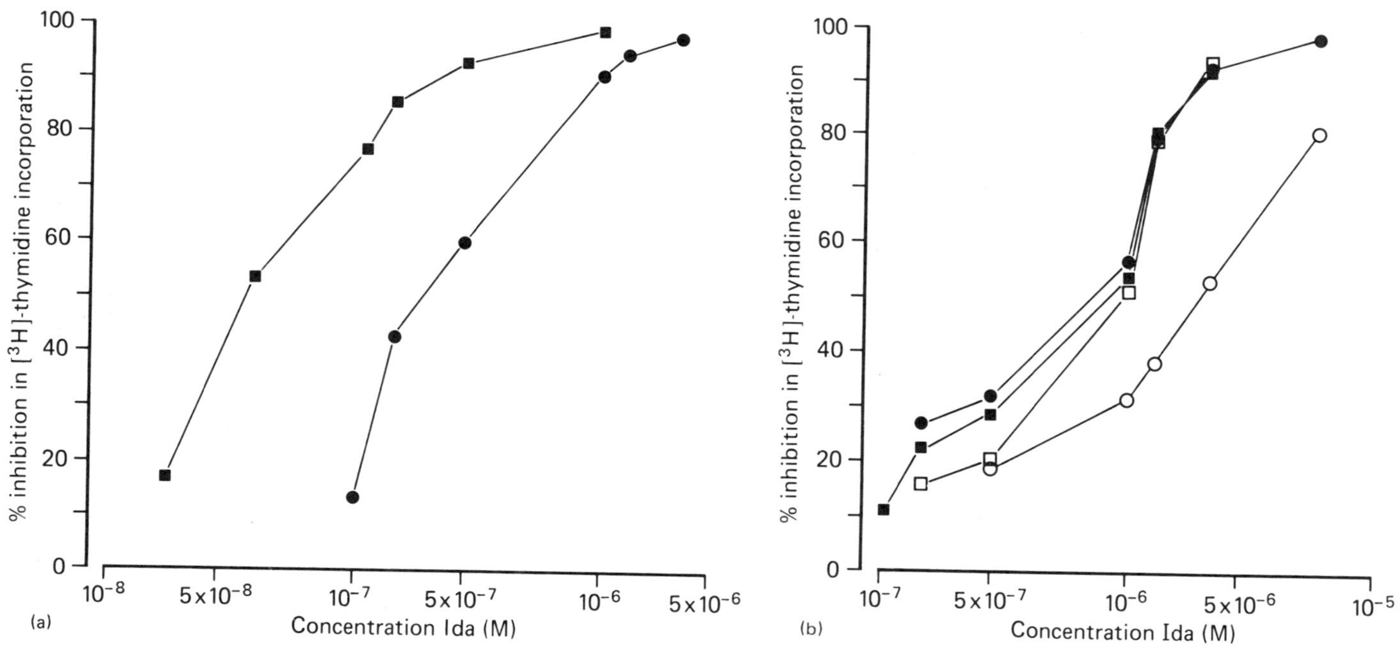

Figure 14 (a) Inhibitory effect of free Ida (■) and Ida-250-30.6 conjugate (●) on COLO 205 target cells in the 24-hour assay; and (b) inhibitory effect of free Ida (■) or Ida-250-30.6 conjugate (●) on antibody reactive cells COLO 205 and of free Ida (□) or conjugate (○) on antibody nonreactive cells (E3) in the 30-minute specificity assay.

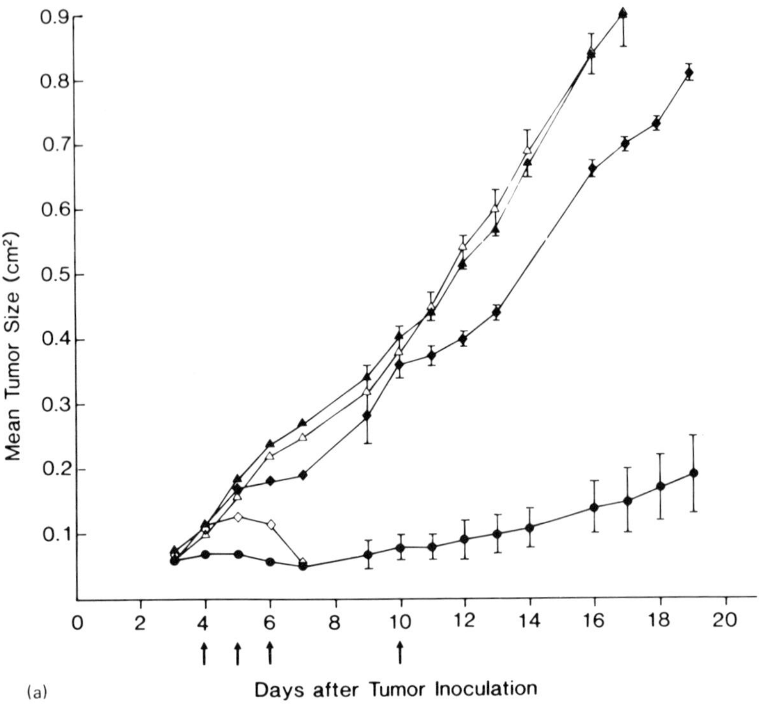
Mean Tumor Size (cm²)
0.9
0.8
0.7
0.6
0.5
0.4
0.3
0.2
0.1
0 2 4 6 8 10 12 14 16 18 20
Days after Tumor Inoculation

(a)

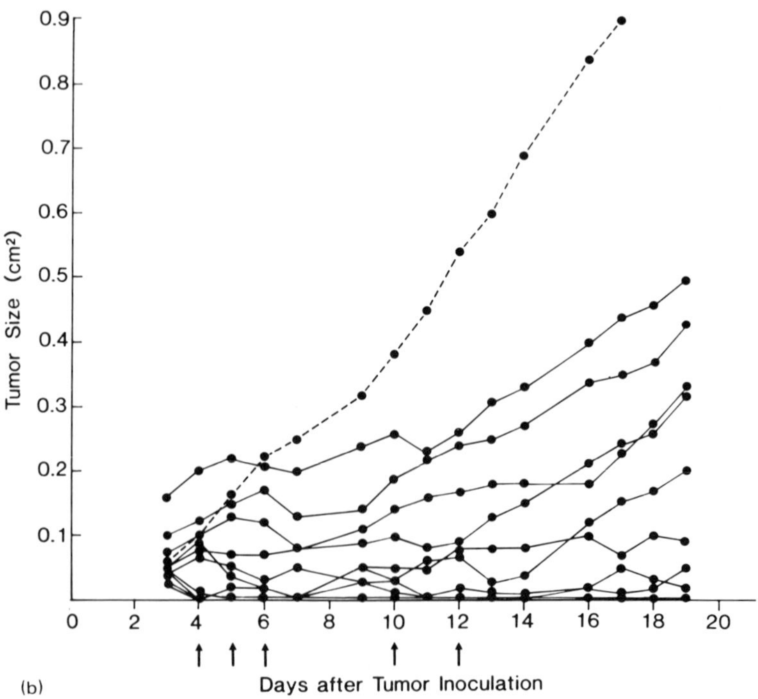
Tumor Size (cm²)
0.9
0.8
0.7
0.6
0.5
0.4
0.3
0.2
0.1
0 2 4 6 8 10 12 14 16 18 20
Days after Tumor Inoculation

(b)

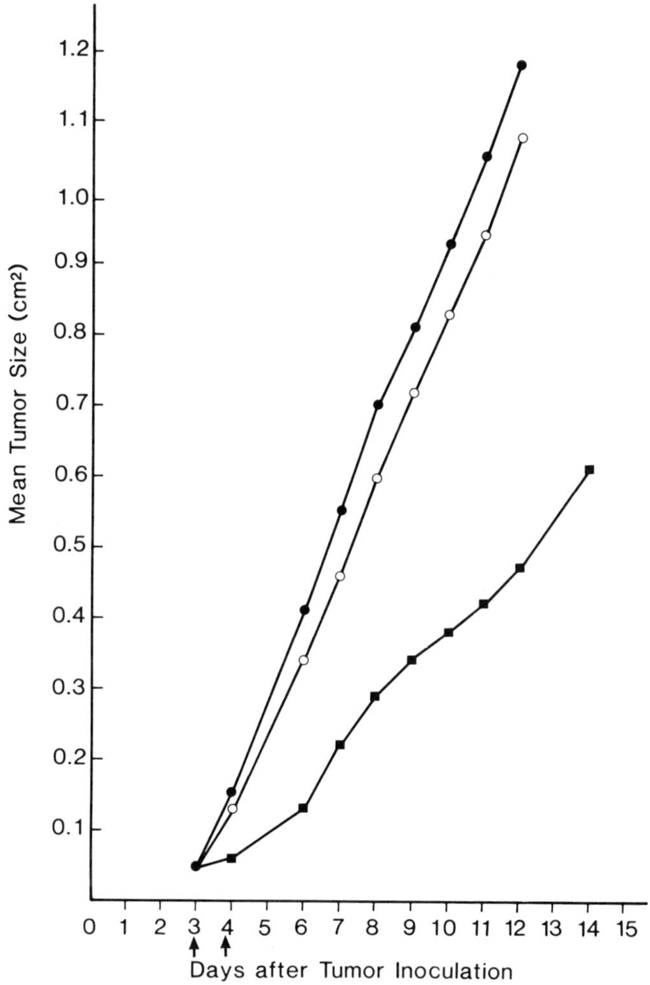

Figure 16 Growth of the murine thymoma ITT(1)75NS E3 in CBF_1 mice injected s.c. with 3 X 10^6 cells. Groups of 10 mice were given treatment i.v., denoted (↑); PBS (●), idarubicin (○), and Ida-anti-Ly-2.1 conjugate (■). Standard error for each point was not more than ± 0.03 cm^2.

Figure 15 Growth of the COLO 205 human tumor xenograft in nude mice injected subcutaneously with 2 X 10^6 cells. (a) Groups of 10 mice were given the following treatments i.v., denoted (↑); PBS (△), free Ida (♦), Ida-250-30.6 conjugate (●), mixture of Ida and 250-30.6 (◇), and 250-30.6 (▲). Error bars represent ± standard error of the mean tumor size and (b) individual tumor growth curves of xenografted nude mice which were treated i.v. (↑) with Ida-250-30.6 conjugate. The broken line represents the mean tumor size of PBS-treated mice.

III. DISCUSSION

Daunomycin and adriamycin are two anthracycline antineoplastic agents widely used for cancer therapy, but their long-term use may be accompanied by cardiotoxicity and by systemic effects common to all cytotoxic drugs. The concept of conveying these drugs specifically to tumors is an attractive one, for in that way *all* side effects would be minimized. In the last decade there have been numerous reports on the use of antibodies for the specific targeting of drugs such as chlorambucil (20), methotrexate (21,22), mitomycin C (23), and vindesine (24) to tumors. Although several reports have appeared on the targeting of danuomycin (7,12), the closely related drug adriamycin has received little attention, presumably due to its relative instability and solubility in comparison to daunomycin. Two anthracyclines were investigated in this study, adriamycin and idarubicin. Idarubicin is a recently introduced analog of daunomycin (25), which is 10 times more toxic than adriamycin in vitro. These potent analogs are useful in the light of the amount of conjugate that localizes to the tumor, where more toxic drugs would be more efficacious with less conjugate. This was shown when conjugates of methotrexate and the more potent analog, aminopterin, were compared in vivo, where the latter conjugates were more efficacious than the former (26).

In this study both antibody and drug activity of the conjugates were monitored in simple experiments, which allowed quantiative comparisons to be made between various adriamycin-antibody conjugates before more difficult and less precise in vivo experiments were commenced. Three different derivatives of adriamycin were made for conjugation to antibody: MPB-Ad, IA-Ad, and Succ-Ad. MPB-Ad and IA-Ad can react with free sulfhydryl groups of antibody introduced by chemical modification (Figs. 2 and 4) or partial reduction but Succ-Ad can only react with antibodies after activation of its carboxyl group (Fig. 3). All derivatives were tested for their in vitro cytotoxicity on tumor cells, which was compared with the activity of free adriamycin; all were found to have a reduced toxicity, although higher doses of conjugates could achieve almost total inhibition of tumor cell growth. The iodoacetyl adriamycin derivative was the most active, being approximately 1/40 as active as free adriamycin (Fig. 7). Nevertheless, if this moiety could be specifically "targeted" the conjugate could be useful.

There are several possible explanations for the loss of adriamycin activity after chemical modification. The accepted mechanism of cytotoxicity of adriamycin is via intercalation to DNA (15), where the hydrogen of the amino group weakly binds to the negatively charged oxygen on the DNA backbone; modification of the basic amino group to a neutral amide by the chemical reactions used herein could conceivably decrease binding and therefore result in lower activity. However, AD32, an adriamycin analog with an amide incapable of binding to DNA, shows a wide spectrum of activity (16). It may also be that the derivatives simply do not enter the cell, or upon entering, the adriamycin does not reach its target. It has recently been suggested that an alternative target for adriamycin is the cell membrane (27), so that an explanation for the activity of IA-Ad, compared to the other derivatives, could be due to cell surface alkylation by the idoacetyl group.

The three analogs MPB-Ad, Succ-AD, and Ad-IA were all successfully conjugated to monoclonal antibodies, but conjugates derived from MPB-Ad and Succ-Ad analogs were devoid of either antibody or drug activity. In addition to Succ-Ad and MBP-Ad analogs had poor activity, and if they were to be made active they would require hydrolysis in the lysosomal compartment; the failure to detect cytotoxicity with these conjugates suggests that insufficient drug is internalized or that there is inefficient hydrolysis of the conjugate.

In contrast to the conjugates made using MPB-Ad and Succ-Ad derivative, the IA-Ad analog yielded an active conjugate, which showed toxicity comparable to the free analog although less toxic than free adriamycin (Figs. 6 and 7). This is an important finding, as it would be expected that IA-Ad, barely larger than free Ad, would surely enter cells more readily than the IA-Ad-antibody conjugate. However, the fact that both are highly toxic must indicate that both enter equally well (by presumably different mechanisms) or, alternatively, that Ad is cleaved from antibody at the cell surface. In this light it should be noted that IA-Ad is bound to antibody by irreversible thio-ether linkages, although liposomal and cell surface enzymes could digest antibody to yield small IA-Ad peptide complexes, which could act either internally or at the cell surface. There is of course, a third explanation—that targeting is occurring in vitro, i.e., that *all* the Ad in the solution binds to the cell via antibody, whereas free Ad or IA-Ad bind only when they randomly hit the cell.

It was also demonstrated that the IA-Ad-antibody conjugate reacted specifically, i.e., conjugate bound only to tumor cells carrying the appropriate antigen, and not to cells lacking the antigen (Fig. 8).

We have therefore succeeded in producing a specific adriamycin-antibody conjugate with acceptable in vitro activity. The activity is clearly less than that of free Ad, but all activity is directed to the target, whereas free Ad can react with all cells. Although these Ad conjugates are active and specific when used in vitro, the in vivo results were not impressive and we decided to approach the synthesis of anthracycline conjugates by conjugation via an alternative site in the anthracycline molecule. Coupling of daunomycin via the C-14 carbon has been reported previously (17,18), and it was decided to use the more potent analog idarubicin. Idarubicin was bound to antibodies via bromoidarubicin and conjugates with up to six residues of Ida/mol antibody were obtained with acceptable protein recovery and antibody activity (Figs. 12,13). Susceptibility of the Ida-MAb conjugates to alkaline conditions indicated that the Ida is most likely to be linked to the MAb via an ester bond (Fig. 11). Assays for inhibition of DNA synthesis of antibody reactive COLO 205 cells on exposure to the Ida-250-30.6 conjugate indicated that conjugates were one fourth as toxic as free Ida (Fig. 14a)—a big improvement when compared to the IA-Ad-anti-Ly-2.1 conjugate, which was only 1/40 as active as free Ad. Furthermore, these conjugates, at least in vitro, were entirely specific (Fig. 14b). However, it should be noted that at high concentrations of the conjugates, there was some nonspecific cell lysis (18)—a phenomenon which occurs only in vitro, as these conjugates in vivo (see below) do not show the side effects seen with Ida. When nude mice bearing a COLO 205 xenograft were treated intravenously with Ida-250-30.6, there was substantial retardation of tumor growth (Fig. 15a) and similar results occurred in the thymoma model (Fig. 16), in both cases using mice with established tumors. Furthermore, histopathological examination of mice receiving up to 2.4 mg/kg in one dose did not show any nonspecific toxic effects (19). It was noted that tumors over a certain size did not seem to respond well to the therapy, and the analysis of recurring tumors for differences in antigenic expression did not show any differences to control tumors. However, these recurrent tumors need to be examined for drug resistance. Ways of increasing the therapy for larger tumors also need to be examined. However, in our hands, Ida-MAb conjugates have been the most efficacious conjugates to date.

As it can be seen from the data, we have investigated a number of approaches to link anthracyclines to MAb. The most efficacious conjugates were found to be those coupled via the C-14 of the anthracycline, but we are currently exploring the possibility of using other functional groups of the anthracyclines as sites to couple antibodies. The comparison of adriamycin conjugates with idarubicin conjugates illustrates the need for more toxic agents for coupling to antibodies and over the years large numbers of antineoplastic agents have been tested and shelved due to the severe toxicity to the host. It is appropriate for these drugs to be examined for the production of potent conjugates with specific antitumor activity.

IV. APPENDIX

A. Materials

1. Chemicals and Suppliers

Adriamycin hydrochloride, idarubicin hydrochloride, and bromoidarubicin hydrochloride (Farmitalia Carlo Erba, Milan, Italy); N-succinimidyl 3-(2-pyridyldithio)propionate (SPDP) and succinimidyl 4-(p-maleimidophenyl) butyrate (SMPB) (Pierce Chemicals Company, IL); Porapak Q (Waters Associates, MA); Sephadex G25 (PD10) columns, DEAE Sephacel and Protein A Sepharose CL-B from Pharmacia Pty. Ltd. (Uppsala, Sweden); [^{3}H]-thymidine (specific activity, 5Ci/m mole) or [^{3}H]-methylthymidine (specific activity, 105Ci/m mole) (The Radiochemical Centre, Amersham, England); newborn calf serum DME and RPMI 1640 (Flow Laboratories, Sydney, Australia); glutamine and penicillin (Commonwealth Serum Laboratories, Sydney, Australia); streptomycin (Glaxo, Melbourne, Australia); Affi-Gel Blue (Bio-Rad, Richmond, CA).

2. Monoclonal Antibodies

Four monoclonal antibodies were used in these studies: (a) The 250-30.6 monoclonal antibody (IgG2b) recognizes an antigen present on normal and malignant human gastrointestinal epithelium (28). (b) Monoclonal anti-Ly-2.1 (IgG2a) reacts with the murine lymphocyte Ly-2.1 alloantigen (29). (c) HuLy-m9 (IgG1), an antibody raised against the human transferrin receptor (30). (d) 17.1 monoclonal antibody recognizes an antigen present on human tumor cells (31). All antibodies were produced in this laboratory. The antibodies were purified from ascites fluid by 40% ammonium sulfate fractionation followed by affinity chromatography on Protein A Sepharose CL-B (anti-Ly-2.1, 17.1) or ion exchange chromatography on DEAE Sephacel (250-30.6) or Affi-Gel Blue (HuLy-m9).

3. Tumor Cells

Human cell lines used were the human colon carcinomas HT29 (32), Colo 205 (33), and the acute T-lymphocyte leukemia CEM (34). The murine cell line used was the thymoma ITT(1)75NS E3 variant (E3) (20). The human and murine cells lines were maintained in vitro in RPMI 1640 and DME, respectively, supplemented with 10% heat inactivated newborn calf serum, 2 mM glutamine, 100 μg/ml streptamycin, and 100 I.U./ml penicillin. The E3 cell line was maintained in vivo by the passaging of cells from ascites fluid produced in (C57BL/6 × BALB/C)F_1 (BCF_1) mice. Ascites were washed in DME and PBS, and a solid tumor developed after the subcutaneous injection into the abdominal wall of mice. Adherent cells were harvested with 0.125% trypsin washed with RPMI 1640 and either used for in vitro assays or injected into the abdominal wall of nude mice. Tumor size was measured daily with a caliper square measuring along the perpendicular axes of the tumors. Data was recorded as mean tumor size (product of two diameters ± standard error).

4. Mice

(C57BL/6 × BALB/c)F_1 mice were produced in this department. Nude mice (Swiss) were obtained from Animal Resources Centre, Western Australia.

B. Methods

1. Synthesis of Adriamycin Analogs for Conjugation

Adriamycin-antibody conjugates were prepared by introducing suitable functional groups into adriamycin and then reacting the activated adriamycin with monoclonal antibodies.

a. *N-(p-Maleimidophenylbutyryl) Adriamycin (MPB-Ad)*: Adriamycin hydrochloride, dissolved in dry N,N-dimethylformamide (DMF) at a concentration of 4.5 mg/ml, was treated with an excess of silver carbonate, shaken for 15 min and then centrifuged at 450 *g* for 10 min. When the supernatant was decanted, a slight molar excess of SMPB added and the mixture was stirred overnight at room temperature. DMF was then evaporated and the residue dissolved in dichloromethane which was washed with water, dried with anhydrous sodium sulfate, and the solvent evaporated. The residue was taken up in dichloromethane and diethyl ether added until precipitation was completed; the precipitate was washed several times with diethyl ether/dichloromethane (2:1), and finally dried and stored at 4°C in the dark. Thin layer chromatography (TLC) on silica gel plates (DC-Plastikfolien Kieselgel 60 F254, Merck), using n-butanol:acetic acid:water at a ratio of 4:1:5, indicated only one spot at Rf.0.71 indicating a pure sample.

b. *Succinylation of Adriamycin (Succ-Ad)*: Adriamycin hydrochloride (8.4 mg) was dissolved in dry DMF (2 ml) and treated with an excess of silver carbonate, mixed, centrifuged, and the supernatant decanted and treated with succinic anhydride (64 μl, 28 mg/ml) in DMF, and stirred for 1 hr. The solvent was removed and the residue treated as above, except for the washing of the organic solution, which was done with a saturated solution of sodium chloride as succinyl adriamycin has low solubility in water; TLC indicated only one spot, Rf.0.59.

c. *N-Iodoacetyl Adriamycin (IA-Ad)*: Adriamycin hydrochloride (7 mg) was dissolved in dry DMF (4 ml) and treated with excess silver carbonate, the mixture centrifuged, and the supernatant treated with one equivalent of succinimidyl iodoacetate. The mixture was stirred overnight, and the solvent then evaporated. The residue was dissolved in chloroform, washed with saturated sodium chloride solution, the organic layer dried with anhydrous sodium sulfate, and evaporated to yield a red solid, which was washed several times with ether and the powder stored at 4°C in the dark. TLC indicated only one spot of Rf.0.72.

2. Introduction of Sulfhydryl (-SH) Groups on the Monoclonal Antibodies

Sulfhydryl (-SH) groups were introduced into antibody molecules by using either SPDP, which introduces -SH groups to the epsilon amino group of the antibody. SPDP (5 mM) in absolute alcohol was added to the antibody in PBS and the mixture stirred intermittently for 30 min at room temperature, unreacted SPDP was then removed by gel filtration using a Sephadex G25 column (PD10), equilibrated with 0.1 M sodium acetate, 0.1 M sodium chloride (35). The eluted antibodies were reduced with dithiothreitol (DTT) (50 mM) and subjected to a second gel filtration step in PBS to remove 2-pyridinethione. The number of SPDP residues introduced into each antibody molecule was quantitated spectrophotometrically by determining the concentration of 2-pyridinethione, released after addition of 100 mM DTT to an aliquot of the protein solution: The absorption at 343 nm was measured where the extinction coefficient for 2-pyridinethione is 8.03×10^3 $M^{-1} cm^{-1}$. In the second method, sulfhydryl groups were exposed by treating antibody (1 ml, 1 mg/ml) with DTT (75 μl, 1 M) for 45 min; the mixture was desalted by gel filtration on a PD10 column equilibrated with deoxygenated 0.01 M Tris-saline buffer, pH 8.6, and the protein collected.

3. Preparation of Adriamycin-Antibody Conjugates

Three different methods of conjugation were used.

Method A: Antibody (1 ml, 1 mg/ml) was thiolated with SPDP and mixed with MPB-Ad (0.4 mg) in DMF (100 μl), and allowed to stand for 3 hr when the mixture was centrifuged to remove a red precipitate, which formed, desalted using a Sephadex G25 (PD10) column, and passed through a Porapak Q column to remove any nonspecifically adsorbed drug (36). The colored fractions were collected, quantitated (see below), and used for biological testing after filtration.

Method B: Succinyl adriamycin (1 mg) was dissolved in DMF (100 μl) and treated with a DMF solution of N-hydroxysuccinimide (17 μl, 10.1 mg/ml) and N,N-dicyclohexylcarbodiimide (37 μl, 8.3 mg/ml) and allowed to stand overnight. Antibody (1 ml, 1 mg/ml) was treated with 10 μl of this mixture, stirred intermittently for 0.5 hr, and then purified as above.

Method C: To a solution of partially reduced antibody (2.5 ml), iodoacetyl adriamycin (0.4 mg) in 100 μl DMF was added and allowed to stand for 2.5-3 hr. The slight precipitate formed was removed by centrifugation and the supernatant purified as above (Method A).

The number of residues (N) of adriamycin molecules bound per immunoglobulin molecule was calculated according to the formula:

$$N = 215{,}000 \times \frac{A_{280}}{(11{,}600 \times A_{280})} - (8{,}600 \times A_{480})$$

where A_{480} and A_{280} are the absorbance of the conjugate at 480 nm and 280 nm, where the extinction coefficients of adriamycin at 480 and 280 nm are 11600 $M^{-1} cm^{-1}$ and 8600 $M^{-1} cm^{-1}$, respectively. The extinction coefficient of immunoglobulin at 280 nm is 215000 $M^{-1} cm^{-1}$.

4. Preparation of Idarubicin-Antibody Conjugates

Antibody (1-2 mg/ml in Borate, pH 8.0) were mixed with molar excesses (0-50) of 14-bromo-4-demethoxydaunorubicin (Br-Ida) dissolved in N,N-dimethylformamide (DMF) at 10 mg/ml. The reaction was maintained at room temperature for 4 hr before centrifuging (400 $g \times 5$ min) to remove any precipitate. Free Br-Ida and other unreacted starting materials were removed by gel filtration chromatography using a Sephadex G25 column (PD10), and the conjugates were then passed through a column of Porapak Q to remove any adsorbed drug (36). The amount of Idarubicin incorporated in drug-antibody conjugates was determined by absorbance spectrophotometry at 498 nm ($E_{483} = 3.4 \times 10^3$ $M^{-1} cm^{-1}$) and protein estimation (37).

5. Testing for Antibody Activity

The titers of free antibody or antibody covalently linked to drugs were measured in a rosetting assay, which detects immunoglobulin bound to target cells using sheep anti-mouse immunoglobulin bound to red cells (38).

6. Testing for Drug Activity

The pharmacological activity of either free drug, drug derivatives, or conjugates was measured by the inhibition of the incorporation of [^{3}H]-methylthymidine or [^{3}H]-thymidine into deoxyribonucleic acid. Two types of assay were performed.

(*a*) *24-Hour Inhibition Assay*: Target cells were suspended in 100 μl medium at 2×10^6/ml in microtiter plates and incubated for 1 hr at 37°C. Free drug and conjugates were filtered sterile, and dilutions were performed in sterile PBS. 50 μl of free drug or conjugate were added to the cells using duplicate wells/sample; control wells received 50 μl of PBS and the cells cultures at 37°C and 7% CO_2 for 24 hr.

(*b*) *30-Minute Inhibition Assay*: 200 μl of cells at 2×10^6/ml were suspended in sterile tubes and sterile drug or conjugate mixed for 30 min at 37°C. Cells were then centrifuged (400 $g \times 5$ min), resuspended in growth medium, and 100 μl aliquots were seeded into a microtiter plate using duplicate wells/sample before an incubation period of 16-24 hr.

In both assays 1 μCi of [^{3}H]-thymidine in 50 μl of medium was added and incubation continued for a further 4-7 hr. Cells were then harvested onto filter paper using an automated cell harvester, the filter papers dried, suspended in 5 ml of scintillation fluid, and counted in a scintillation counter. The results were recorded as the percentage inhibition of incorporation of [^{3}H]-thymidine relative to cell controls: all assays were performed in duplicate, and the standard error for any point did not exceed 5% for any given experimental point. When adherent cell lines HT29 and COLO 205 were used, cells were exposed to 100 μl of 0.125% trysin for 10 min prior to harvesting. In a number of different studies, it was found that the inhibition of [^{3}H]-thymidine was equivalent to cell cytotoxicity measured by the uptake of Trypan blue. The two assays are used to give some measure of specificity; in the short (30 min) assay, nonreactive materials were washed away.

ACKNOWLEDGMENTS

The authors thank Farmitalia Carlo Erba for grant support and samples of anthracyclines. We also thank Mimi Morgan, Ruth Godding, and Antoinette Gentile for excellent secretarial assistance.

REFERENCES

1. Ehrlich, P. (1913) Chemotherapy, Proc. 17th Int. Congr. Med. (1913) 1914. In *The Collected Papers of Paul Ehrlich* (F. Himmelweit, Ed.) Vol. III, p. 510. Pergamon Press, Oxford, 1960.
2. Ghose, T., Blair, A. H., and Kulkarni, P. (1983) Preparation of antibody linked cytotoxic agents. *Methods Enzymol. 93*:280-333.
3. Zalcberg, J. R., Thompson, C. H., Lichtenstein, M., and McKenzie, I. F. C. (1984) Tumour immunotherapy in the mouse with the use of ^{131}I-labeled monoclonal antibodies. *J. Natl. Cancer Inst. 72*:697-704.
4. Frankel, A. E., Houston, L. L., and Issell, B. F. (1986) Prospects for immunotoxin therapy in cancer. *Ann. Rev. Med. 37*:125-142.
5. Ford, C. H. J., and Casson, A. G. (1986) Antibody-mediated targeting in the treatment and diagnosis of cancer: an overview. *Cancer Chemother. Pharmacol. 17*:197–208.
6. Young, R. C., Ozols, R. F., and Myers, C. E. (1981) The anthracycline antineoplastic drugs. *N. Eng. J. Med. 305*:139-153.
7. Hurwitz, E., Levy, R., Maron, R., Wilchek, M., Arnon, and Sela, M. (1975) The covalent binding of daunomycin and adriamycin to antibodies with retention of both drug and antibody activities. *Cancer Res. 35*:1175-1181.
8. Latif, Z. A., Lozzio, B. B., Wust, C. J., Krauss, S., Aggio, M. C., and Lozzio C. B. (1980) Evaluation of drug-antibody conjugates in the treatment of human myelosarcomas transplanted in nude mice. *Cancer 45*:1326–1333.
9. Varga, J. M., Asato, N., Lande, S., and Lerner, A. B. (1977) Melanotropin-daunomycin conjugate shows receptor-mediated cytotoxicity in cultured murine melanoma cells. *Nature 267*:56-58.
10. Kitao, T., and Hattori, K. (1977) Concanavalin A as a carrier of daunomycin. *Nature 265*:81-82.
11. Kaneto, Y. (1981) Thyrotropin-daunomycin conjugate shows receptor-mediated cytotoxicity in cultured thyroid cells. *Horm. Metab. Res. 13*: 110-114.
12. Tsukada, Y., Bischof, W. K-D., Hibi, N., Hirai, H., Hurwitz, E., and Sela, M. (1982) Effect of a conjugate of daunomycin and antibodies to rat α-fetoprotein on the growth of α-fetoprotein-producing tumor cells. *Proc. Natl. Acad. Sci. USA 79*:621-625.
13. Pimm, M. V., Jones, J. A., Price, M. R., MIddle, J. G., Embleton, M. J., and Baldwin, R. W. (1982) Tumor localization of monoclonal antibody against a rat mammary carcinoma and suppression of tumor growth with adriamycin-antibody conjugates. *Cancer Immunol. Immunother. 12*:125-134.

14. Ghose, T., Ramakrishnan, S., Kulkarni, P., Blair, A. H., Vaughn, K., Nolido, H., Norvell, S. T., and Belitsky, P. (1981) Use of antibodies against tumor-associated antigens for cancer diagnosis and treatment. *Transp. Proc. 13*: 1970-1972.
15. Neidle, S. (1979) The molecular basis for the action of some DNA binding drugs. *Prog. Med. Chem. 16*:156-221.
16. Israel, M., Modest, E. J., and Frei, E. (1975) N-Trifluoroacetyl adriamycin-14-valerate, an analog with greater experimental antitumor activity and less toxicity than adriamycin. *Cancer Res. 35*:1365-1368.
17. Zunino, F., Gambetta, R., Vigevani, A., Penco, S., Geroni, C., and Di Marco, A. (1981) Biologic activity of daunorubicin linked to proteins via the methylketone side chain. *Tumori 67*:521-524.
18. Gallego, J., Price, M. R., and Baldwin, R. W. (1984) Preparation of four daunomycin-monoclonal antibody 79IT/36 conjugates with anti-tumor activity. *Int. J. Cancer 33*:737-744.
19. Pietersz, G. A., Smyth, M. J., and McKenzie, I. F. C. (1986) Immunochemotherapy of a murine thymoma with the use of Idarubicin-monoclonal antibody conjugates. *Cancer Res.* (in press).
20. Smyth, J. J., Pietersz, G. A., Classon, B. J., and McKenzie, I. F. C. (1986) The specific targeting of chlorambucil to tumors with the use of monoclonal antibodies. *J. Natl. Cancer Inst. 76*:503-510.
21. Garnett, M. C., Embleton, M. J., Jacobs, E., and Baldwin, R. W. (1983) Preparation and properties of a drug-carrier-antibody conjugate showing selective antibody-directed cytotoxicity in vitro. *Int. J. Cancer 31*:661-670.
22. Kanellos, J., Pietersz, G. A., and McKenzie, I. F. C. (1985) Studies of methotrexate-monoclonal antibody conjugates for immunochemotherapy. *J. Natl. Cancer Inst. 75*:319-332.
23. Kato, Y., Tsukada, Y., Hara, T., and Hirai, H. (1983) Enhanced antitumor activity of mitomycin C conjugated with anti-α-fetoprotein antibody by a novel method of conjugation. *J. Appl. Biochem. 5*:313-319.
24. Embleton, M. J., Rowland, G. F., Simmonds, R. G., Jacobs, E., Marsden, C. H., and Baldwin, R. W. (1980) Selective cytotoxicity against human tumour cells by a vindesine-monoclonal antibody conjugate. *Br. J. Cancer 47*:43-49.
25. Berman, E., Wittes, R. E., Leyland-Jones, B. et al. (1983) Phase I and clinical pharmacology studies of intravenous and oral administration of 4-demethoxydaunorubicin in patients with advanced cancer. *Cancer Res. 43*: 6096-6101.
26. Kanellos, J., Pietersz, G. A., Cunningham, Z., and McKenzie, I. F. C. (1986) Anti-tumor activity of aminopterin-monoclonal antibody conjugates; in vitro and in vivo comparison with methotrexate-monoclonal antibody conjugates. *Immunol. Cell Biol.* (in press).
27. Tritton, T. R., and Yee, G. (1982) The anticancer agent adriamycin can be actively cytotoxic without entering cells. *Science 217*:248-250.
28. Thompson, C. H., Jones, S. L., Pihl, E., and McKenzie, I. F. C. (1983)

Monoclonal antibodies to human colon and colorectal carcinoma. *Br. J. Cancer 47*:595-605.
29. Hogarth, P. M., Edwards, J., McKenzie, I. F. C., Goding, J. W., and Liew, F. Y. (1982) Monoclonal antibodies to murine Ly-2.1 cell surface antigen. *Immunology 46*:135-144.
30. Panaccio, M., Zalcberg, J. R., Thompson, C. H., Leyden, M. J., Sullivan, J. R., Lichtenstein, M., and McKenzie, I. F. C. (1986) Heterogeneity of the human transferrin receptor and use of anti-transferrin receptor antibodies: Heterogeneity of the TFR and use to detect tumors in vivo. *Immunol. Cell. Biol.* (in press).
31. Thompson, C. H., Jones, S. L., Whitehead, R. H., and McKenzie, I. F. C. (1983) A human breast tissue-associated antigen detected by a monoclonal antibody. *J. Natl. Cancer Inst. 70*:409-419.
32. Fogh, J., and Trempe, G. (1975) New human tumor cell lines. In *Human Tumor Cells in Vitro* (Fogh, J., Ed.). Plenum Press, New York, pp. 115-120.
33. Semple, T. U., Quinn, L. A., Woods, L. F., and Moore, G. E. (1978) Tumor and lymphoid cell lines from a patient with carcinoma of the colon for a cytotoxicity model. *Cancer Res. 38*:1345-1355.
34. Foley, G. E., Lazarus, H., Farber, S., Geren Uzman, B., Boone, B. A., and McCarthy, R. E. (1965) Continuous culture of human lymphoblasts from peripheral blood of a child with acute leukemia. *Cancer 18*:522-529.
35. Carlsson, J., Drevin, H., and Axen, R. (1978) Protein thiolation and reversible protein-protein conjugation. *Biochem. J. 173*:723-737.
36. Niederwieser, A. (1971) Adsorption on neutral polystyrene resin-A simple method for extraction of 2,4-dinitrophenyl derivatives from aqueous solution and for decoloration of protein hydrolysates. *J. Chromatog. 54*:215-223.
37. Bradford, M. M. (1976) A rapid and sensitive method of quantitation of microgram quantities of protein utilizing the principle of protein-dye binding. *Anal. Biochem. 72*:248-253.
38. Parish, C. R., and McKenzie, I. F. C. (1978) A sensitive rosetting method for detecting subpopulations of lymphocytes which react with alloantisera. *J. Immunol. Methods 20*:173-183.

3

KS1/4-DAVLB, a Monoclonal Antibody-Vinca Alkaloid Conjugate for Site-Directed Therapy of Epithelial Malignancies

THOMAS F. BUMOL, A. LEROY BAKER, ERIC L. ANDREWS, SONJA V. DeHERDT, STEPHEN L. BRIGGS, MARSHALL E. SPEARMAN, and LYNN D. APELGREN

Lilly Research Laboratories, Indianapolis, Indiana

I. INTRODUCTION

The hybridoma technology of Kohler and Milstein can be utilized to construct monoclonal antibodies with high specificity and affinity for human tumor cells (1-6). In most cases, monoclonal antibodies define "tumor-associated antigens" (TAA) rather than tumor-specific antigens, but these tumor-associated gene products frequently have limited normal tissue distribution. In some cases, as will be described below for the KS1/4 monoclonal antibody, TAAs often have properties of differentiation antigens of the normal tissue of origin of the malignancy.

Monoclonal antibodies have already been utilized extensively in investigations into the cell/tumor biology of human solid tumors (7-10). These antibody probes which define TAAs are also being explored for the in vitro diagnosis and classification of tumors (11,12). Monoclonal antibodies have also been constructed to oncogene products of human tumors and, coupled with the techniques of molecular biology may help classify tumors and explore the biology of transformation (13-15). These applications of the monoclonal antibody technology are well established and will lead to better understanding of human tumors.

As first suggested by Ehrlich, antibodies with appropriate specificities may be targeting vehicles for site-directed drug therapy (16). This idea, first proposed with the use of polyclonal antisera is now being explored again with the monoclonal products of the hybridoma technology. Certain properties of the TAAs defined by monoclonal antibodies suggest that these gene products may be appropriate targets for site-directed therapy of human solid tumors. Initially these properties might include but may not be restricted to (1) cell surface topography of the TAAs, (2) high surface density of the TAA molecules on target malignancies, and (3) limited normal tissue distribution as determined by extensive immunoperoxidase screening of frozen normal tissues with the monoclonal antibody. Practical considerations include (1) the ability to produce large quantities of the monoclonal antibody product, (2) the in vivo molecular stability of the antibody molecule, and (3) the appropriate conjugation chemistry to modify the monoclonal antibody with a therapeutic agent while not compromising the antibody's "targeting" properties for a novel strategy at site-directed tumor therapy. This last point remains the most critical step in the evolution of monoclonal antibody conjugates for tumor therapy in man.

Many research efforts are in place to explore possible therapeutic monoclonal antibody conjugates. These efforts include the conjugation of isotopes, catalytic toxins of plant and microbial origin, and conventional chemotherapeutic agents to monoclonal antibodies (17-23). The efforts of these laboratories have focused on the use of conventional chemotherapeutic drugs in conjugates with monoclonal antibodies. Chemotherapeutic agents in clinical use have several advantages over other agents such as an extensive data base of clinical information on pharmacokinetics, tumor efficacy, and dose-limiting toxicology. These agents will also typically have extensive preclinical pharmacology and toxicology studies. This information can be important in the preclinical and clincal development of a monoclonal antibody conjugate with this agent. In addition, a number of highly active antitumor agents have been discovered which are too toxic as free drugs in early clinical testing but have excellent antitumor spectrums in preclinical models. These agents are also candidates for conjugation and site directed therapy strategies.

The primary goal of the preclinical development of a monoclonal antibody-drug conjugate for tumor therapy is to demonstrate that the conjugate provides an advantage over free drug therapy. An improvement in the preclinical therapeutic index (the ratio of a maximum tolerated toxic dose/minimum effective efficacy dose in preclinical animal models) is one criteria. These studies typically involve extensive animal testing for antitumor efficacy as well as toxicology. This chapter will summarize some of the preclinical studies of KS1/4-DAVLB (Lilly Research Laboratories serial number LY256787). KS1/4-DAVLB is a covalent conjugate of the monoclonal antibody KS1/4 (24), which recognizes a human adenocarcinoma/epithelial antigen and deacetylvinblastine, a derivative of the vinca alkaloid vinblastine. These results will include details on the purification of the monoclonal antibody, conjugation chemistry, biochemical characterization, preclinical efficacy models and biodistribution studies.

II. RESULTS FROM THE PRECLINICAL DEVELOPMENT OF KS1/4-DAVLB

A. Biochemical Characterization of KS1/4-DAVLB

Details of the purification process of the KS1/4-S2 monoclonal antibody fraction and conjugation to deacetylvinblastine are described in the text and supplemental figures in the Appendix section. These conjugates were routinely subjected to a variety of biochemical analyses, which include sodium dodecyl sulfate polyacrylamide gel electrophoresis (SDS-PAGE) and high resolution isoelectrofocusing (IEF) analysis. An example of an SDS-PAGE analysis of a KS1/4-DAVLB conjugate is shown in Figure 1. Typically, under reducing conditions, the heavy and light chain components of the purified KS1/4-DAVLB fraction migrate more slowly than the components of the unmodified monoclonal antibody fraction. These data suggest that both light and heavy chains are modified with a vinca alkaloid species. This result was confirmed by an independent investigation conjugating a [^{3}H]-DAVLB compound to the KS1/4-S2 species. SDS-PAGE analysis of this conjugate followed by fluorography revealed the covalent incorporation of vinca alkaloid species into both heavy and light chain fractions (data not shown). Heavily conjugated monoclonal antibodies (conjugation ratios exceeding 8 moles of vinca/mole of monoclonal antibody) demonstrate increasingly slower migration of heavy and light chain components and often are present with aggregate fractions not resolved under reducing conditions. SDS-PAGE analysis under nonreducing conditions and size exclusion chromatography can also be utilized to characterize aggregate fractions in conjugates. An example of an IEF analysis of the KS1/4-DAVLB conjugate is shown in Figure 2. IEF analysis provides a "fingerprint" profile of a monoclonal antibody species, which can be examined postconjugation to examine the effects of drug modifications on the isoelectric points of the glycoproteins. Figure 2 demonstrates that the unmodified KS1/4-S2 species displays six prominent bands in the pI range of 6.5-7.35. The KS1/4-DAVLB conjugate demonstrates a shift in these species, indicating that drug modification indeed changes the IEF profile of the monoclonal antibody. The combination of these techniques can be utilized to reject conjugate lots which do not have appropriate analytical profiles as predetermined with biologically active reference standard monoclonal antibody and conjugates with defined profits.

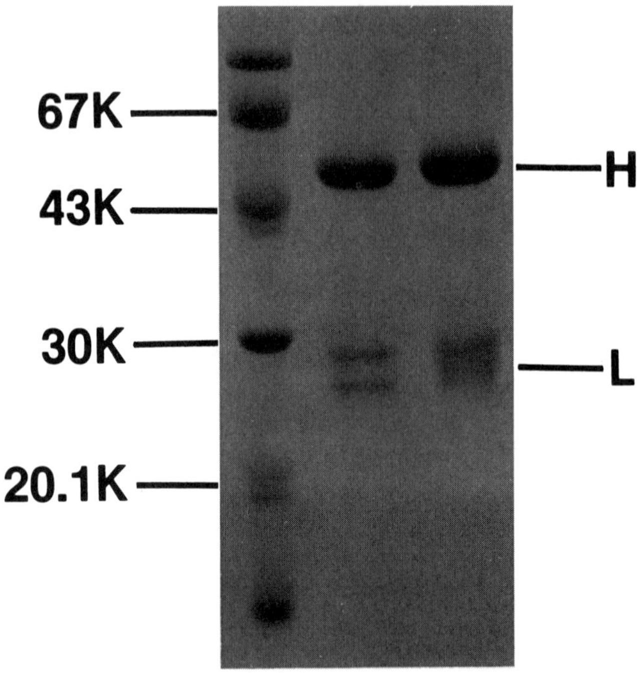

Figure 1 SDS-PAGE analysis of monoclonal antibody KS1/4 and KS1/4-DAVLB. The second lane depicts the SDS-PAGE profile of unmodified KS1/4 monoclonal antibody under reducing conditions in a 12.5% acrylamide gel with designation of heavy chain (H) and light chains (L) indicated. The third lane depicts the migration of the KS1/4-DAVLB conjugate under identical conditions. Migration of molecular weight standards is also indicated.

B. In Vitro Analyses of the KS1/4-DAVLB Conjugates

1. Immunoreactivity Assay

Several techniques have been utilized to examine the antigen-binding activity of KS1/4-DAVLB conjugates for target tumor cells including flow cytometry (25), immunofluorescence, and enzyme-linked immunoadsorbent essays (ELISA). The routine assay utilized for rapid analysis of monoclonal antibodies and covalent monoclonal antibody-drug conjugates in these laboratories is the ELISA assay described in the Appendix. While the described assay does not measure a true immunoreactive fraction of antibody molecules in antigen excess, it provides a rapid analytical assay for monitoring deleterious changes in the monoclonal antibody's capacity to bind target tumor cells. In addition, the use of repeti-

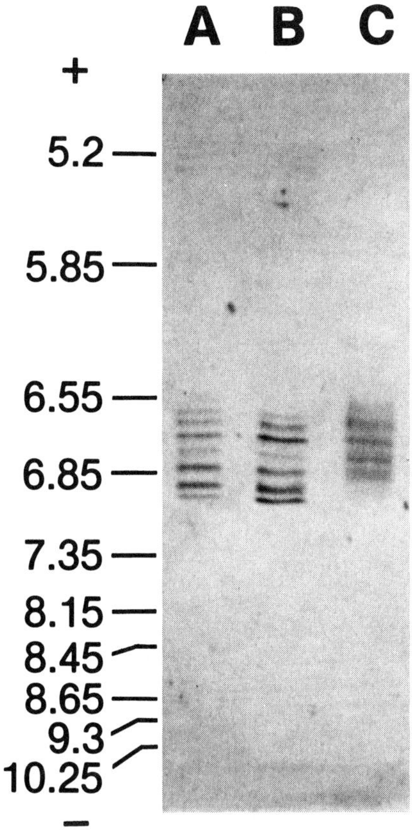

Figure 2 Isoelectricfocusing analysis of KS1/4 and KS1/4-DAVLB. Lanes A and B indicate the IEF profile of unmodified KS1/4 monoclonal antibody, while Lane C indicates the IEF profile of KS1/4-DAVLB. Migration of various pI standards is indicated.

tive absorptions by fixed target tumor cells followed by measurement of murine monoclonal antibody in the supernatant can provide a parallel immunoreactive fraction assay. Table 1 presents a typical summary of ELISA analysis of KS1/4-DAVLB conjugates with different conjugation ratios of vinca alkaloid species. As the drug molar ratio increases, the ratio of ELISA potency/protein content decreases in these conjugates. Unmodified KS1/4-S2 antibody will typically have an ELISA potency/protein content ratio of greater than 0.90. Based on a number of experiments comparing in vitro and in vivo analyses of KS1/4-DAVLB conjugates, KS1/4-DAVLB conjugates exceeding an average molar ratio

Table 1 ELISA Analysis of KS1/4-DAVLB Conjugates

Sample	C.R.[a]	Protein (μg/ml)	ELISA potency (μg/ml)	Ratio (ELISA/protein)
KS1/4-DAVLB	1.8	440	330.2	.75
KS1/4-DAVLB	4.8	190	125.3	.67
KS1/4-DAVLB	5.5	600	348.6	.58
KS1/4-DAVLB	7.4	170	48.8	.28

[a]Designates molar conjugation ratio of vinca alkaloids/monoclonal antibody.

of 7.0-8.0 generally have a poor ELISA profile corresponding with poor in vivo antitumor activity by assays described below. Conjugates which display a ELISA potency/protein content ratio exceeding 0.5 demonstrate good in vivo antitumor activity.

2. In Vitro Drug Potency Assays

A number of assays exist to examine the in vitro potency of oncolytic drugs and corresponding conjugates. These assays might include biosynthetic proliferation assays, growth curve analysis, and soft agar anchorage-independent growth assays. An assay in use in these laboratories for this purpose is the MTT colorimetric assay. MTT [3,(4,5-dimethyl-thiazoyl-2-yl)2,5-diphenyltetrazolium bromide] is a dye metabolized by viable cells to an easily measured colorimetric product. While this assay must be tailored to each particular cell line being studied (see details in the Appendix), it can provide a rapid measurement of the relative potency of free drugs and corresponding conjugates. Antigen-mediated effects of the conjugates are less easily addressed as most human tumor cells secrete a variety of proteins into the spent tissue culture media which appear capable of degrading monoclonal antibody-drug conjugates (unpublished observations) in long-term incubations. However, the effects of derivatizing drugs for conjugation purposes can be assessed in this assay as well as comparing parenteral drugs to covalent monoclonal antibody conjugates. Table 2 documents a typical experiment in which free vinblastine (VLB) and KS1/4-DAVLB were assayed by the MTT assay. In this experiment, VLB has an Inhibition concentration$_{50\%}$ (IC_{50}) of less than 1.5 ng/ml. In contrast, KS1/4-DAVLB

Table 2 In Vitro Potency Analysis of Vinblastine (VLB) and KS1/4-DAVLB

Drug	Concentration (μg/ml)	% Inhibition vs. control
VLB	.00015	0
VLB	.0015	80
VLB	.015	87
KS1/4-DAVLB	.1	8
KS1/4-DAVLB	.25	38
KS1/4-DAVLB	.5	71
KS1/4-DAVLB	2.5	84

As determined by the MTT proliferation assay as described in the Appendix utilizing the P3-UCLA human lung adenocarcinoma cell line with a 72-hour exposure to drug or monoclonal antibody-drug conjugate. All concentrations are in terms of vinca alkaloid content.

has an IC_{50} between 250 and 500 ng/ml demonstrating that the conjugated vinca alkaloid species has a significant drop in potency compared to the VLB.

C. In Vivo Antitumor Activity of KS1/4-DAVLB in Preclinical Models

1. Results of the Tumor Initiation Xenograft Model

The predominant xenograft model initially developed was based on the cell line initially used to construct the KS1/4 monoclonal antibody, the P3-UCLA human lung adenocarcinoma (22). A series of experiments were conducted which established a treatment schedule where unmodified KS1/4 monoclonal antibody treatment groups did not mediate antitumor activity (data not shown). This schedule utilized three intravenous doses of conjugate or free VLB on days 2, 5 and 8 after subcutaneous tumor implantation. Figure 3 summarizes such

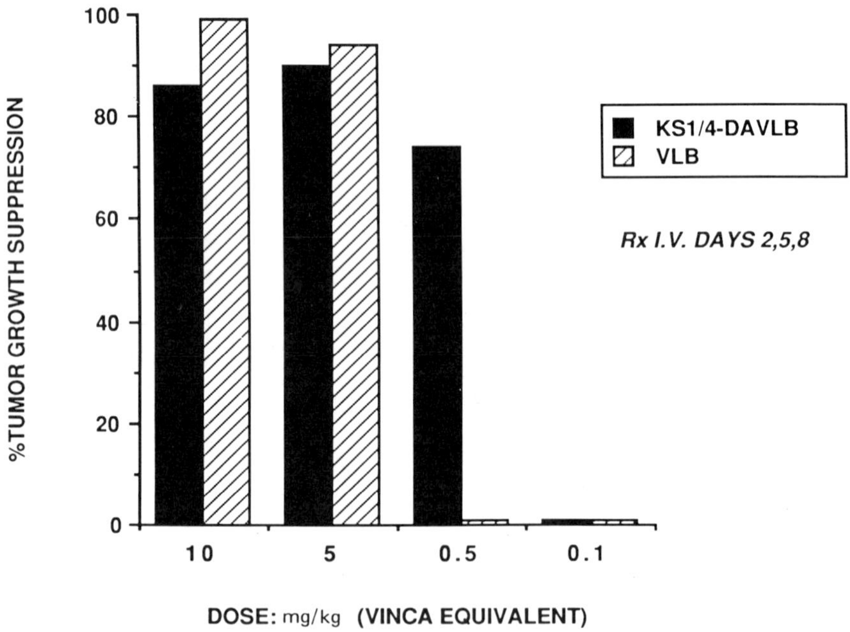

Figure 3 In vivo tumor initiation model for evaluating the efficacy of KS1/4-DAVLB. Nude mice with 48-hour established P3-UCLA human lung adenocarcinoma xenografts were treated with either KS1/4-DAVLB or VLB on the schedule with dose groups indicated. The % tumor growth suppression data is based on average tumor mass estimates of untreated control animals (n = 10) on day 14 of tumor growth.

an experiment examining a dose-response of KS1/4-DAVLB and VLB. Despite a significant drop in measurable in vitro potency as an antiproliferative agent compared to VLB, KS1/4-DAVLB demonstrated 87% and 90% inhibition in tumor growth at the 10 and 5 mg/kg dose groups with no observed toxicities. VLB treatment groups demonstrate similar profiles at the 10 and 5 mg/kg groups but with observed toxicities at the 10 mg/kg group. Significant antitumor activity is still observed at the 0.5 mg/kg group for KS1/4-DAVLB treatment groups while the parallel VLB group's effect is nonsignificant. In subsequent experiments it was established that the maximum tolerated vinblastine dose under this schedule is between 10 and 11.5 mg/kg, suggesting a narrow therapeutic index for vinblastine. Under the described schedule, KS1/4-DAVLB has comparable in vivo antitumor activity to VLB without significant toxicity. These observations have been confirmed by toxicological investigations of KS1/4-DAVLB in several species, indicating that conjugated vinca alkaloid species are considerably less toxic than free vinblastine or related vinca alkaloids (G. Todd, unpublished observations).

Additional experiments were performed to document that the observed antitumor effects were not simply due to a "carrier" effect of the monoclonal antibody protein for the vinca alkaloid species. Figure 4 depicts the result of an experiment in which an irrelevant murine myeloma protein, S1, was conjugated with VLB and utilized in the tumor initiation xenograft model just described. This conjugate, S1-DAVLB, was completely inactive as an antitumor agent even at 10 mg/kg vinca equivalent dose in this three-dose protocol. In contrast, KS1/4-DAVLB demonstrates significant antitumor activity even at a day 21 tumor measurement after a three-dose protocol on days 2, 5, and 8. This experiment strongly suggests that the observed effects of the KS1/4-DAVLB conjugate are target antigen-mediated through a functional monoclonal antibody.

2. Results of the Established Tumor Model

The previously described xenograft model examined the effects of the KS1/4-DAVLB conjugate on 48 hour subcutaneously implanted tumors. The P3-UCLA human lung adenocarcinoma xenograft system at this time point provides a minimum tumor burden to the nude mouse. A second model was established which allowed the P3-UCLA tumors to grow for at least 16 days. These well-established tumors can typically vary in size from 100-500 mg at this juncture prior to immunotherapy. Figure 5 summarizes a typical experiment examining the effects of KS1/4-DAVLB on established P3-UCLA xenograft tumors. Animals treated with unmodified KS1/4 at antibody equivalent doses to the KS1/4-DAVLB doses indicated demonstrated progressively growing tumors which paralleled the growth of no treatment controls. Animals receiving free VLB treatments at 10 mg/kg demonstrate a plateau in average tumor mass through day 23 but with an LD_{100} after this first tumor measure-

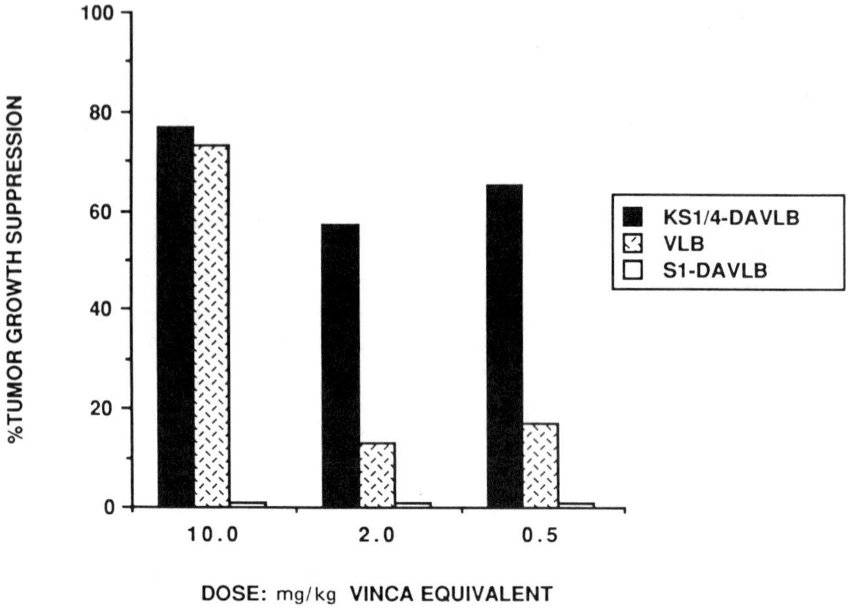

Figure 4 In vivo tumor initiation model for comparing the efficacy of KS1/4-DAVLB and an irrelevant non-tumor binding myeloma protein conjugate, S1-DAVLB. Nude mice with 48-hour established P3-UCLA xenografts were treated with either KS1/4-DAVLB, VLB, or S1-DAVLB on a three-dose schedule (Rx i.v. days 2, 5, and 8) at the dose indicated. The % tumor growth inhibition data is based on average tumor mass estimates of untreated control animals (n = 10) on day 21 of tumor growth.

ment point on this treatment schedule. In contrast, KS1/4-DAVLB-treated animals demonstrate an initial retardation of growth through day 23 followed by an actual tumor regression through day 30 without toxicity. These experiments demonstrate that the KS1/4-DAVLB conjugate can mediate antitumor effects on well-established P3-UCLA xenograft tumors.

3. Results of an Experimental Metastases Model

A third model was established which produced multifocal, multiorgan systemic tumor growth in irradiated nude mice of the P3-UCLA human lung adenocarcinoma (T. F. Bumol et al., manuscript submitted). Nude mice with such experimental metastases demonstrate rapid systemic tumor growth and death, which allow the possibility of survival analysis for KS1/4-DAVLB therapy experiments. Figure 6 depicts the results of an initial experiment in which several

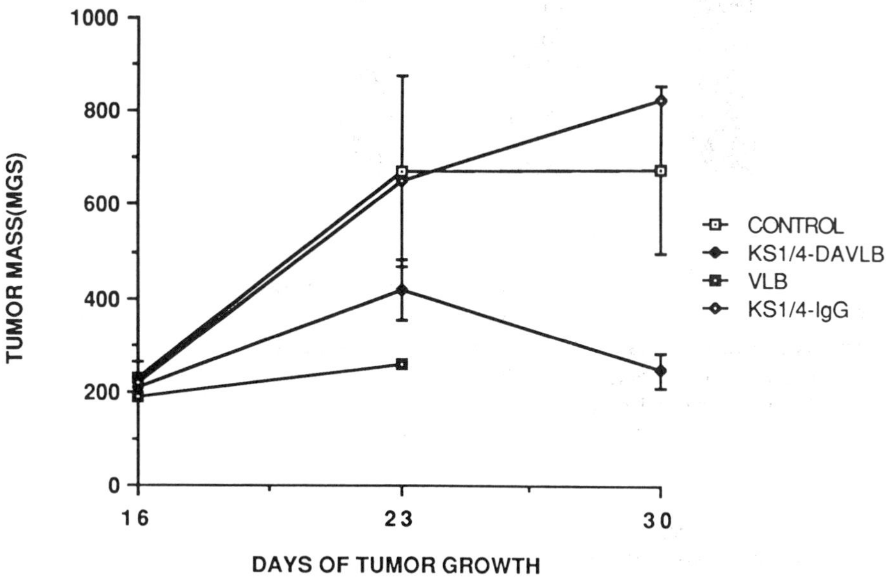

Figure 5 In vivo established tumor model for examining the antitumor efficacy of KS1/4-DAVLB conjugates. Nude mice with 16-day established P3-UCLA xenograft tumors were treated by intravenous administration with KS1/4-DAVLB, VLB, or unmodified KS1/4-IgG on days 16, 18, 20, 22, 24, 27, and 30 at 10 mg/kg vinca alkaloid equivalent doses or corresponding antibody content (KS1/4 IgG group). Tumor mass estimates are plotted with time and include the standard error terms for control and KS1/4-DAVLB treatment groups. Regressions are observed in the KS1/4-DAVLB treatment group.

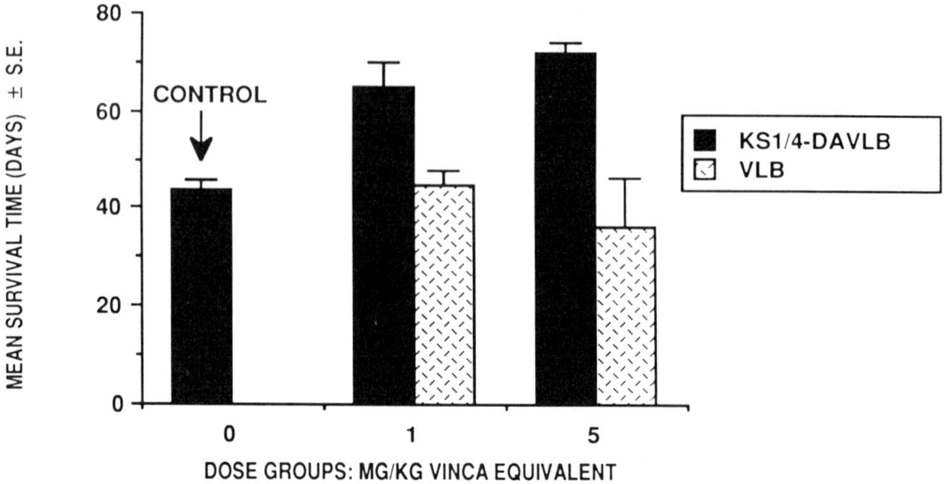

Figure 6 In vivo experimental metastases models for examining the antitumor efficacy of KS1/4-DAVLB conjugates. Nude mice were treated by intravenous administration with KS1/4-DAVLB or VLB on days 2, 6, 10, 14, and 18 following an intravenous injection of viable P3-UCLA lung adenocarcinoma cells to establish experimental metastases. The mean survival time and standard error are indicated for various experimental groups.

groups of mice received either KS1/4-DAVLB or VLB treatments on days 2, 5, 8 11, and 14 after initiation of intravenous tumor inoculations. Control animals had a mean survival time of 44 days in this experiment. VLB treatment groups at 1 and 5 mg/kg dose levels demonstrated no survival advantage. In contrast, KS1/4-DAVLB treatment groups at 1 and 5 mg/kg vinca equivalent doses demonstrate significant increases in the average mean survival time for these mice. Macroscopic observations of conjugate-treated animals demonstrate overall lower tumor burden even at death, suggesting that KS1/4-DAVLB treatment can have antitumor effects at many tumor sites systemically in this preclinical model. Unmodified KS1/4 treatment groups, as in the two previously described models, had no significant effect on survival (data not shown). The lack of any antitumor effects from VLB treatment groups must be viewed in terms of the model in which nude mice are heavily irradiated prior to the establishment of experimental metastases. Hematological analysis of similarly treated animals suggest that conditions of severe leucopenia are present which might artificially exaggerate the toxicities of free vinca alkaloid species and limit observable efficacy. Despite this irradiation-induced toxicity, KS1/4-DAVLB treatment groups demonstrate increased survival. Optimization and extension of treatment schedules are currently underway in an effort to further extend the survival time of

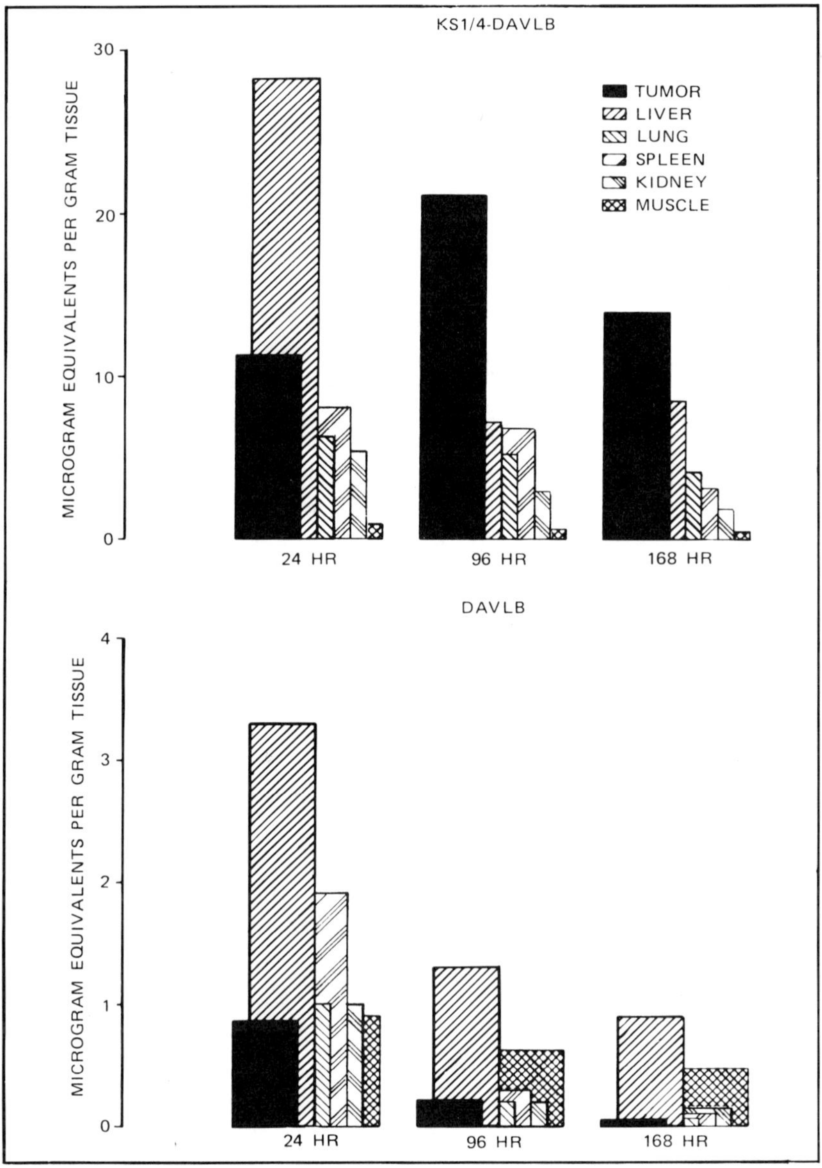

Figure 7 In vivo biodistribution analysis of KS1/4-[^{3}H]-DAVLB and [^{3}H]-DAVLB in P3-UCLA xenograft-bearing nude mice. Nude mice with established P3-UCLA xenografts were administered a single i.v. dose of KS1/4-[^{3}H]-DAVLB and [^{3}H]-DAVLB at 5 mg/kg vinca alkaloid equivalent doses. Animals were sacrificed at the time points indicated and microgram equivalents determined for all tissues. Select normal tissues and tumor tissue results are indicated for three timepoints.

these experimental animals. The data suggest that KS1/4-DAVLB treatment is effective on micrometastatic multiorgan tumor growth in this prelinical model which might extend to an application in human clinical trials.

D. Biodistribution Studies

Studies were initiated which compared the biodistribution of unconjugated vinca alkaloid as [^{3}H]-DAVLB to KS1/4-[^{3}H]-DAVLB in P3-UCLA tumor-bearing nude mice. Figure 7 summarizes such an experiment in which the concentrations of KS1/4-[^{3}H]-DAVLB and [^{3}H]-DAVLB radioequivalents are shown for several normal tissues and the P3-UCLA human lung adenocarcinoma xenograft tumor. With the free [^{3}H]-DAVLB (Fig. 7, lower panel), a rapid initial elimination phase resulted in low concentrations in many tissues. Tumor tissue concentrations of the unconjugated drug were maximal at the initial time points. No accumulation of drug in tumor tissue was observed with the concentrations of drug being greater in several normal tissues sampled at the time points listed. In contrast with these data, the initial redistribution/elimination phase with KS1/4-[^{3}H]-DAVLB was of a small magnitude (Fig. 7, upper panel). Concentrations of KS1/4-[^{3}H]-DAVLB radioequivalents were found to increase to a maximum at 96 hours after dosing. As can be observed, the concentrations were greater in tumor tissue than other normal tissues. The area under the curve (AUC) values were approximately 80 and 3200 microgram equivalents*hr/g tumor tissue after dosing with [^{3}H]-DAVLB and KS1/4-[^{3}H]-DAVLB, respectively. Radioequivalent concentrations measured after dosing similar tumor-bearing animals with an irrelevant MAb-[^{3}H]-DAVLB conjugate which was not reactive with the tumor were comparable to the data found with [^{3}H]-DAVLB (data not shown) demonstrating that the observed drug targeting with KS1/4-[^{3}H]-DAVLB was indeed target antigen-mediated. In addition, these data suggest that the antitumor efficacy observed with KS1/4-DAVLB cannot be attributed simply to pharmacokinetic changes in circulating concentrations of vinca alkaloid species at the tumor site.

III. DISCUSSION

These data summarize several preclinical studies that demonstrate that KS1/4-DAVLB is a monoclonal antibody-drug conjugate effective as a site-directed therapy agent against a model human lung adenocarcinoma. Despite a significant loss in potency compared to free vinca alkaloid species as measured by in vitro techniques, this agent was effective in treating nude mice with low animal tumor burdens (Tumor Initiation Model), established tumors, and an experimental metastases model. These effects appear to be antibody-mediated and can be correlated with an actual accumulation of drug at the tumor site by biodistribution studies. KS1/4-DAVLB does not demonstrate typical vinca alkaloid-mediated toxicities in the xenograft models as well as in studies in rats and primates (G. Todd, unpublished observations), suggesting that this agent is a candidate for human clinical testing.

While these preclinical results are promising, human clinical trials face additional theoretical issues not present in the preclinical studies which include (1) the vascular permeability barriers for human tumors, (2) inadequate drug potency, (3) innocent bystander-targeted tissue toxicology (i.e., normal tissues which cross-react with KS1/4 MAb), (4) tumor antigenic heterogeneity, and (5) the host immune response to the murine monoclonal antibody and potentially to "haptenic" drug substituents. Of these points, the immunogenicity issue of murine proteins has already been evident in early clinical testing of monoclonal antibody-based cancer therapy. Multiple dose clinical trials must be designed to safely and adequately test the potential efficacy of an agent like KS1/4-DAVLB. This clinical research will synergize with ongoing preclinical research efforts underway in many of the "issue" areas to dampen or eliminate potential problems associated with this first-generation monoclonal antibody-drug conjugate. Second-generation conjugates are currently under extensive preclinical testing as well with alternative conjugation chemistry strategies and novel oncolytic agents. The ultimate goal of this site-directed therapy program would be to develop combination immunotherapeutic approaches with agents of different oncolytic mechanisms. If monoclonal antibodies can consistently alter the pharmacokinetics and tumor localization of these oncolytic agents with an increased therapeutic index over conventional chemotherapy, those biotechnology products could be the basis of a new pharmacology in cancer and potentially many other disease applications.

IV. APPENDIX–MATERIAL AND METHODS

A. Cell Lines

The KS1/4 hybridoma was maintained as previously described (24). Various tissue culture and ascites-sourced materials have been utilized to purify the relevant monoclonal antibody fractions from this hybridoma as described below. Monoclonal antibody KS1/4 defines an adenocarcinoma-associated antigen by immunoperoxidase reactivity (24), which with additional analysis appears to be antigen-associated with epithelial malignancies and certain normal epithelial surfaces (T. F. Bumol et al., submitted for publication). The P3-UCLA human lung adenocarcinoma was obtained from Dr. Les Walker, Scripps Clinic and Research Foundation, La Jolla, CA, and maintained as an adherent culture in Dulbecco's Modified Eagle's medium supplemented with 10% fetal bovine serum (GIBCO), 0.2 mM L-glutamine and gentamycin sulfate at 5 μg/ml (this media is referred to as DMEM-Complete). All cells utilized in these experiments were greater than 90% viable by dye exclusion assays.

B. Enzyme-Linked Immunoabsorbent Assay (ELISA)

A functional enzyme-linked immunoabsorbent assay has been developed to monitor the reactivity of KS1/4 and KS1/4 monoclonal antibody drug conjugates. The target antigens for this assay are P3-UCLA human lung adenocarcinoma cells which have been air-dried onto 96-well microtiter plates (Falcon). When cultured P3-UCLA cells reach 80-90% confluency by microscopic examination the cells are harvested with trypsin/EDTA (GIBCO). Previous studies have documented that the antigen recognized by KS1/4 is not sensitive to this treatment (unpublished observations). After the cells are harvested by centrifugation, they are resuspended in DMEM-Complete and incubated for one hour at 37°C on a cell rocker to reduce aggregation.

The cell suspension is washed three times with phosphate buffered saline, pH 7.2 (PBS), resuspended in PBS by pipetting and filtered through 100 uM nylon mesh. Cells are enumerated and adjusted to 2×10^6 viable cells/ml in PBS. Fifty μl is plated per well of flexible U-bottom 96-well plates followed by an overnight incubation at 37°C. The air-dried antigen plates are sealed with parafilm and can be stored for at least 30 days at ambient temperature for use in ELISA assays.

Prior to starting an ELISA protocol, the P3-UCLA coated plates are rehydrated with ELISA wash buffer (0.2% Tween-20, 0.01% Thimeroal in PBS) for two minutes. This procedure is then repeated and the buffer removed prior to sample dilution. All standard and sample dilutions are prepared at room temperature using ELISA diluting buffer (0.1% bovine serum albumin (SIGMA, RIA grade) in ELISA wash buffer). KS1/4 monoclonal antibody which has been diluted to 1 mg/ml in PBS is utilized to prepare a standard curve for each 96-well plate. The standard curve consists of 10 concentrations of antibody and an eleventh point consisting of diluting buffer. The 1 mg/ml KS1/4 reference standard is diluted to 5000 ng/ml. Twofold serial dilutions are carried out to obtain concentrations from 2500 ng/ml to 2.4 ng/ml. A positive and negative control sample is included with each plate. From unknown samples' protein estimates, five twofold serial dilutions are made from an initial dilution, such that the most dilute sample woudl have a protein concentration of 25-50 ng/ml. All standards, controls, and unknowns are run in quadruplicate with one replicate/plate quadrant (a quadrant consisting of three eight-well plate columns).

Fifty μl of all of the dilutions described above are added/well and the plates incubated initially at ambient temperature for thirty minutes. This incubation step is followed by two washing steps with ELISA wash buffer and a second incubation with peroxidase conjugated goat anti-mouse IgG and IgM (TAGO, 1:500 dilution, 50 μl/well) for thirty minutes. After this incubation the plates are washed three times with ELISA wash buffer and 50 ul of substrate solution added. Substrate solution is freshly made by adding 4 mg o-phenylenediamine

(SIGMA) and 3 ul of 3% hydrogen peroxide to 10 ml of 80 mM citrate phosphate buffer pH 5.0. After a thirty minute incubation protected from light, the reaction is quenched by adding 25 ul of 4N sulfuric acid to each well. Plates are then evaluated in an ELISA reader using a double wavelength setting; Reference wavelength 570 nm, Test wavelength 490 nm. Data is subsequently stored in a Lilly Interface Microcomputer and transferred to a main frame VAX computer (Digital Corp.) for analysis using RIASYS, a program written and copyrighted by W. C. Smith and E. D. Suckstorff, Lilly Research Laboratories. The RIASYS program lists and sumarizes data for review, estimates a standard curve using a four parameter logistic model and estimates weighted mean potencies for unknown samples from each plates' individual standard curve. The ELISA Potency/Protein Content provides the ratio for monitoring the effects of conjugation on KS1/4 antibody performance.

C. Purification of the KS1/4 Monoclonal Antibody

Chromatographic matrices S-Sepharose Fast Flow, Q-Sepharose Fast Flow, Phenyl Sepharose Fast Flow, Phenyl Sepharose CL-4B, and Sephadex G-25 were purchased from Pharmacia Fine Chemicals. Mouse ascites cultures of the KS1/4 hybridoma were obtained from Charles River and Lilly Research Laboratories; hollow fiber culture supernatants, microencapsulated culture supernatants and large-scale suspension cultures were obtained by contract research and hybridoma fermentation efforts at Eli Lilly and Company. All chemicals were of reagent grade quality.

KS1/4 is a dual secreting hybridoma cell line observed to express an irrelevant myeloma protein IgG_1, presumably from the myeloma fusion partner. Varying amounts of the irrelevant IgG_1 myeloma protein are secreted by the KS1/4 hybridoma dependent on the culture technique and continuous culture generation time. Therefore, purification strategies for the desired spleen cell antibody product, an IgG_{2a}, must address the objective of removing irrelevant immunoglobulin as well as other contaminants associated with particular culture techniques. Figure 8 exhibits the heterogeneity of pure immunoglobulin, obtained from mouse ascites culture of KS1/4 by procedures described below, upon gradient elution from a column of cation exchanger S-Sepharose Fast Flow. The protein peak labeled S-1 is a nonfunctional (nonantigen-reactive) IgG_1. Peaks S-2a, S-2b, and S-2c are all immunoreactive and contain IgG-2a heavy chain and the correct kappa light chains. Peaks S-2a and S-2b are mixtures of molecular hybrids, displaying both myeloma and spleen cell character.

Table 3 outlines entry of product from various culture techniques into a three-column purification process for KS1/4 antibody. An initial cation exchange step is used to increase the purity of a relatively crude, serum-supplemented suspension culture broth from as low as 0.5% to >25% antibody. This 25% pure fraction, as well as antibody of comparable quality from (a) either

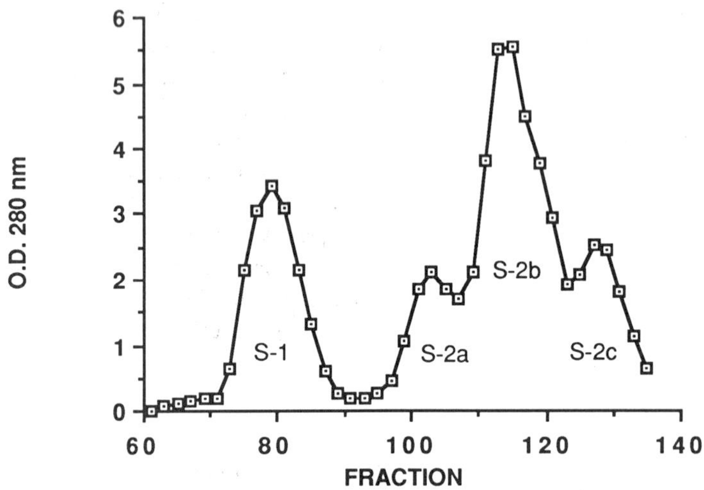

Figure 8 The heterogeneity of immunoglobulin from the KS1/4 hybridoma. Purified immunoglobulin from ascites culture of KS1/4 is resolved into inactive (S-1) and immunoreactive (S-2 complex) fractions upon chromatography on cation exchanger S-Sepharose Fast Flow. See text for details.

Table 3 A Purification Process For KS1/4 Monoclonal Antibody and Its DAVLB Conjugate

Chromatographic sequence	Raw materials	
	Culture technique	% Antibody purity
Cation exchange	Serum-supplemented, suspension	0.5
Anion exchange	Hollow fiber or micro-encapsulated	25
	Defined media, suspension	
	Ascites	
Cation exchange or Hydrophobic interaction		50
	–Conjugation–	95
Reverse phase purification		

hollow fiber or microencapsulated entrapment culture, (b) defined media suspension culture, or (c) in vivo mouse ascites culture can be increased to >50% purity by anion exchange chromatography. Final resolution of inactive from active antibody is achieved on either cation exchange or hydrophobic interaction chromatography.

The outlined process has been employed on several laboratory and preparative scales, lot sizes ranging from milligrams to hundreds of grams of antibody. Overall yields of active antibody, as measured by ELISA assay, exceed 50%. A detailed procedure for preparing 500 mg of purified antibody from suspension culture broth follows.

Twenty liters of spent, serum-supplemented KS1/4 suspension culture broth (containing approximately 50 μg/ml antibody and 3 mg/ml total protein) is concentrated by ultrafiltration to a volume of 1 l. The concentrate is acidified to pH 4.5 with the dropwise addition of glacial acetic acid and, after stirring one hour, is clarified by centrifugation at 27,000 X g for 30 minutes. The supernatant is diluted with an equal volume of water to result in a conductivity of less than 10 millimohs. The pH of the diluted solution is checked and readjusted, if necessary, to 4.5.

The above solution is chromatographed on a 4.4 X 70 cm column of S-Sepharose Fast Flow, previously equilibrated in 170 mM acetate buffer, pH 4.5. Flow rate is maintained at 4 ml/min. Following sample application the column is washed with 500 ml of 170 mM acetate buffer, pH 4.5, and 500 ml of 160 mM sodium chloride in the acetate buffer. The column is eluted with a 7 liter linear gradient of sodium chloride, from 160 to 400 mM, in the acetate buffer. Fractions are collected during gradient elution of the column and are evaluated for antibody by ELISA assay and overall purity by conventional polyacrylamide gel electrophoresis analysis (26). Fractions containing active antibody, eluting between 240 and 300 mM sodium chloride in the gradient, are pooled for further processing. The 1.3 l pool (containing 600 μg/ml antibody and 2.5 mg/ml total protein) is carefully neutralized with 1 M triethanolamine solution and concentrated by ultrafiltration to a volume of 100 ml. The concentrate is solvent exchanged into 50 mM triethanolamine buffer, pH 8.0, by either diafiltration in the ultrafiltration cell or gel filtration on Sephadex G-25.

Following clarification by centrifugation, the solvent exchange antibody solution is chromatographed on a 2.2 X 30 cm column of Q-Sepharose Fast Flow, previously equilibrated in 50 mM triethanolamine buffer, pH 8.0. Flow rate is maintained at 1 ml/min. Following sample application the column is washed with 50 ml of 50 mM triethanolamine buffer, pH 8.0, and 50 ml of 70 mM sodium chloride in the triethanolamine buffer. The column is eluted with a 1000-ml linear gradient of sodium chloride, from 70 to 210 mM, in the triethanolamine buffer. Fractions are collected during gradient elution of the column and are evaluated for purity by conventional polyacrylamide gel electrophoresis analysis. Fractions containing essentially pure immunoglobulin, eluting between 120 and 150 mM sodium chloride in the gradient, are pooled. The 200-ml pool contains 3 mg/ml antibody and 4 mg/ml total protein.

The pH of the Q-Sepharose pool is adjusted to 4.5 with acetic acid. The pool is chromatographed on a 2.2 × 30 cm column of S-Sepharose Fast Flow, previously equilibrated in 170 mM acetate buffer, pH 4.5. Flow rate is maintained at 1 ml/min. Following sample application the column is washed with 30 ml of 170 mM acetate buffer, pH 4.5, and 50 ml of 180 mM sodium chloride in the acetate buffer. The column is eluted with a 900-ml linear gradient of sodium chloride, from 180 to 300 mM, in the acetate buffer. Fractions are collected during gradient elution of the column and are evaluated for antibody activity by microelisa assay. Fractions containing active antibody, eluting between 240 and 300 mM sodium chloride in the gradient, are pooled. The 310-ml pool, containing 1.7 mg/ml active antibody, is neutralized and concentrated approximately 12-fold by ultrafiltration. The concentrate is solvent exchanged into 340 mM borate buffer, pH 8.0, prior to conjugation. Alternately, the Q-Sepharose pool can be adjusted to 1 M in ammonium sulfate and chromatographed on a 2.2 × 30 cm column of Phenyl Sepharose Fast Flow, previously equilibrated with 1 M ammonium sulfate in 100 mM phosphate buffer, pH 7.0. Flow rate is maintained at 1 ml/min. Following sample application the column is washed with 50 ml of 1 M ammonium sulfate in 100 mM phosphate buffer, pH 7.0. The column is eluted with a 1000-ml linear gradient from 1 to 0 M ammonium sulfate in the phosphate buffer. Fractions are collected during gradient elution of the column and are evaluated for antibody activity by the ELISA assay. Fractions containing active antibody, eluting between 600 and 400 mM ammonium sulfate in the gradient, are pooled. The pool is concentrated and solvent exchanged into the borate buffer as described above.

D. Preparation of the KS1/4-DAVLB Conjugate

The S2-fraction described above for KS1/4 is coupled to succinoyl desacetyl vinblastine N-hydroxysuccinimide (DAVLB-HS-NS) by a variation of a procedure originally developed for the conjugation of vindesine to murine monoclonal antibodies (27). Briefly, KS1/4-S2 is diluted to a concentration of 20 mg/ml in 0.34 M borate buffer, pH 8.6 and then reacted with a 8:1 molar ratio of DAVLB-HS-NS in distilled dimethylformamide (DMF) supplied by the laboratory by Dr. B. Laguzza, Lilly Research Laboratories. The final DMF concentration is 7.4% for the reaction which stirs at ambient temperature for 30 minutes. The reaction at this stage is complete, and the conjugate is then purified as described below.

Estimates of conjugation ratio (moles DAVLB/mole antibody) are determined spectrophotometrically according to a previously described method (27) and can be defined as follows:

$$\text{conjugation ratio} = 15.1\ \frac{(P - 0.840\ Q)}{(Q - 0.904\ P)}$$

where P and Q are absorbances at 270 nm and 280 nm, respectively.

The conjugation of DAVLB-HS-NS to antibody is presumed to occur primarily through the epsilon amino groups of lysine. As there are over 80 residues of lysine per mole of antibody, it is not surprising that the product of conjugation is quite heterogeneous. A reverse phase chromatographic purification procedure, exploiting the hydrophobic character added to the antibody by the DAVLB moieties, was developed to allow control over the degee of conjugation in the final product by eliminating both unmodified and heavily derivatized antibody. The details of a 1-gram scale are described.

The conjugation reaction solution is neutralized and diluted with two volumes of 100 mM phosphate buffer, pH 6.2. After stirring one hour, the solution is clarified by centrifugation at 27,000 X *g* for 30 minutes. The clear supernatant is chromatographed on a 1.6 X 25 cm column of Phenyl Sepharose CL-4B, previously equilibrated in 100 mM phosphate buffer, pH 6.2. Flow rate is maintained at 1 ml/min. Following sample application the column is washed with 50 ml of the phosphate buffer and then eluted with an 800-ml linear gradient of acetonitrile, from 0 to 30% (v/v), in the phosphate buffer. Fractions are collected throughout the development of the column and assayed spectrophotometrically for protein concentration and conjugation ratio (Fig. 9). Fractions exhibiting satisfactory conjugation ratios are pooled, solvent exchanged into phosphate buffered saline on Sephadex G-25, and concentrated by ultrafiltration to approximately 5 mg/ml. The final solution is sterile filtered and stored at 4°C.

E. Isoelectricfocusing (IEF) Analysis

IEF analysis was performed utilizing a LKB slab multiphor device cooled by a Lauda refrigerated circulating bath according to the manufacturers suggested procedures. Precast IEF slab gels were purchased from LKB. Samples of monoclonal antibodies and conjugates and pI standard proteins (LKB) were absorbed onto 4 X 4 mm filter paper squares and placed on the pre-equilibrated IEF gel. Focusing was performed at 10°C for 95 minutes at 60 watts constant power. The IEF gels were stained in Coomassie Blue (0.5%) in methanol/acetic acid. Following destaining, photographs were taken to record the results.

F. MTT In Vitro Cytotoxicity Assay

In vitro cytotoxicity of various drug species and conjugates were assessed by use of the MTT assay. P3-UCLA cells were harvested by trypsinization and plated at a initial cell density of 5 X 10^4 viable cells/well in 96 well microtiter plates. Various dilutions of drugs and monoclonal antibody drug conjugates were added to the cultures after 24 hours of initial culture. After a second 24 hour incuba-

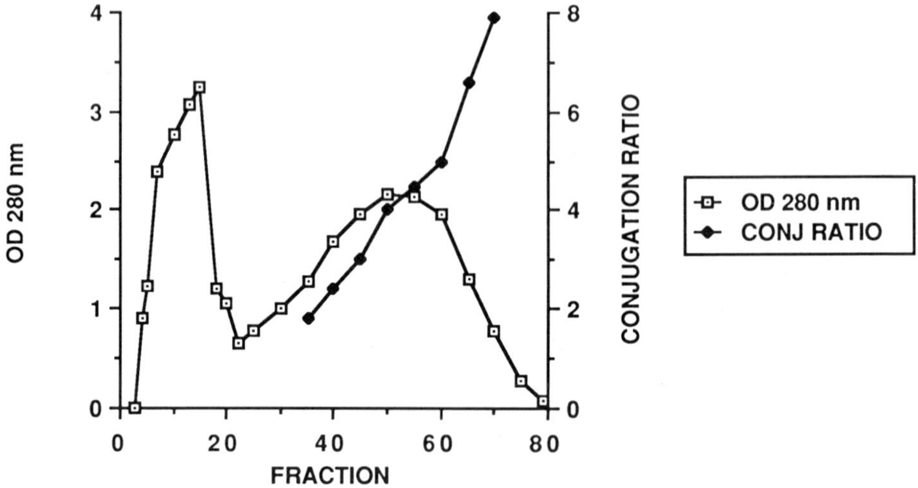

Figure 9 The heterogeneity of the KS1/4-DAVLB conjugate. The degree of DAVLB derivatization of the KS1/4 monoclonal antibody can be partially controlled by reverse phase chromatography of the conjugation reaction mixture on Phenyl Sepharose CL-4B. See text for details.

tion, 20ul of the MTT dye stock (5 mg/ml in PBS, pH 7.4) is added followed by a thirty minute incubation at room temperture. The plates were then centrifuged at 1000 X g for ten minutes and an acid alcohol dye solubilization reagent added (acidified isopropyl alcohol). The % cytotoxicity is calculated from the following calculation:

$$\% \text{ cytotoxicity} = 1 - \frac{\text{O.D. drug or conjugate treated cells}}{\text{O.D. untreated control cells}} \times 100$$

G. In Vivo Xenograft Models for Efficacy Experiments

In the Tumor Initiation Model, P3-UCLA human lung adenocarcinoma cells (10^7 viable cells) were implanted subcutaneously in groups of 8-10-week-old 18-22-g athymic nude mice (Charles River). Intravenous tail vein injections of the KS1/4 MAb, KS1/4-DAVLB, or vinblastine sulfate (VLB) at the doses indicated in the results were utilized in all xenograft immunotherapy experiments. In the tumor initiation model, treatments occurred on days 2, 5, 8. All doses of KS1/4-DAVLB and VLB are expressed in terms of mg/kg with respect to drug content. Treatment doses of KS1/4 are with respect to protein content in mg/kg. Tumor mass estimates were determined from tumor volume measurements made with electronic digital calipers (Material Control Inc.) interfaced with a Hewlitt-Packard Personal Computer utilizing a previously described formula (28). Data processing for comparative analyses of experimental groups and control groups examining tumor growth suppression was achieved utilizing a program developed by Mr. John Wrozalla, Lilly Research Laboratories.

The above-described procedure was extended to an established tumor model by allowing the implanted tumors to grow for 14-17 days prior to the initiation of treatment. The treatment schedule utilized for this assay was to administer KS1/4-DAVLB I.V. at the doses indicated in the text on days 16, 18, 20, 22, 24, 27, and 30.

An experimental metastases model was also developed. In this model, nude mice were initially sublethally irradiated with 400 rad and then given an intravenous injection of deaggregated viable P3-UCLA human lung adenocarcinoma cells (10^7). In this model, treatment was initiated within 24-48 hours after tumor implantation The animals develop multifocal/multiorgan system metastatic foci ultimately resulting in the animal's death. In these experiments, KS1/4-DAVLB was administered on days 1, 6, 10, 14, and 18. The animals were monitored for at least 100 days and the mean survivial times calculated and compared statistically utilizing the R SURV program developed and utilized at Lilly Research Laboratories.

H. Biodistribution Methods

Distribution and pharmacokinetic studies were conducted in male P3-UCLA human lung adenocarcinoma tumor-bearing nuce mice with KS1/4-[^{3}H]-DAVLB, [^{3}H]-DAVLB, and a nonimmunoreactive MAb-[^{3}H]-DAVLB conjugate. Equimolar doses of 5 mg/kg of vinca alkaloid (equivalent of 150 mg/kg of antibody drug conjugate) were injected intravenously and animals sacrificed at the indicated time points. Tissues were dissected, combusted in a Packard sample oxidizer, and radioactivity was determined by liquid scintillation counting with external standard quench correction curves. The area, under the tissue concentration versus time curve (AUC) was calculated from Simpson's trapezoidal rule.

REFERENCES

1. Kohler, G, and Milstein, C. (1975) Continuous cultures of fused cells secreting antibody of predefined specificity. *Nature 256*:455-457.
2. Bumol, T. F., and Reisfeld, R. A. (1982) A unique glycoprotein-proteoglycan complex defined by monoclonal antibody on human melanoma cells. *Proc. Natl. Acad. Sci. USA 79*:1245-1249.
3. Colcher, D., Hand, P. H. Nuti, M., and Schlom, J. (1981). A spectrum of

monoclonal antibodies reactive with human mammary tumor cells. *Proc. Natl. Acad. Sci. USA 78*:3199-3203.
4. Herlyn, M., Steplewski, Z., Herlyn, D., and Koprowski, H. (1979) Colorectal carcinoma-specific antigen detection by means of monoclonal antibodies. *Proc. Natl. Acad. Sci. USA 76*:1438-1452.
5. Muraro, R., Wunderlich, D., Thor, A., Lundry, J., Noguchi, P., Cunningham, R., and Schlom, J. (1985) Definition by monoclonal antibodies of a repertoire of epitopes on carcinoembryonic antigen differentially expressed in human colon carcinomas versus normal adult tissue. *Cancer Res. 45*:5769-5780.
6. Bjorn, M. J., Ring, D., and Frankel, A., (1985). Evaluation of monclonal antibodies for the development of breast cancer immunotoxins. *Cancer Research 45*:1214-1221.
7. Reisfeld, R. A., Harper, J. R., and Bumol, T. F. (1984) Human tumor antigens defined by monoclonal antibodies. *CRC Crit. Rev. Immunol. 5*:27-53.
8. Bumol, T. F., Walker, L. E., and Reisfeld, R. A. (1984) Biosynthetic studies of proteoglycans in human melanoma cells with a monoclonal antibody to a core glycoprotein of chondroitin sulfate proteoglycans. *J. Biol. Chem. 259*: 12733-12741.
9. Cheresh, D. A., Harper, J. R., Schulz, G., and Reisfeld, R. A. (1986) Localization of the gangliosides GD_2 and GD_3 in adhesion plaques and on the surface of human melanoma cells. *Proc. Natl. Acad. Sci. USA 81*:5767-5771.
10. Edwards, D. P., Grzyb, K. T., Dressler, L. G., Mansel, R. E., Zava, D. T., Sledge, G. W., Jr., and McGuire, W. L. (1986). Monclonal antibody identification and characterization of a Mr 43,000 membrane glycoprotein associated with human breast cancer. *Cancer Res. 46*:1306-1317.
11. Hellstrom, K. E., Hellstrom, I., and Brown, J. P. (1984) Diagnostic and therapeutic use of monoclonal antibodies to human tumor antigens. *Med. Oncol. Tumor Pharmacother. 3*:140-147.
12. Herlyn, M., Blaszczyk, M., Sears, H. F., Verrill, H., Lindgren, J., Colcher, D., Steplewski, Z., Schlom, J., and Koprowski, H. (1983) Detection of carcinoembryonic antigen and related antigens in sera of patients with gastrointestinal tumors using monoclonal antibodies in double-determinant radioimmunoassays. *Hybridoma 2*:329-339.
13. Thor, A., Horan-Hand, P., Wunderlich, D., Caruso, A., Muraro, R., and Schlom, J. (1984) Monclonal antibodies define differential ras gene expression in malignant and benign colonic diseases. *Nature 311*:562-565.
14. Young, H. A., Klein, R. A., Shib, T. Y., Morgan, A. C., and Schroff, R. W. (1986) Detection of the intracellular ras p21 oncogene product by flow cytometry. *Anal. Biochem. 156*:67-71.
15. Gentry, L. E., and Lawton, A. (1986) Characterization of site-specific antibodies to the ErbB gene product and EGF receptor: inhibition of tyrosine kinase activity. *Virology 152*:421-431.
16. Ehrlich, P. (1909) In *Beiträge zur experimentellen Pathologie and Chemotherapie*. Akademische Verlagsgesellschaft, Leipzig, pp. 167-202.
17. Miller, R. A., Oseroff, A. R., Stratte, P. T., and Levy, R. (1983) Monoclonal

antibody therapeutic trials in seven patients with T-cell lymphoma. *Blood 62*:988-995.

18. Sears, H. F., Mattis, J., Herlyn, D., Hayry, P., Atkinson, B., Ernst, C., Steplewski, Z., and Koprowski, H. (1982) Phase-1 clinical trial of monoclonal antibody in treatment of gastro intestinal tumors. *The Lancet 318*:762-763.
19. Shawler, D. L., Miceli, M. C., Wormsley, S. B., Royston, I., and Dillman, R. O. (1984) Induction of in vitro and in vivo antigenic modulation by the anti-human T-cell monoclonal antibody T101. *Cancer Research 44*:5921-5927.
20. Houghton, A. N., Mintzer, D., Cordon-Cardo, C., Welt, S., Fliegel, B., Vadhan, S., Carswell, E., Melamed, M., Oetigen, H. F., and Old, L. J. (1985). Mouse monoclonal IgG_3 antibody detecting Gd_3 ganglioside: A phase I trial in patients with malignant melanoma. *Proc. Natl. Acad. Sci. USA 82*:
21. Goodman, G. E., Beavmier, P., Hellstrom, I., Fernyhough, B., and Hellstrom, K. E. (1985) Pilot trial of murine monoclonal antibodies in patients with advanced melanoma. *Clin. Oncol. 3*:340-352.
22. Baldwin, R. W. (1985) Monoclonal antibody targeting of anti-cancer agents: Mihlbock memorial lecture. *Eur. J. Can. Clin. Oncol. 21*:1281-1285.
23. Arnon, R., and Sela, M. (1982) In vitro and in vivo efficacy of conjugates of daunomycin with anti-tumor antibodies. *Immunol. Rev. 62*:5-27.
24. Varki, N. M., Reisfeld, R. A., and Walker, L. E. (1984) Antigens associated with a human lung adenocarcinoma defined by monoclonal antibodies. *Cancer Research 44*:681-686.
25. Marder, P., Apelgren, L. D., and Bumol, T. F. (1987). Comparative analysis of monoclonal antibody-drug conjugate binding by flow cytometry. *J. Immunol. Methods 96*:165-170.
26. Laemmli, U. K. (1970) Cleavage of structural proteins during the assembly of the head of bacteriophage T4. *Nature 277*:680-685.
27. Rowland G. F., Axton, C. A., Baldwin, R. W., Brown, J. P., Corvalan, J. R. F., Embleton, M. J., Gore, V. A., Hellstrom, I., Hellstrom, K. E., Jacobs, E., Marsden, C. H., Pimm, M. V., Simmonds, R. G., and Smith, W. (1985) Antitumor properties of vindesine monoclonal antibody conjugates. *Can. Immunol. Immunother. 19*:1-7.
28. Anderson, J. C., Fugmann, R., Stofli, R. L., and Martin, D. S. (1974) Metastatic incidence of a spontaneous murine mammary adenocarcinoma. *Cancer Research 34*:1916-1920.

4

Synthesis and Testing of Antibody-Antifolate Conjugates for Drug Targeting

TARUNENDU GHOSE
Dalhousie University and Victoria General Hospital, Halifax, Nova Scotia, Canada

A. HUNTLEY BLAIR, JAROSLAV KRALOVEC, and MOLLY MAMMEN
Dalhousie University, Halifax, Nova Scotia, Canada

P. O. UADIA
University of Port Harcout, Port Harcourt, Nigeria

I. INTRODUCTION

A. The Basis of the Choice of Antifolate-Antibody Conjugates for Investigation

In spite of advances in cancer chemotherapy, most agents have a low therapeutic index (1), i.e., they damage normal proliferating cells as well as neoplastic cells (2). The rationale for the use of antibodies against tumor-associated antigens as selective carriers of cancer chemotherapeutic agents for increasing their chemotherapeutic index is based on observations by us and others that anti-TAA antibodies or their immunologically reactive fragments do indeed selectively localize in tumors in vivo (3). Furthermore, we have demonstrated that the $F(ab')_2$ fragments of anti-TAA antibodies are capable of crossing the "blood-brain" barrier and localizing in tumors of the central nervous system. Our reviews (4-7) cover the current status of preparation and assay of drug-antibody conjugates and evidence for their effectiveness against cancer in vitro, in rodent tumors and in human tumor xenografts. Before we discuss antifolates, we shall briefly consider the four different approaches to cancer therapy based on anti-TAA antibodies and give our reasons for focusing on antibody-linked chemotherapeutic agents (especially antifolates).

1. Antibodies Alone as Tumor Inhibitors

Our experience (8,9) and that of others (10,11) in experimental models and results of recent phase 1 clinical trials of anti-TAA MAb alone have been disappointing (12-15) although, in an occasional patient, results were dramatic (16). Antibodies themselves are not inherently cytotoxic, and their binding to a target cell does not affect growth except in rare instances (9,17). This confirms the necessity for linkage of cytotoxic agents to anti-TAA antibodies (18-26).

2. Antibody-bound Toxins (Immunotoxins)

Toxins that have been conjugated to antibodies include gelonin, pokeweed antiviral protein, abrin, ricin, diphtheria toxin, and Pseudomonas exotoxin (5,6). Tumor inhibition has been demonstrated in leukemias and solid tumors but, in general, immunotoxins have shown less consistent antitumor action than drug conjugates (5). The very high potency of toxins (27,28) makes specificity even more stringent. Approaches for eliminating nonspecific binding include removal of the B chain prior to conjugation or the use of single-chain toxins. However, there is a problem of internalization of antibody-linked A chains in the absence of B chains (5). The clinical trial of immunotoxins has been confined mainly to the elimination of leukemia/lymphoma cells or T cells from bone marrow in vitro prior to bone marrow transplantation. Results are still too preliminary for evaluation (5); however, in vitro depletion of T cells from grafts prior to transplantation inhibits the acceptance of grafted bone marrow (29).

3. Antibody-linked Radionuclides (Immunoradiotherapy)

Isotope-carrying antibodies can deliver radiation to adjacent cells that may lack the target antigen (30). We demonstrated that injections of ^{131}I-labeled antibodies could prolong the survival and produce cure in a proportion of tumor-bearing mice (19,23). Further evidence of tumor regression has been obtained with antibody-bound ^{131}I after local administration, e.g., in ovarian cancer, ascites tumors, and some liver tumors (31-33). However, responses were transient and the amounts of radioactivity necessary for tumor eradication may be unacceptably high.

4. Antibody-linked Chemotherapeutic Agents (Immunochemotherapy). The Advantages of Antifolate Drugs for Investigating the Feasibility of Antibody-mediated Targeting

For reasons above, chemotherapeutic agents appear to have the greatest potential (4-6). A number of factors have led us to extensively study the antimetabolite MTX and, lately, its gamma aspartate derivative. MTX is in widespread clinical use; its structure-action relationships, modes of action, induction of drug resistance, and reversibility of its toxicity with compounds such as leucovorin are well elucidated (34). Also, a number of antifolates, exemplified by MTX, possess certain advantages for studies on conjugate synthesis and testing. They can form complexes with the target enzyme DHFR in a virtually stoichiometric relationship, although an excess is required intracellularly for effective cytotoxic action (35). Furthermore, MTX exhibits a characteristic absorption spectrum, which is useful for analysis of fractions during purification and for determination of extent of incorporation in conjugates. This drug is also available in tritium-labeled form, either in the glutamate or p-aminobenzoyl moieties, which also facilitates these analyses and provides a means of studying the mode of action and catabolism of the conjugated drug in vitro and in vivo (36-38).

MTX was the subject of early attempts to synthesize drug-antibody conjugates (4,39,40). Conjugates obtained in these attempts using a diazo reaction were not assayed for retention of drug and antibody activities and the method was not reproducible in our hands. As far as conjugation chemistry is concerned, MTX and some of its derivatives possess both amino and carboxyl groups, so there are several possible ways of linkage to immunoglobulins. Modification of the carboxyl groups is less likely to interfere with inhibition of DHFR (41). We have developed methods for linkage of MTX to antibodies through these moieties, e.g., by amide bonds, with preservation of drug and antibody activities.

Methods for conjugating MTX to antibodies should maximally retain drug and antibody activities without substantial increase in the size of the conjugate. The first two characteristics are the basis of therapeutically useful targeting with antibodies. Furthermore, substantial increases in the size of the conjugate as a result of using macromolecular carriers (that might allow greater drug incorporation) is likely to alter the pharmacokinetics of the conjugate. There may be interference with its passage through capillary walls to reach the target or with its subsequent endocytosis by target cells. Also, such a conjugate may exhibit increased susceptibility to phagocytosis. The linkage of antifolates directly to antibody molecules (or their reactive fragments) without the use of intermediaries obviates the complications associated with large conjugates.

II. STUDIES WITH MTX AND MTX-gamma-ASP

A. MTX

1. Direct Conjugation of MTX to Intact IgG

We have evaluated several methods of conjugating MTX to IgG (41). These methods include coupling via water-soluble carbodiimides and via reactive intermediate derivatives of MTX, e.g., active esters formed by reaction with N-hydroxysuccinimide, hydrazides, and a mixed anhydride reported by Burstein and Knapp (42) to be formed by reaction with acetic anhydride. Conjugates (4,41) retaining drug and antibody activity were produced using active esters, hydrazides, and ECDI. Model studies with anti-BSA IgG comparing the active ester and ECDI methods showed that the active ester method was more effective with respect to recovery of antibody activity and yield of conjugated protein. Ten moles of MTX per mole of IgG could be incorporated with retention of 90% of the anti-BSA activity of an equimolar amount of unconjugated IgG and with recovery of 70% of the original protein (41). MTX conjugated by the active ester method retained 25-45% of its ability to inhibit DHFR and was shown to be effective in inhibiting the murine EL4 lymphoma and human melanoma xenografts (4,41,43) (see below). Some recent studies have been directed toward linking antifolate hydrazides to the carbohydrate moieties of IgG to determine whether drug loading and antitumor effect can be improved compared to linkage to amino acid residues (see below).

a. Active Ester-mediated Synthesis of Conjugates The active ester-mediated synthesis entails two steps. In the first, MTX (I) is reacted with NHS in the presence of DCC to form the corresponding NHS active ester (II) (scheme 1). In the second stage, the active ester is reacted with the IgG in an aqueous buffered medium to yield the conjugate.

Generally speaking, good results are achieved using an active ester method, one of the most common techniques for activation of carboxyl groups. NHS active ester derivatives often can be isolated and purified and are stable to extended storage. The NHS moiety is a sufficiently good leaving group so that reaction with free amino groups occurs readily. The relative stability of the anion of NHS is of great importance in this regard. Another important feature is that active esters generally inhibit racemization during the course of the reaction. In this section we discuss some of the factors that influence the reaction. The detailed procedures for active ester-based conjugation are given in the appendix.

i. Synthesis of active ester intermediates. Synthesis of carboxy derivatives of MTX must take into account the fact that this drug possesses two carboxyl groups than can react with DCC and so the range of products formed comprises two monoesters and the diester. The derivative expected to lead to the most active drug in conjugate form is the gamma monoester. To restrict synthesis mainly to monoesters, the ratio of antifolate:DCC:NHS should be maintained at 1:1:1. The yield of active ester was measured by reactivity toward an amino group containing gel (41) or by using TLC.

ii. Formation of conjugates by reaction of the active ester intermediate with an immunoglobulin. In the case of MTX, the active ester derivatives are difficult to purify, and we have used DMF solutions of the active ester directly for conjugation to IgG at pH 7. Also, a limited amount of DMF is introduced into the IgG solution prior to the MTX to increase the solubility of the drug derivative in the aqueous reaction mixture. Using an IgG concentration of 4-10 mg/ml (27-67 μM), incorporation ratios as high as 30 moles of drug per mole of IgG

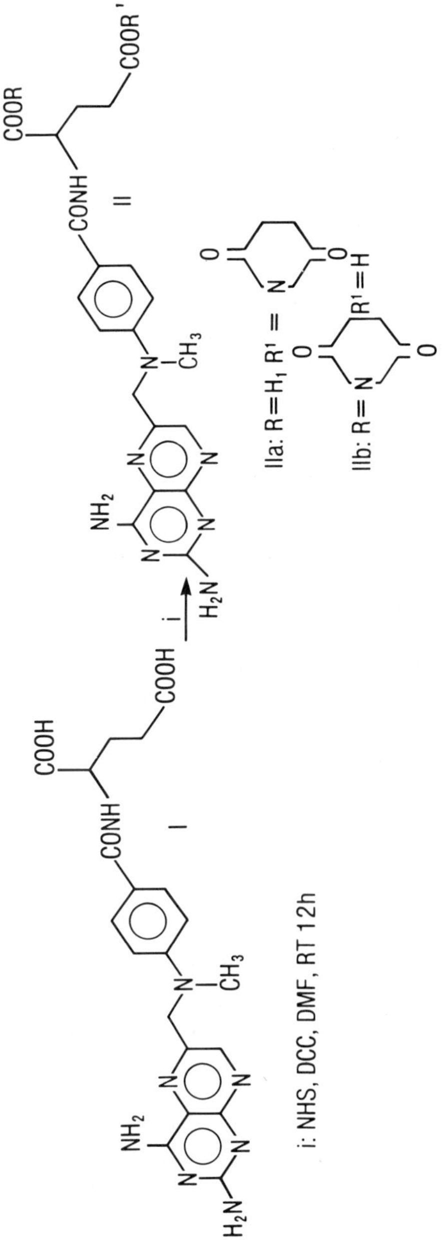

Scheme 1

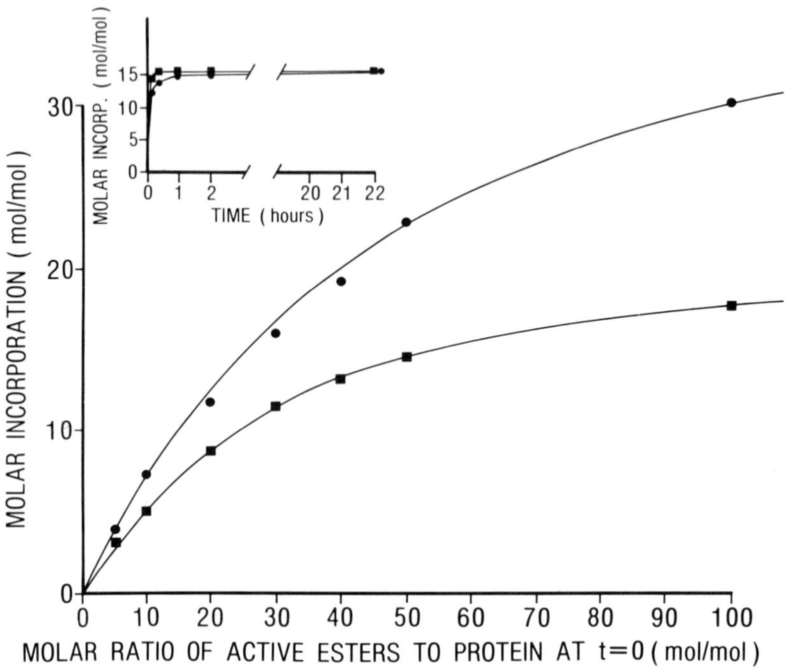

Figure 1 Incorporation of MTX and MTX-gamma-ASP into IgG as a function of the molar ratio of active ester to IgG in the reaction mixture. Reaction mixtures contained: MTX (●) or MTX-gamma-ASP (■) at the molar ratio indicated; IgG, 10 mg (66.7 nmol); DMF, 0.5 ml; PBS, 4.5 ml; in a total volume of 5 ml. Antifolates ranged from 333 nmol to 6.63 μmol and were added in 100 μl of DMF. Inset shows time course of MTX-NRG and MTX-gamma-ASP-NRG coupling using a 25-fold molar excess of MTX-AE and a 50-fold molar excess of MTX-gamma-ASP-AE.

can be obtained. Figure 1 shows the incorporation ratio as a function of the molar ratio of active ester to IgG in the reaction mixture at an IgG concentration of 2 mg/ml. A 25-fold molar excess of MTX with the protein concentration maintained at 5-10 mg/ml has consistently led to incorporations of 10-12 moles of drug per mole of IgG with recoveries of protein approaching 90%.

One potential disadvantage of using unpurified active esters is that small amounts of unreacted DCC are likely to be present during conjugation. This could result in cross-linkage of the protein amino and carboxyl groups by residual unreacted DCC, leading to loss of antibody activity and denaturation particularly at low protein concentrations. The ratio of 1:1:1 for antifolate:DCC: NHS specified above for active ester synthesis with MTX is likely to result in the least side reactions when the active ester is used without isolation. In an early experiment where the protein concentration was 4 mg/ml and the synthesis ratio was 1:5:2, the recovery of protein in the subsequent conjugation reaction was only 45%, compared to 65-70% for a ratio of 1:1:1.

iii. Retention of drug and antibody activities. Apart from evaluating their effect in mice bearing tumors, the following assay systems yield valuable information regarding the properties of conjugates and their mode of action. Retention of drug activity when the drug is bound to IgG depends upon not introducing steric hindrance due to the change in drug structure produced by the linkage groups or as a result of interference with the interaction between bound drug and its target molecules by the adjacent region of the IgG. However, loss of ability of conjugated MTX to inhibit DHFR in an in vitro assay does not necessarily indicate lack of antitumor effect in vivo, since catabolism in vivo may give products that regain drug activity. If catabolism occurs in the milieu of the target tumor, the conjugate may display cytotoxic action toward tumor cells in culture or in tumor-bearing animals.

Retention of drug activity in intact conjugates can be conveniently assessed by inhibition of target DHFR. A partially purified beef liver DHFR can be obtained commercially from Sigma. Our assay procedure for this enzyme is based on that of Peterson et al. (44), which spectrophotometrically measures the conversion of DHFA to THFA along with the concomitant conversion of NADH to NAD^+. DHFR inhibition by conjugated MTX is substantially less than by the free drug and has varied with different conjugate and DHFR preparations. Typical values range between 15 and 25% of the effectivenes of free MTX. At incorporation ratios between 15 and 30 moles of drug per mole of IgG, the inhibition drops to 10-12% of that by the free drug. It may be possible to improve the retention of drug activity by regiospecific conjugation, e.g., selective linkage by a particular carboxyl group so as to obtain a single structural isomer in the conjugate. A fraction (isolated by gel filtration) containing catabolic fragments of conjugate resulting from the action of a cell homogenate gave inhibition approximately equal to the conjugate from which the fraction was derived. The conjugate used in this experiment had an incorporation ratio of 5-6 moles per mole and the bound drug was approximately half as effective as free MTX. It remains to be established whether catabolism can lead to small fragments (or free MTX) with restored DHFR inhibitory capacity.

A better approach for assessing antitumor antibody conjugates would be to use DHFR from target tumor cells. We have been purifying DHFR from EL4 and CLL cell lines that are used to measure the antitumor effect of our conjugates. Assay conditions may require modification to deal with enzymes from different sources. For example, the optimal pH for CLL DHFR is 7.5, a value substantially higher than for the beef liver enzyme, and MET is required in the assay system.

Retention of antibody activity in intact conjugates depends upon not blocking the antigen-binding site by incorporated drug and upon not producing any conformational alterations as a result of drug loading anywhere in the IgG that interfere with antigen binding. To evaluate loss of antibody activity after conjugation, we usually carry out pilot experiments using a polyclonal rabbit IgG against BSA (41,45). Radial immunodiffusion in this system provides a rapid and reliable method for assay of antibody activity (41). We realize that each MAb may behave differently after linkage, but a rapid screening using the BSA-antiBSA system can help in weeding out methods that result in gross denaturation. Methods for determination of activity of anti-TAA-IgG conjugates include inhibition of binding of ^{125}I-labeled unconjugated anti-TAA IgG to target cells in vitro (46).

iv. Effect of conjugated MTX on target cells in culture. Two different assay methods are used for determining the effectiveness of the conjugates, i.e., inhibition of proliferation and a clonogenic assay. In assays involving inhibition of proliferation, free MTX is more potent than MTX-antibody conjugates, but MTX conjugated to the antibody is more potent than MTX conjugated to nonspecific IgG. For example, the IC_{50} of MTX for M21 cells was 0.015 μg/ml, whereas the IC_{50} values for MTX conjugated to rabbit antimelanoma IgG, antimelanoma MAb 225.28S, and NRG were 0.38, 0.26, and 0.96 μg/ml, respectively.

b. Synthetic Approaches Based on Water-soluble Carbodiimides and a Mixed Anhydride Water-soluble carbodiimides have found wide use for conjugation in spite of the inherent limitation due to reactivity toward the protein, which can lead to cross-linkage and precipitation. We produced active conjugates by this procedure but in lower yield than with the active ester method (41). MTX conjugated by the ECDI method retained its ability to inhibit DHFR to approximtely the same extent as when conjugated by the active ester method. When tested in EL-4 lymphoma-inoculated mice, at equimolar drug dosages, MTX-AELG conjugates synthesized by the ECDI method were as potent tumor inhibitors as those synthesized by the active ester method (41).

A paper appeared several years ago giving a conjugation method for MTX in which the drug was first treated with acetic anhydride, the intent being to form a mixed anhydride product that could then be reacted with the IgG (42). (This approach is related to earlier chloride methods.) In our hands, the mixed anhydride procedure failed to incorporate more than 2 to 3 moles of MTX per mole of IgG (as measured by tritium labeling), even when high molar ratios of anhydride to IgG were incubated together (42). The conjugate inhibited neither DHFR nor tumor cells in vitro. Moreover, it was found that the product obtained by treating MTX with acetic anhydride was not capable of being hydrolyzed at pH 8 to regenerate a compound capable of inhibiting DHFR. Its spectral properties also differed from those of MTX, the peak at 270 nm being shifted to 340 nm.

c. Linkage of Antifolate Hydrazides to the Carbohydrate Moieties of Immunoglobulins We have been investigating the potential of carbohydrate moieties of IgG as linkage sites for MTX and MTX-gamma-ASP. Immunoglobulin molecules of all classes contain carbohydrate attached mainly to the constant region of heavy chains (47,48). The content varies from 2.5 to 12% (49). The major oligosaccharide present in rabbit IgG is attached to an asparagine residue at position 297 in the Fc region (50). It comprises five glucosamine, two galactose, five mannose, and approximately one fucose and one sialic acid residue. A second carbohydrate group containing galactosamine, galactose, and two residues of sialic acid is present in about 40% of rabbit H chains. This oligosaccharide is bound via galactosamine to threonine 225 in the hinge region of just one H chain, so it disturbs an element of symmetry (51). In about 15% of rabbit IgG H chains, a third carbohydrate group containing only glucosamine has been found. It is probably localized in the V_H segment of the molecule (52).

The rationale of using carbohydrate moieties for linkage is based on the fact that they are infrequent in the antigen-binding sites, and their use for linkage reduces the risk of loss of antibody activity. Also, there will not be an increase in the size of the carrier. On the other hand, they may be sterically hindered by their presence between heavy chains in the Fc region and incapable of supporting the anticipated increase in incorporation. The question that we have addressed is whether MTX can be incorporated in amounts higher than or even equal to that achieved by the active ester method with greater preservation of the antibody activity. The linkage chemistry we have chosen to investigate first is based on periodate oxidation of the carbohydrate moiety in IgG to produce multiple aldehyde groups that can form hydrazones with hydrazide groups introduced into the antifolate (4-6). Hydrazone conjugates could be used directly or stabilized by reduction with borohydride. The difference in stability of the linkage could have an effect on cytotoxicity.

The reaction scheme (scheme 2) may be divided into steps as follows: i) generation of aldehyde groups from the carbohydrate moieties of immunoglobulins; ii) formation of hydrazones; iii) stabilization of the immino bond via reduction.

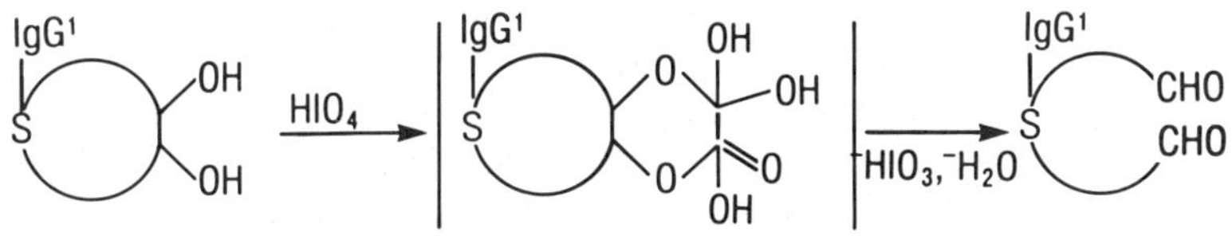

Scheme 2

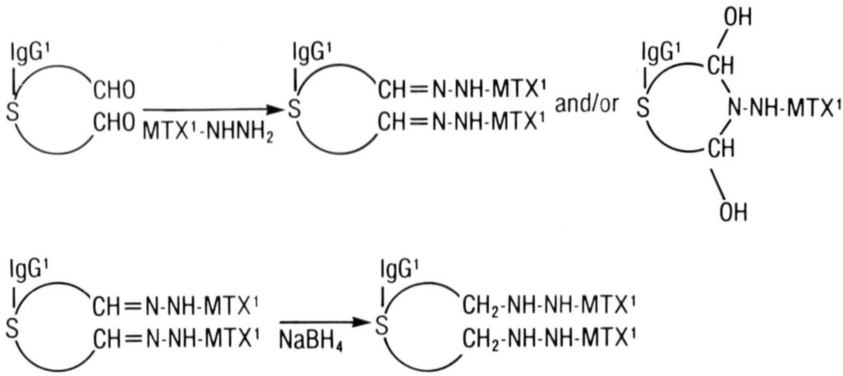

where IgG'...polypetide portion of IgG
S...carbohydrate moiety of IgG
MTX'...remainder of MTX molecule

Scheme 2 (Continued)

i. The oxidation of IgG by periodate to form polyaldehyde-IgG. A molecule containing appropriate free neighboring hydroxyl groups, such as the glycoprotein IgG, is easily oxidized with periodate, most workers carrying out the reaction at pH value between 4 and 5.6 (49,53-56). The univalent, nonhydrated metaperiodate ion (IO_4^-) is responsible for most of the vicinal hydroxyl cleavage activity of the salt (57,58), and its concentration is substantial in this pH range. In contrast, alpha-amino alcohols are oxidized most rapidly at pH 7.5. The periodate concentration range used in the oxidation of glycoproteins is generally 0.005-0.1 M (59-61), since concentrations greater than these (e.g., 0.5 M) can promote nonspecific oxidation (62). Also, to suppress nonspecific oxidation, temperatures of 0-4°C (63,64) are recommended.

Periodate oxidation is one of the simplest reactions to carry out, but when applied to a glycoprotein it can be also one of the most difficult to interpret unambiguously (64). For example, certain amino acids that contain alpha-amino alcohol groupings may be oxidized by periodate, e.g., threonine and serine (65-67). Also, hydroxyproline, proline, tryptophan, cyst(e)ine, and particularly methionine react with periodate readily at room temperature (68,69), albeit usually more slowly than sugars (70-72). To evaluate the kinetics of periodate consumption during the oxidation of immunoglobulins we have used a spectrophotometric method modified from that of Fields and Dixon for the microdetermination of periodate (73). This assay is based on the excellent reactivity of the dihydrobenzoins of the type represented by 1,2-bis-(p-dimethylaminophenyl) ethane-1,2-diol toward periodate ion.

Our experiments at room temperature using 0.05-0.1 M sodium acetate buffers with rabbit IgG shows that a 30-fold molar excess of periodate in the pH range 4-6 results in an extent of reaction equivalent to 19-25 oxidative sites formed in 1 hr. The rate of oxidation increased with decreasing pH (Fig. 2) and with increasing molar excess of periodate (Fig. 3). Small variations in the number of oxidative sites (e.g., 21-25) at pH 4.5 were seen in different batches of IgG. The kinetics of oxidation also varied depending on the IgG concentration. Imidazole buffer was found to be unsuitable for carrying out these oxidations, in keeping with the reported presence of a reducing agent as an impurity (74). We found that incubation of periodate with 0.04 M imidazole buffer led to total inactivation after 4 hr at 4°C.

In this treatment of IgG, the objective is to obtain maximal oxidation of sugar residues without oxidation of amino acid residues and without loss of antibody activity. To differentiate between the sensitivity of the sugar moieties and amino acid residues to periodate under our experimental conditions, we compared the behavior of BSA, a nonglycosylated protein, and a rabbit IgG anti-

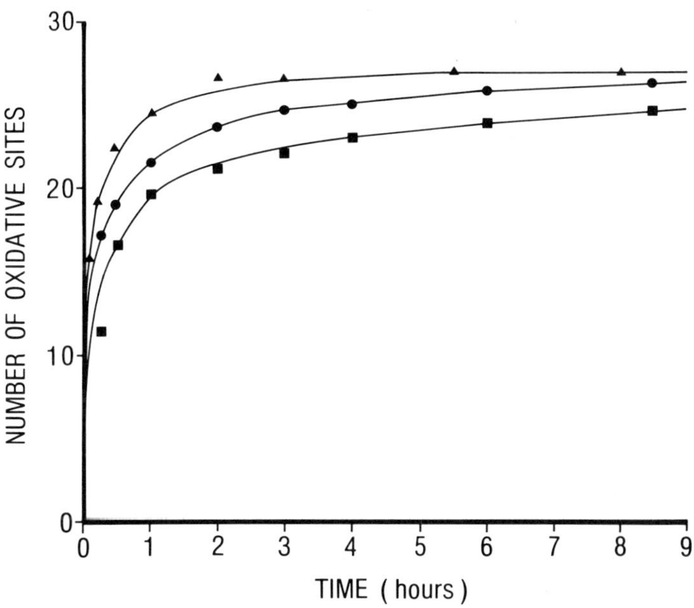

Figure 2 Kinetics of oxidation of NRG by sodium periodate at a 30-fold molar excess of oxidant at 4°C. The reaction mixtures contained: 2.0 μmol sodium periodate (0.1 ml of a 20 mM solution in water); 10 mg (0.067 μmol) NRG; 0.2 M sodium acetate buffer pH 4.0 (▲), pH 4.4 (●), or pH 5.6 (■) in a total volume of 2.1 ml.

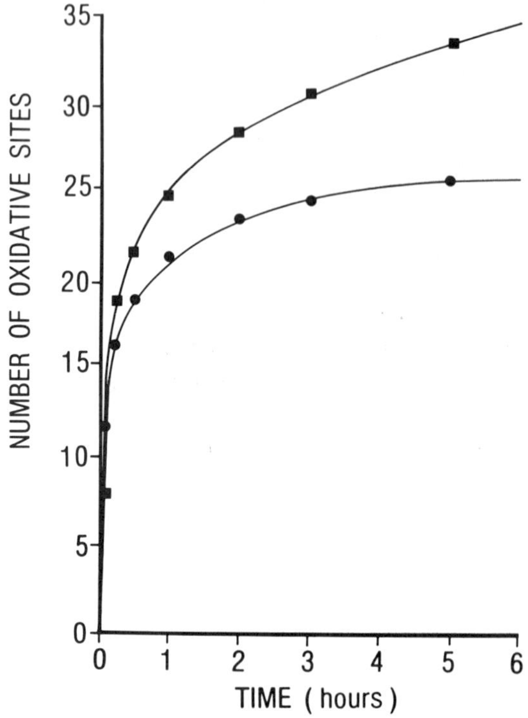

Figure 3 Kinetics of oxidation of NRG by sodium periodate at 30- and 60-fold molar excesses of oxidant at 4°C. The reaction mixtures contained: 2.0 (●) or 4.0 (■) μmol sodium periodate; 10 mg (0.067 μmol) NRG; 0.2 M sodium acetate buffer, pH 4.4 in a total volume of 2.2 ml.

body, i.e., anti-BSA IgG, toward periodate oxidation. At pH 7, BSA showed a relatively low rate of oxidation of amino acid residues; 6 moles of periodate were consumed in 3 hr compared to 22 moles for the IgG. To limit side reactions, we have limited the periodate concentration to a 25 to 30-fold molar excess.

Tests were carried out on retention of antibody activity of the anti-BSA IgG as a function of the pH at which oxidation was carried out and its duration. Full activity was retained between pH 6 and 7 (Table 1). The duration of exposure of the antibody to periodate did not appear to have any effect on its antibody activity. Similarly high recoveries of antibody activity were also obtained when the molar excess of periodate was 60-fold. Other workers have found that retention of antibody activity was dependent on protein concentration. Murayama and co-workers (56) found that 50% activity was retained when the concentration of human IgG was 10 mg/ml, whereas only 25% was retained when the

Table 1 Retention of Antibody Activity in Anti-BSA IgG after Periodate Oxidation

pH of incubation mixture[a]	Duration of incubation (min)					
	5	15	30	60	120	180
4.0	88	92	99	99	92	89
5.0	90	91	91	94	88	88
6.0	100	97	99	97	100	100
7.0	100	100	100	100	100	100

[a]The antibody concentration was 5.0 mg/ml and the periodate excess was 30-fold. Assays were carried out by single radial immundiffusion as described in the Appendix.

concentration was 5 mg/ml. In this study at pH 4.5-8.5, the molar ratios of IgG to periodate were not given.

In summary, our data indicate that approximately 19-25 periodate-susceptible sites are available in rabbit IgG when a 30-fold molar excess of periodate is used, and, that after oxidation, the IgG retains antibody activity. Our results are in agreement with theoretical predictions (53-74) regarding effect of pH, concentration, and temperature on periodate oxidation of glycoproteins.

ii. Formation of conjugates by reaction of MTX-hydrazide with polyaldehyde-IgG. Human and rodent IgG contains 20-25 moles of monosaccharide per mole of IgG, and our periodate consumption data indicate the presence of 19-25 oxidative sites, each of which will theoretically yield two aldehyde groups capable of reacting with a hydrazide. Thus, it may be possible to achieve incorporations in excess of 20 moles per mole of IgG. However, the incorporation ratios may be limited by steric hindrance and possible side reactions of aldehydes such as formation of hemiacetals with hydroxyl groups, aldol condensations or intramolecular formation of imine groups from amino groups. Determination of the exact number of available aldehyde groups is difficult because there is still no reliable method for assay of carbonyl groups and other oxidized sites in biomolecules. Methods used up to the present to "trap" aldehyde groups in biopolymers (e.g., by reaction with nucleophiles) (74b) do not yield reliable results because of steric hindrance and the side reactions referred to above. Preliminary trials of periodate oxidation of the carbohydrate moiety in anti-BSA IgG, followed by the attachment of ethylene diamine, then $NaBH_4$ reduction of the resulting imines indicated oxidation of approximately 20 carbohydrate sites per mole of IgG with retention of 70-80% of antibody activity. Coupling of a model hydra-

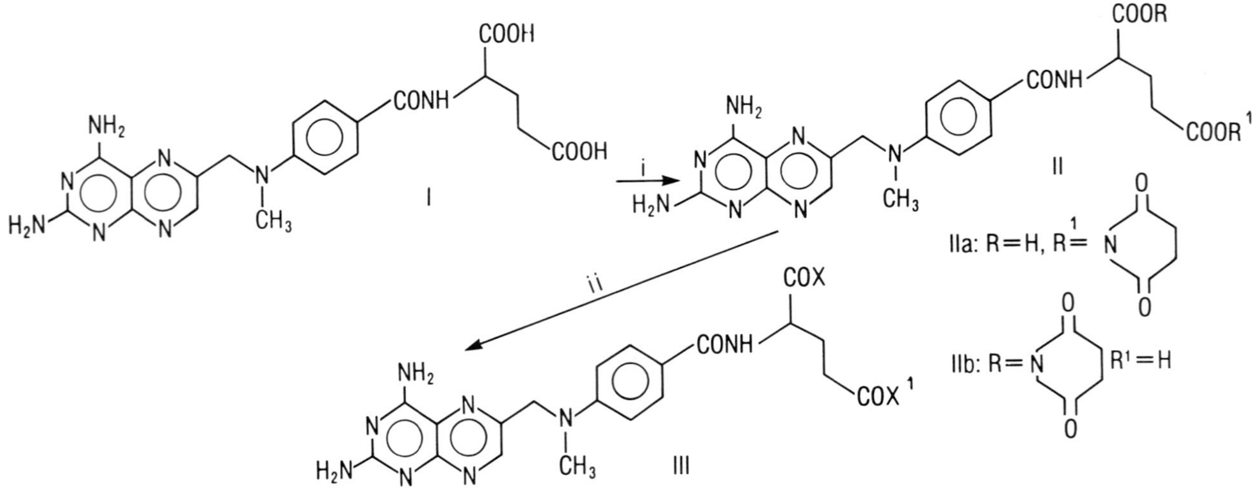

IIIa: $X=OH$, $X^1=NHNH_2$

IIIb: $X=NHNH_2$, $X^1=OH$

i: NHS, DCC, DMF, RT 12h

ii: NH_2NH_2, RT 24h

Scheme 3

zide containing compound, INH, to oxidized anti-BSA IgG was then carried out to establish the extent to which the reactivity of the putative aldehyde sites could be taken advantage of for our application. Incorporation was assayed using trichloracetic acid to cleave the hydrazone linkage, followed by spectrophotometric analysis with trinitrobenzene sulfonic acid. Incorporation varied from 6-9 moles INH/mole IgG. These rather modest incorporation ratios suggested that this application of the hydrazone method may be limited by the high degree of steric hindrance accompanying reactions between the low molecular weight hydrazine and the protein and possible unfavorable equilibria between hydrazides and protein sites. Further complications could arise from the intramolecular cross-linkage reactions involving carbonyl groups alluded to above. To determine the practical limits on antifolate incorporation, we have carried out a study with MTX-hydrazide.

Generally speaking, the best method for preparation of hydrazides is to react carboxylic acid esters with hydrazine (75-77), and this approach has been used with MTX (78). However, much better results are frequently achieved by the simple modification of reacting hydrazine with active esters or amides (77-81). We developed a synthesis based on NHS esters of MTX since we have already prepared MTX-AE for direct coupling to amino groups in IgG and because of the general capability of NHS esters (82) to inhibit possible racemization during the course of the reaction. Methotrexate (I) was transformed to its active form (II) by means of N-hydroxysuccinimide in dry DMF in the presence of DCC. II was then treated with hydrazine to yield the product (II) (Scheme 3). Both steps were carried out at room temperature. This product was purified by DEAE-52 cellulose column chromatography using gradient elution (78).

Addition of a hydrazide group to a carbonyl function follows the pattern established for other nucleophiles with formation of a carbinolamine. The reaction has been the subject of extensive study, notably by Jencks (83-85). The general pattern showing the entire mechanism is given in Scheme 4.

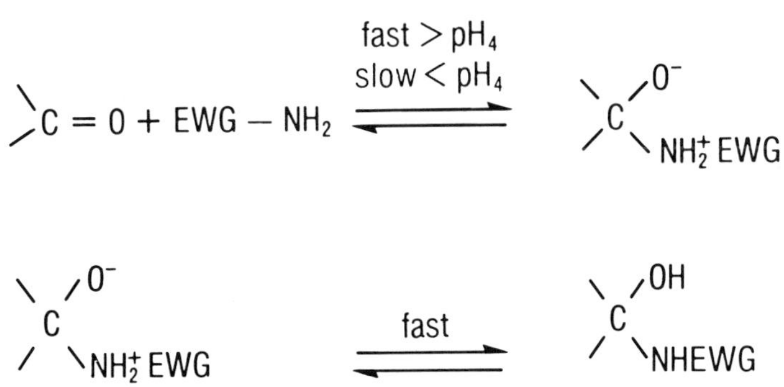

Scheme 4

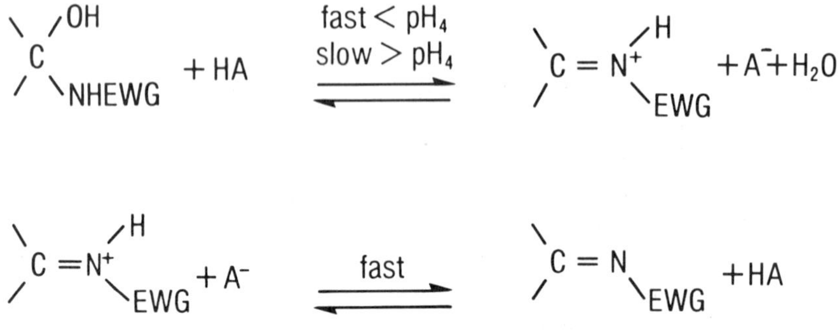

EWG....electron withdrawing group

Scheme 4 (Continued)

We have investigated the coupling of MTX-hyd to polyaldehyde-NRG at pH values ranging from 8.5 down to 4.5. The polyaldehyde-NRG had 25 oxidized sites, and we employed a 50-fold molar excess of MTX-hyd. Reactions were carried out at 4°C and stopped after 12 hr. At pH 8.0, the resulting conjugates had molar incorporations ranging from 3 to 6 moles of MTX per mole of IgG. The molar incorporation at these alkaline pH values may be limited by a combination of steric and electronic effects that are dependent on pH and result in an unfavorable equilibrium. Better results were obtained under slightly acidic conditions. The highest molar incorporation achieved was at pH 5.6, i.e., 10 to 12 moles of free drug per mole of IgG with protein recoveries of 79-88%. Control experiments, in which MTX-hydrazide was incubated with unoxidized IgG or in which MTX itself was incubated with periodate-oxidized IgG, showed incorporations of 1.0 moles per mole of IgG or less.

MTX-hydrazide conjugates were inhibitory toward beef liver DHFR. A conjugate containing 7 moles of drug per mole of IgG was 15% as effective as the free drug whereas one containing 3 moles of drug per mole of IgG was 19% as effective. Retention of anti-BSA activity in hydrazide conjugates was 88-94%. We also tested the stability of the linkage formed by comparing the molar incorporation in the original MTX-NRG hydrazone conjugates and their corresponding reduced forms prepared according to Scheme 2. A sample of MTX-IgG hydrazone conjugate (e.g., with 10 moles of drug per mole of IgG) was treated with 0.10 M sodium borohydride at 4°C for 4 hr. The reduced conjugate was subjected to dialysis against PBS for 48 hr. The molar incorporation remained unchanged. The molar incorporation of an unreduced sample of this conjugate was lowered from 10 to 8 by this dialysis treatment.

One would expect higher retention of antibody activity at equimolar incorporations via carbohydrate moieties compared to direct conjugation to protein residues. Results from our and other laboratories have shown that when MTX or chlorambucil are linked to antibodies using a carbodiimide, there is a rapid decline in antibody activity at molar incorporation above 10. The use of carbohydrate moieties for drug coupling described here indicates that drug loadings substantially above those observed using active ester-based conjugation cannot be attained under the reaction conditions used so far. However, the total number of carbohydrate residues may vary from one MAb to another depending on factors that include their class and subclass. Studies are in progress to investigate the number of linkage sites in different MAb by assay of periodate-produced aldehydes and compare the antitumor effect of conjugates prepared by hydrazide-based linkage (with and without borohydride reduction) with those prepared by active ester-based linkage. As stated above, the difference in stability of the linkage could have an effect on cytotoxicity.

2. Inhibition of Ascites Tumors of Mice

MTX was rendered selectively toxic to tumor cells when covalently coupled by the active ester or carbodiimide methods to a rabbit IgG antibody against a TAA on the surface of mouse EL4 lymphoma cells; the specific conjugates inhibited tumor growth more effectively in vivo than did equivalent amounts of free MTX, unconjugated antibody, MTX followed by antibody, or MTX linked to normal rabbit IgG (41). In this study, eight of eleven mice treated with the specific active ester-based conjugate survived tumor-free for an observation period of 90 days, whereas control animals died at 17 ± 2.5 days after tumor inoculation (41). An up-to-date summary of our data using active ester-based conjugates in this mode is given in Table 2. Results show: (1) Although free MTX, AELG, and MTX-NRG had some antitumor effect, only MTX-AELG at the 4 or 5 mg/kg dose levels consistently produced long-term tumor-free survivors (more than 200 days). (2) Compared to free MTX, both MTX-AELG and MTX-NRG exhibited greater systemic toxicity. However, MTX-NRG failed to produce any long-term survivors even at the LD_{30} doses (7.5 mg/kg for MTX as MTX-NRG and 5 mg/kg for MTX as MTX-AELG). MTX-AELG preparations were not toxic at the 4 mg/kg dose at which they showed maximal tumor inhibitory effect. Administration of 4 mg/kg MTX followed by AELG prolonged survival compared to untreated controls. Only MTX-AELG produced long-term survivors.

3. Inhibition of Human Tumors Xenografted in Nude Mice

We are using human tumor xenograft models that are more pertinent to the clinical setting than ascites tumor models. This is because cells in xenografts of a "solid" human tumor are not as readily accessible to intravenously administered MTX-antibody conjugates as are free-floating tumor cells in rodent ascites tu-

Table 2 Survival of EL4 Lymphoma-bearing C57BL/6J Mice after Treatment with MTX Conjugated to Anti-EL4 IgG

Agent injected[a]	Total no. of mice	Toxic death	Cure	Tumor death with mean survival (days)
No treatment	28	–	–	28/28 (16.9 ± .31)
MTX (4 mg/kg)	10	0	0	10/10 (19.2 ± 1.8)
MTX (5 mg/kg)	6	0	0	6/6 (20.3 ± 1.5)
MTX (50 mg/kg)	11	1	0	10/11 (23.2 ± 6.7)
AELG (100 mg/kg)	5	0	0	5/5 (24.0 ± 3.4)
AELG (200 mg/kg)	5	0	0	5/5 (26.0 ± 2.5)
Free MTX (4 mg/kg) plus AELG (100 mg/kg) unlinked	10	0	0	10/10 (24.2 ± 3.8)
MTX (4 mg/kg) as AELG conjugate	27	0	17	10/27 (29.3 ± 6.6)
MTX (5 mg/kg) as AELG conjugate	21	9	6	6/21 (27.8 ± 3.3)
MTX (4 mg/kg) as NRG conjugate	18	0	0	18/18 (24.2 ± 3.8)
MTX (5 mg/kg) as NRG conjugate	5	0	0	5/5 (25.1 ± 3.9)
MTX (7.5 mg/kg) as NRG conjugate	6	3	0	3/6 (31.7 ± 2.1)

[a]Starting 24 hr after i.p. inoculation of 10^4 /EL4 cells/mouse, the mice were injected with different agents on days 1, 4, and 7.

mors or leukemia models after intraperitoneal or intravenous injection of conjugates. We have shown that i.v. injected ^{131}I-labeled MAb 225.28S selectively localizes in human melanoma xenografts in nude mice (26). Also, sera from melanoma-bearing mice did not obstruct binding of the specific MAb to melanoma cells. With two different MAb, against human melanoma, tumor to normal tissue ratios of localization in M21 xenografts varied directly with the proportion of immunoreactive molecules in the radiolabeled MAb preparation (determined by the method of Lindmo et al. (86)) and their titer of binding to M21 cells. Figure 4 shows the inhibition of the growth of human melanoma in xenograft-bearing mice by MTX conjugated to antimelanoma MAb. Intravenous injections of MTX-MAb 225.28S inhibited the tumor more effectively than MAb alone, free drug, drug linked to normal mouse IgG, or a mixture of MTX and

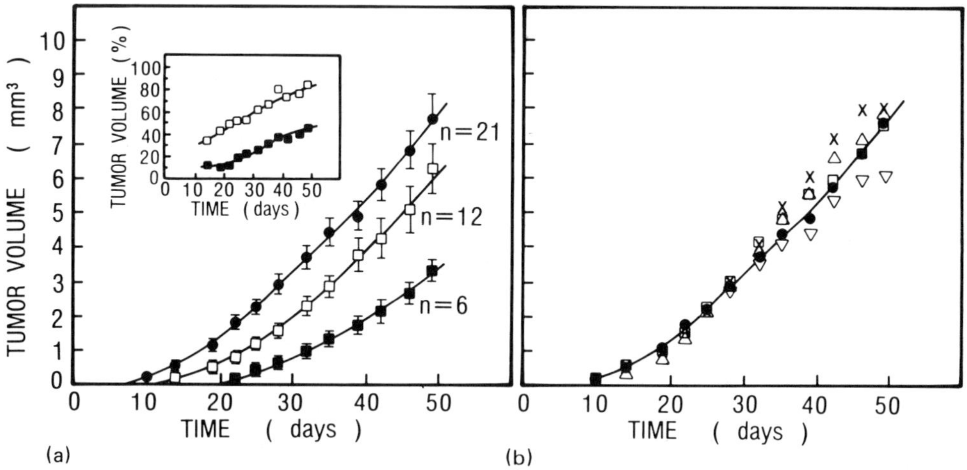

Figure 4 Growth of M21 melanoma in untreated (●) nude Balb/C mice and in mice treated with (a): MTX-RAMG (□) or MTX-MAb 225.28S (■); and (b): MTX (■, $n = 7$), MAb 225.28S (△, $n = 6$), MTX plus the MAb unlinked (X, $n = 8$), MTX-NMG (▽, $n = 9$). Nude Blab/C mice (20 g) were inoculated s.c. with 2×10^6 trypan blue impermeable tumor cells. Five i.v. injections of agents were given on days 1, 4, 7, 10, and 14 starting 24 hr after tumor inoculation. The dose was 5 mg/kg for free and conjugated MTX and 150 mg/kg for free MAb 225.28S. Conjugates contained 5 to 6 moles of MTX per mole of IgG. Diameters were measured in three dimensions by caliper and the volume of expressed as $0.53\ d_1 d_2 d_3$. Inset: Inhibition of tumor growth by MTX-MAb (■) and MTX-RAMG (□). The mean volume of tumors in treated animals on a given day is expressed as a percentage of the mean volume of tumors in untreated animals on the same day. On E-Toxate assay (Sigma, St. Louis, MO) all conjugates were free of endotoxin.

MAb. MTX conjugated to a rabbit antimelanoma IgG was less tumor inhibiting than the MAb conjugate (43).

Kanellos et al. (87) have used the active ester method to conjugate MTX to a monoclonal IgG2b against a human colon carcinoma antigen and a monoclonal IgG1 against the human transferrin receptor. Incorporations obtained were similar to those of Kulkarni et al. (41), i.e., 8 and 13 moles of MTX per mole of protein with retention of most of the antibody activity. Both conjugates inhibited uptake of tritiated deoxyuridine by target cells but not by cells lacking antigen. This specific cytotoxic action was inhibited by unconjugated antibodies. Conjugated MTX was of the order of 20-fold less toxic toward target cells than the free drug. Growth of xenografts of human colon carcinoma HT-29 in nude mice could be inhibited approximately 50% by the specific conjugate. A mixture of equivalent amounts of MTX and antibody, unlinked, was without effect.

4. Pharmacokinetics, Tumor Uptake, and Catabolism of MTX-IgG Conjugates

We have studied the pharmacokinetics, tumor uptake, and catabolism of MTX-IgG conjugates in relation to their mechanism of action. Our results show that reasons for the increased effectiveness of anti-TAA-linked MTX include high uptake followed by slow sustained catabolism, so giving prolonged maintenance of intracellular active derivatives at a level higher than that of DHFR, the target of MTX (36).

a. Pharmacokinetics Studies in ascites EL4 lymphoma-bearing mice have confirmed higher tumor uptake of AELG-conjugated MTX than MTX given as a NRG conjugate or free (37). Ig-conjugated MTX was retained in all tissues, including EL4 cells, much longer than free MTX. MTX conjugated to AELG was retained longest in the tumor cells at levels above DHFR. Amounts of MTX taken up by EL4 cells in vitro correlated well with its uptake in vivo and with the therapeutic effectiveness of the test agents, i.e., antibody conjugate > nonspecific Ig conjugate < free drug.

b. Internalization of Conjugates When EL4 cells were incubated in vitro, they took up the MTX-AELG conjugate more slowly than free MTX, but the net uptake of conjugated MTX later exceeded that of the free drug (or drug linked to nonspecific Ig) (38). When M21 cells were incubated with MTX, free or conjugated to various antimelanoma IgG, the amount of uptake of conjugated MTX corresponded to the amount bound at equilibrium at 0°C and the titer of the antibody. More MTX was endocytosed when linked to antibodies than when linked to a nonspecific Ig or free. MAb 225.28S was more efficient for internalization of MTX than our rabbit antimelanoma IgG. Furthermore, the efflux of conjugated MTX was much slower than that of free MTX, resulting in prolonged high intracellular levels of MTX. We had previously demonstrated that more Chlorambucil was taken up by EL4 cells in vitro when the drug conjugated to an antibody than when conjugated to a nonspecific IgG (88).

Preliminary results showing uptake of antimelanoma antibodies have been obtained by electron microscopy. M21 cells were incubated with rabbit antimelanoma IgG, permeabilized with paraformaldehyde/saponin, and probed with ferritin-labeled goat antirabbit IgG. Cells were then postfixed with 2% glutaraldehyde. In comparing electron micrographs of cells treated with specific antibody and cells treated with nonspecific rabbit IgG, it was found that 10% of the cells treated with specific antibody showed the presence of much greater amounts of ferritin-labeled second antibody. The ferritin was distributed outside and beneath the plasma membrane, in invaginations of the plasma membrane, throughout the cytoplasm, and on the surface of cellular organelles.

c. Catabolism by Whole Cells and Homogenates Studies in our laboratory, especially those of Dr. P. Uadia (3,38,38a), have also been directed toward the characterization of catabolites of MTX conjugates. Incubation of an MTX-NRG conjugate with homogenates of EL4 lymphoma cells or mouse liver produced a low molecular weight fraction which, on Bio-Gel P100 chromatography, emerged slightly ahead of the position of a sample of free MTX (38). The proportion of MTX-containing low molecular weight catabolites after incubation with liver homogenate for 28 hr increased from 51% at pH 5.6 to 74% at pH 4.6 but did not increase further at pH 4.0. The catabolic activity of the homogenates was also increased by their dialysis overnight in DTT-containing buffer but was inhibited by leupeptin, pepstatin, antipain, N-alpha-p-tosyl-L-lysine chloromethyl ketone, and iodacetate. Calcium chloride and EDTA had no effect on the catabolic activity of the homogenates (Table 3). An attempt was made to characterize the low molecular weight fraction(s) by adsorption on DEAE-cel-

Table 3 Effect of Inhibitors and Activators of Lysosomal Enzymes on the Breakdown of an MTX-NRG Conjugate by Liver Homogenates

Inhibitors	Concentration (mM)	Percent of original radioactivity in low MW peak	Inhibition (%)
Control	–	49	–
Leupeptin	0.092	23	53
Pepstatin	0.092	34	31
Antipain	0.094	23	53
Nα-p-tosyl-L-lysine chloromethyl ketone	0.86	20	59
Calcium chloride	0.64	49	–
Iodoacetate	0.64	33	33
EDTA	0.64	49	–
EDTA + Dithiothreitol	0.64	62	27[a]
Dithiothreitol	0.64	59	20[a]

[a]Activation.

Freshly removed liver (2.2 g wet weight) from an adult female C57BL/6J mouse was homogenized in 10 ml of 0.1 M sodium acetate buffer, pH 4.6. Reaction mixtures contained: 2 mg MTX–NRG conjugate, 0.5 ml liver homogenate; test compounds as indicated and 1.2 ml of 0.1 M sodium acetate buffer, pH 4.6 in a total volume of 2.2 ml. The reaction mixture was incubated at 37°C for 28 hr. The mixture was centrifuged and 1 ml of the supernatant was passed through a Biogel P100 column (1 × 20 cm) and eluted with 0.1 M acetate buffer pH 4.6. Fractions (1 ml) were collected and counted for radioactivity in a Beckman Model LS 7000 scintillation counter.

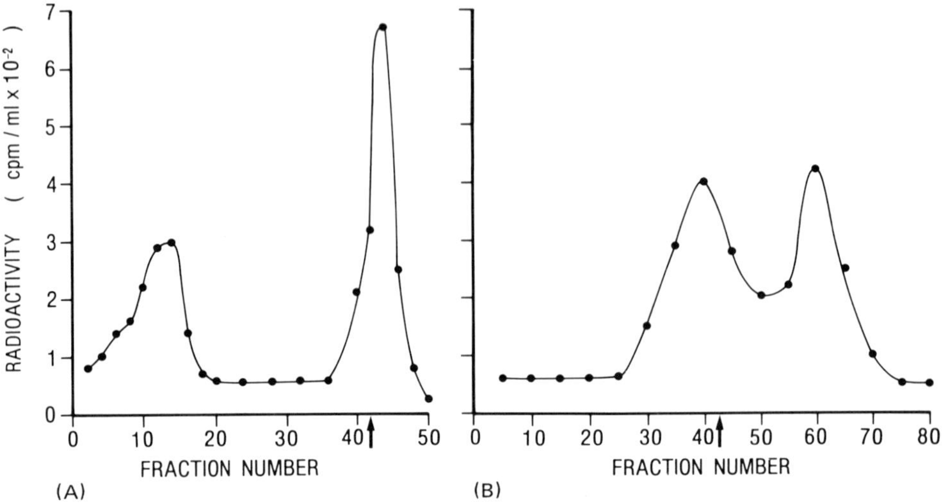

Figure 5 DEAE-cellulose chromatography of MTX-containing low molecular weight catabolites of MTX-antibody conjugates. (A) The MTX-NRG conjugate was incubated with a mouse liver homogenate (conditions as in the legend to Table 3). A low molecular weight MTX-containing fraction was isolated by Bio-Gel P100 column chromatograph (38). This was adsorbed on a column (1.2 × 30 cm) of DEAE-cellulose equilibrated with 5 mM phosphate buffer (pH 7.0) and eluted with a linear gradient of 1 liter of 5 mM phosphate buffer in the mixing chamber and 1 liter of 0.5 M NaCl in the same buffer in the reservoir. Fractions of 19 ml were collected and measured for radioactivity. The arrow indicates the position at which free MTX elutes. (B) The low molecular weight fraction was obtained from the efflux medium of M21 cells previously loaded with an MTX-antimelanoma IgG conjugate (38). It was subjected to DEAE-cellulose column chromatography as described for Figure 5A.

lulose and elution with a linear ionic strength gradient. This resulted in the emergence of a peak that eluted at approximately the same ionic strength as free MTX (Fig. 5A). When subjected to thin layer chromatography, using 0.1 M glycine containing 2% EDTA, pH 9.0, as the solvent system, this eluted fraction migrated with an R_f of 0.4, while MTX had an R_f of 0.63 and the conjugate remained at the origin.

When M21 melanoma cells were preloaded with an MTX-antimelanoma IgG conjugate for 7.5 hr and then incubated in conjugate-free medium for 9.5 hr, gel chromatography revealed low molecular weight MTX-containing fragments both in the cell homogenate and efflux medium. The low molecular weight fraction from the efflux medium was further resolved into 2 peaks by DEAE-cellulose chromatograph (Fig. 5B). Both peaks migrated on thin layer chromatography with an R_f of 0.63 and the conjugate remained at the origin. All low molecular weight MTX-containing fractions either obtained after incubation with mouse liver homogenate or derived from M21 cells preloaded with conjugate were capable of inhibiting DHFR to an extent approximately equal to that for the intact conjugate and less than half that for free MTX.

To further investigate the possible role of lysosomal enzymes in catabolism of drug-antibody conjugates, M21 cells were incubated with the MTX-antibody conjugate with and without 100 μM chloroquine or 100 μM leupeptin. At 7.5 hr, the cells incubated in the presence of chloroquine had taken up 148 pmol MTX/mg protein and those incubated in its absence had taken up 154 pmol MTX/mg protein. In the presence of 100 μM leupeptin, the cells took up 152 pmol MTX/mg protein, but in its absence, they took up 177 pmol MTX/mg protein. When the cells in medium containing chloroquine were allowed to efflux for 9 hr, 127 pmol MTX/mg protein (86% of the initial value) remained cell-associated, whereas 92 pmol MTX/mg protein (60% of the initial value) remained in the cells that were preloaded and allowed to efflux in medium without chloroquine. With cells in medium containing leupeptin, 83.5 pmol MTX/mg protein (55% of the initial value) remained cell-associated after efflux and 54 pmol MTX/mg protein (31% of the initial value) remained in the cells that were preloaded and allowed to efflux in medium without leupeptin. Thus, the intracellular catabolism of MTX-antibody conjugates was inhibited both by chloroquine and leupeptin.

5. Action of MTX and Its Conjugates in Relation to the Cell Cycle

Our studies have demonstrated that both free and Ig-conjugated MTX cause arrest of the exposed cells in the S phase. (S phase-specific inhibition of cells by MTX is well known.) M21 cells were exposed in vitro to 1.0 μg/ml and 5.0 μg/ml of MTX, free or conjugated to NRG or rabbit antimelanoma IgG. Flow cytometric analysis (Fluorescence Activated Cell Sorter Model III, Cg, Becton Dickinson) showed that with free MTX, cells were arrested in the S region only at 5.0 μg/ml whereas cells treated with both concentrations of MTX conjugated to NRG or antibody showed distinct peaks at the S region. The height of the peaks varied with the concentration of the drug in the incubation mixture. Thus, the mechanism of inhibition of cells by MTX conjugated to anti-TAA IgG or nonspecific IgG appears to be the same as that of free MTX but at equimolar concentrations, IgG-conjugated MTX appears to be more potent.

6. Direct Conjugation of MTX to the $F(ab')_2$ Fragment of IgG

As commented upon before, substantial increase in the size of drug-antibody conjugates might affect their pharmacokinetics, i.e., impede their passage through the capillary wall and access to extravascular tumor cells, reduce their diffusion in tissue spaces, and impede endocytosis by target cells. Susceptibility to phagocytosis by reticuloendothelial cells may also be increased. A way of reducing the size of drug-antibody conjugates is the use of immunologically reactive $F(ab')_2$ fragments instead of the intact IgG molecule as the carrier. An advantage of $F(ab')_2$ over smaller reactive fragments is its divalency, which allows capping and endocytosis. Also, removal of the Fc moiety reduces antigenicity and susceptibility to ingestion by phagocytic cells that possess Fc receptors. The circulating half-life of the $F(ab')_2$ moiety is adequate (though less than that of the parent IgG) for antitumor action in vivo of the linked MTX. It is likely that smaller carriers [e.g., $F(ab')_2$] will have too short a half-life for therapeutic effectiveness.

The isolation procedure for $F(ab')_2$ (43,45) is described in the Appendix and conjugation procedures applicable to this fragment are similar to those described for IgG. MTX was first conjugated to anti-BSA IgG or its $F(ab')_2$ fragment to define conditions for retention of drug and antibody activities. With identical drug:protein molar ratios, incorporation in the $F(ab)_2$ fragment was lower than in intact anti-BSA, an observation consistent with analysis of the number of lysine residues (22 in $F(ab')_2$ compared to 40 in antiBSA) (45). In either case, up to approximately 10 mol MTX could be incorporated per mole protein, with recovery of 70% of the protein. (In contrast, the use of multivalent intermediaries, such as PLL, should allow higher incorporations, since a restricted number of sites in the protein will be utilized for linkage with either carrier.) MTX-anti-BSA and MTX-$F(ab')_2$ anti-BSA were equally potent in vitro inhibitors of DHFR. At an incorporation ratio of 6 mol MTX per mol protein, MTX-anti-BSA retained 100% of antibody activity and MTX-$F(ab')_2$ anti-BSA retained 75%.

We have found that faster and higher tumor:normal tissue ratios of localization are achieved with the $F(ab')_2$ fragment of an MAb compared to its parent IgG (89). However, the absolute amount and the fraction of the administered dose of an $F(ab')_2$ that localized in tumors was small. Conjugates prepared from AELG and from $F(ab')_2$-AELG significantly increased survivial in EL4 lymphoma-bearing mice compared to mice receiving equal amounts (5 mg MTX/kg) of free MTX, MTX linked to the $F(ab')_2$ fragment of normal rabbit IgG, or a simple mixture of MTX and $F(ab')_2$-AELG. $F(ab')_2$-linked MTX was less effective in tumor inhibition and less toxic in vivo compared to equivalent amounts of MTX linked to the parent immunoglobulin molecule (45). This may be due to the faster clearance from the body of $F(ab')_2$-linked MTX compared to the parent IgG-linked MTX referred to above. We have yet to compare the tumor inhibitory effects of equitoxic doses of $F(ab')_2$-linked and IgG-linked MTX. It can be predicted that with the $F(ab')_2$ moiety of high affinity antitumor antibodies, it may be possible to achieve high tumor:blood (or other sensitive tissues) ratios of localization of $F(ab')_2$-linked MTX with resulting increase in chemotherapeutic index of the drug.

7. Conjugation of MTX to Intact IgG via Intermediaries

Increased incorporation of chemotherapeutic agents into IgG can be achieved by multivalent intermediaries (4-6). However, conjugates produced with MTX using intermediaries have shown substantial loss of either antibody or drug activity. For example, the use of thioether-linked HSA to incorporate approximately 100 moles of MTX per mole of MAb resulted in a loss of 65-70% of antibody activity (90,91). In the method reported by Manabe et al. (92-94) using dextran, not only was there incorporation of only 9 moles of MTX per mole of IgG (which could have been achieved by direct linkage), but there was also 54% loss of drug activity (probably as a result of linkage via amino groups of the pteridine moiety (41)), and the conjugate did not exhibit any selective toxicity toward target cells. The limited effectiveness of these conjugates may possibly be due to loss of antibody activity (91) and altered pharmacokinetics of ternary conjugates containing more than one MTX-loaded HSA molecule each (91), leading to diversion from the target tissue.

It may be more appropriate to use oligopeptides and oligosaccharides of limited size as multivalent intermediaries to increase drug loading without unduly increasing the size of the resulting ternary conjugate. To preserve drug activity, the linkage of the binary drug-intermediary conjugate should be limited to a small number of sites in the IgG. A further elaboration in this approach for achieving high ratios of maximally active drug to antibody without a large increase in size would be regiospecific conjugation using oligopeptide or oligosaccharide multivalent intermediaries. Linkage of intermediaries carrying multiple drug molecules to a very limited number of sites in the IgG should yield active ternary antibody conjugates with greater drug incorporation.

Using PLL as an intermediary, we have produced binary MTX-PLL and ternary MTX-PLL-IgG conjugates by the linkage of MTX-PLL to IgG or by the linkage of MTX to PLL-IgG (E. Kendall, Thesis, Dalhousie University, 1983). Carbodiimide coupling incorporated as many as 40 molecules of MTX into a ternary (MTX_n-PLL)-IgG. Both binary and ternary conjugates were capable of inhibiting DHFR in vitro. MTX-PLL binary conjugates were the most potent inhibitors of growth of EL4 cells, followed, in order, by free MTX and MTX-PLL-IgG ternary conjugates. These active conjugates provide a model for the production of MTX-PLL-tumor-specific-IgG-antibody conjugates with high incorporation of MTX.

B. MTX-gamma-ASP

1. Rationale for Its Use

MTX-gamma-ASP as the free drug has a much higher Km of influx into cells than MTX and is therefore less likely to be taken up by nontarget cells if dissociated from a conjugate in vivo (36,37). This means that any free MTX-gamma-ASP that is released from a conjugate in vivo will be much less cytotoxic than a corresponding amount of MTX. This property may facilitate the investigation of conjugated drug in tumor models and may allow administration of higher doses of conjugated drug than is possible with MTX.

2. Active Ester-mediated Synthesis of Conjugates

As Figure 1 shows, MTX-AE exhibits greater susceptibility toward attack by nucleophilic centers in IgG than does MTX-gamma-ASP-AE. At similar molar ratios of active ester to IgG, there was greater drug incorporation in the conjugate with MTX-AE than with MTX-gamma-ASP-AE. The highest incorporation achieved with the latter derivative was 18-20 when the molar ratio of MTX-gamma-ASP-AE to IgG was 100. A 50-fold molar excess of MTX-gamma-ASP-AE with the protein concentration maintained in the region of 10 mg/ml has consistently led to incorporations of 10-12 moles of drug per mole of IgG with recoveries of protein approaching 90%. The gamma aspartate derivative has three carboxyl groups that would favor the formation of less reactive anhydride species during the reaction with NHS and DCC. Possibly, this 5-membered ring cyclic anhydride results in a certain degree of inactivity toward the weak nucleophilic functions present in the protein. The greater solubility of MTX-gamma-ASP in polar solvents compared to MTX may also play a significant role in conjugation reactions. The retention of DHFR inhibitory capacity in conjugated MTX-gamma-ASP was similar to conjugated MTX, i.e., 15-25% of the capacity of the free drug.

III. CONCLUDING STATEMENT

The effectiveness of MTX and MTX-gamma-ASP depends upon prolonged intracellular maintenance of the active form at a level exceeding that of DHFR (36). The MTX-IgG conjugates produced by present methods of linkage and their intracellular catabolites are only partially active in inhibiting DHFR compared to free MTX (4,41). Therefore, the potency of "first-generation" conjugates can be improved upon by achieving targeting of more active drug to tumor cells. At present, effectiveness is limited by loss of drug activity and by the adverse effect of drug loading on antibody activity (4). Possible approaches to improving linkage methods include regiospecific conjugation, conjugation via multivalent intermediaries, protection of the antigen-binding site of carrier antibodies or their

$F(ab')_2$ fragments during conjugation, and coupling by other linkage groups, e.g., hydrazones involving carbohydrate moieties in the IgG as described in this chapter or lysosomotropic spacer moieties. Certain of these are potentially complementary. For example, protection of the antigen-binding site may be combined with a regiospecific approach to conjugation to give additive improvement. In parallel with the development of methods for the optimal preservation of drug activity, there has also been substantial progress in defining the optimal characteristics of a carrier antibody. Furthermore, recombinant DNA and allied technologies have now made it possible to construct chimeric antibody molecules that not only have defined specificity and high affinity but also have tailor-made Fc moieties that are endowed with therapeutically useful attributes, e.g., reduced antigencity or affinity toward receptors on certain cell types. Methods are also becoming available for the construction of myeloma transfectants that secrete $F(ab')_2$ or monovalent Ig fragments, either completely lacking the Fc moiety or in which the C_H2 and C_H3 domains are substituted (5). Thus it is quite possible that in the future we will obtain myeloma transfectants that secrete antibodies that have high anti-TAA specificity and affinity, are capable of being endocytosed after capping, and have incorporated in the Fc moiety a polypeptide with a sequence that allows optimal linkage of MTX (or other agents). Comparison of the cytotoxic and antitumor effect of these conjugates in conjunction with their pharmacokinetics and catabolism will provide a further foundation for design of linkages that facilitate drug action at the target site.

IV. EXPERIMENTAL PROTOCOLS

A. Purification and Isolation of MAb

Our procedure for isolation of pure MAb varies from preparation to preparation even within an individual Ig subclass. For example, while some IgG1 MAb are retained on a staphylococcal protein A column at pH 8, others will pass right through (95). As each step may have to be altered, depending on the MAb being isolated, it is desirable to use a purification scheme starting with a preparation that is least contaminated by other proteins, e.g., supernatant from serum-free hybridoma cultures. Several of our hybridoma clones were readily adapted to continuous growth in DME/F-12 medium (Sigma) supplemented with insulin, transferrin, selenite, and ethanolamine. Suspension cultures grown in spinner flasks can be centrifuged free of cells and concentrated by ultrafiltration with a low-absorption Amicon YM 100 membrane. MAb are then precipitated with ammonium sulfate at 40-50% saturation as required. At this stage SDS-PAGE is routinely used to check that there is substantially only a single Coomassie Blue stained band migrating at the same Mr as standard IgG. Isoelectric focusing in polyacrylamide gel slabs using ampholytes with a pH range between 3.5 and 10 can be used to demonstrate MAb homogeneity. Retention of antigen-binding activity is assayed by ELISA on viable cell monolayers using appropriate enzyme-linked antiglobulin and on cells by membrane immunofluorescence (96).

B. Production and Isolation of $F(ab')_2$

$F(ab')_2$ fragments of antibodies of the mouse and rabbit Ig subclasses are prepared by limited pepsin digestion (97). Preliminary digestion experiments are carried out with each MAb, since variation among individual proteins of an IgG subclass precludes generalization as to the time and pH of digestion yielding maximum $F(ab')_2$. SDS-PAGE is used to assess the relative amounts of whole IgG and $F(ab')_2$ in a digest. The relative amounts of antigen binding activity present as whole IgG and as $F(ab')_2$ can be determined by immunoassay using anti-$F(ab')_2$ to measure the sum of active IgG and $F(ab')_2$, using anti-Fc to measure active IgG alone, and calculating active $F(ab')_2$ as the difference. ELISA is routinely used in our laboratory for these assays (96). Once the optimum pepsinization procedure has been settled upon and carried out for a particular MAb, the $F(ab')_2$ fragment is separated from whole IgG, pepsin, and peptides on a Sephadex G-200 column. Any traces of intact IgG which remain can be removed if necessary with a DE-52 DEAE cellulose column at pH 8.0 in 5 mM phosphate buffer. After concentration by ultrafiltration and immediately before derivatization or conjugation, the $F(ab')_2$ should be tested for purity, e.g., by SDS-PAGE and for ability to bind antigen, e.g., by ELISA.

C. Active Ester-based Conjugates

1. Purification of MTX and MTX-gamma-ASP

MTX(trihydrate-Sigma) and MTX-gamma-ASP (sesquihydrate, gift from Dr. J. R. Piper) were used without any additional purification. Drying of the commercial MTX for 48 hr under high vacuum at 70°C did not appreciably affect the incorporation ratio, protein recovery or DHFR inhibition.

2. Synthesis of MTX-AE and MTX-gamma-ASP-AE

A solution of MTX (4.5 mg; 0.01 mmol) or MTX-gamma-ASP (6 mg; 0.01 mmol), DCC (2.27 mg; 0.011 mmol), and NHS (1.27 mg; 0.011 mmol) in dry DMF (0.2 ml) is stirred at room temperature for 12 hr (monitored by TLC chloroform/DMSO 3:2). The reaction flask is covered with aluminum foil to protect the reaction mixture from light. To complete precipitation, the reaction flask is kept at −20°C for 30 min. Then the precipitate is filtered off and washed with cold DMF (0.2 ml). The filtered solution is used directly in the next step without any effort at crystallization because of the general lack of crystallinity of MTX derivatives.

3. Synthesis of MTX-IgG and MTX-gamma-ASP-IgG Conjugates by Reaction of Active Ester Derivatives with IgG

To a solution of IgG (10 mg; 66.7 nmol in 2 ml of PBS), DMF (0.2 ml at 4°C is added dropwise over a 5-min period and stirring continued for 20 min. Then a cold solution of MTX-AE (1.67 umol) in DMF (75 μl) is added dropwise over a 2-min period. The cold solution of active ester should also be slowly added to the IgG solution with stirring to avoid denaturation. The reaction mixture is stirred for an additional 1 hr and then centrifuged and dialyzed against PBS over 48 hr. After centrifugation, the required MTX-IgG conjugate is obtained with 79-86% protein recovery and incorporation of 10-12 moles of drug per mole of protein. The procedure for MTX-gamma-ASP-AE differs only in that 3.34 μmol is added to the IgG solution. The recovery of protein is 85-92% and the molar incorporation ratio ranges from 10 to 13.

D. Conjugation to Oxidized Carbohydrate Moieties

1. The Oxidation of IgG by Periodate—A General Procedure

a. Oxidation Procedure To a solution of IgG (10 mg, 66.7 nmol) in acetate buffer (2 ml 0.2 M, pH 5.6), sodium periodate (0.1 ml 20 mM) in distilled water is added at 4°C over a 5-min period. The course of the reaction is monitored spectrometrically at 352 nm. The reaction is stopped by adding ethyleneglycol and reaction mixture is dialyzed against PBS for 48 hr at 4°C.

b. Assay for Periodate Consumed Small aliquots are removed from reaction mixtures containing periodate and mixed with 2.0 ml of a 10 mM solution of DMAPE in assay buffer (0.1 M glycine · HCl, pH 2.55). Aliquots are removed in order to provide a concentration of periodate in cuvettes of 1-25 μM. This is in the linear range of a standard curve for periodate assay. The product of the reaction, p-dimethylamino benzaldehyde, is a chromophore with a molar extinction coefficient of 50,000 $mol^{-1}\,cm^{-1}$ at 352 nm (73). The absorbance of DMAPE at 352 nm is not appreciable. This method is convenient for our analyses because of its sensitivity in the range of 1-25 μM. The number of oxidative sites was calculated according to the following equation:

$$OS = \frac{Csp - A_{352}/E}{C_{protein}}$$

where Csp = molar concentration of sodium periodate at time zero, E = molar extinction coefficient for p-dimethylamino benzaldehyde, and $C_{protein}$ = molar concentration of protein.

In establishing conditions for the assay, it was shown that, in the absence of protein, samples taken either from a reaction mixture or from a blank solution containing the same periodate concentration gave the same value. The change in concentration of IO_4^- ion in the reaction mixture is taken to be the number of oxidized sites in the IgG molecule.

2. Synthesis of MTX-Hyd

To a stirred dimethylformamide solution of MTX-AE, freshly prepared from MTX (100 mg, 0.2 mmol; see above), hydrazine (1 ml) is slowly added. The reaction is continued at room temperature for a total of 24 hr. Then 0.5% NH_4HCO_3 (5 ml) is added and the resulting precipitate is removed by filtration. The product is purified by DEAE-cellulose column chromatography (Whatman DE-52) using a linear NH_4HCO_3 gradient from 0.05 to 0.4 M, yielding 69-78 mg of MTX-hyd eluted in a single peak. Small-scale separations of MTX-hyd and MTX have also been carried out using an RP-8 (5 μm) HPLC column run with 0.01 M sodium phosphate: CH_3CN = 9: 1.

3. Formation of Conjugates by Reaction of Hydrazide Derivatives with IgG

To a stirred polyaldehyde-IgG solution (10 mg; 66.7 nmol) in 2 ml of 0.2 M sodium acetate buffer, pH 5.6, cold DMF (0.2 ml) is portionwise added during a period of 5 min. After 20 min of additional stirring, MTX-hyd (3.34 mg, 6.67 μmol calculated from the formula weight of the monohydrazide containing 3 moles of water) in DMF (0.2 ml) is added during 2 min, the stirring continued for an additional 2 hr at 4°C and then for 23 hr at room temperature. The pH of the reaction mixture is finally adjusted to 7 and dialyzed against PBS for 48 hr. Centrifugation gave conjugates with incorporation ratios of 8-12 moles of MTX per IgG and with 75-81% protein recovery.

4. Reduction of the Hydrazone Double Bond in MTX-IgG Conjugates

A 0.1 M solution of sodium borohydride (50 μl, 5 umol) in distilled water was slowly added to a solution of the MTX-IgG hydrazone conjugate (e.g., with 10 moles of drug per mole of IgG; 55 nmol) in sodium borate buffer (2 ml, 0.1 M, pH 8.0) at 4°C and the stirring continued for 4 hr. After 48 hr dialysis against PBS and centrifugation, the molar incorporation remained unchanged.

E. Determination of Drug Activity by DHFR Inhibition Assay

DHFR assay is based on the method of Peterson (44). To a 5.0-ml cuvette, reagents and test samples are added to the required volume of distilled water in the order as given: 1.0 ml of 1.5 m sodium acetate buffer, pH 6.0 (1.0 ml, 1.5 M); KCl (1.0 ml, 1.8 M); NADPH (Sigma) (150 μl, 1.0 mM); 0-100 μl of MTX-containing sample in 0.01 M PBS (2.2×10^{-5} M and 2.2×10^{-6} M with respect to MTX); 0.01 unit of beef liver DHFR (Sigma: diluted appropriately with distilled water just before use). The DHFR is introduced and mixed with a teflon adder-mixer and incubated at 22°C for 1 to 3 min. The reaction is initiated by the similar addition of DHFR (Sigma) (100 μl, 1 mM). The change in absorbance per min at 340 nm is calculated from the recorder tracings during a 3-min period and at least four concentrations of each test sample are assayed. IC_{50} values may conveniently be obtained from semilogarithmic plots of percent DHFR activity as a function of MTX (free or conjugated) concentration. IC_{50} values for free MTX can vary with different batches of enzyme so we include control inhibitions by the free drug with each set of assays. This variation could arise from contaminating folate-binding proteins in the partially purified DHFR.

The substrate DHFA is a relatively unstable compound, being susceptible to oxidation in air (98-100). We have found that 2-mM stock "solutions" of DHF either in distilled water or in water containing 0.005 M HCl and 14 mM MET can be kept for at least 2-3 weeks at 4°C in airtight containers. Working solutions prepared by dilution to 1.0 mM in water containing 10 mM HCl and 28 mM MET are usable over the course of a day; a solution prepared by dilution in sodium acetate buffer, pH 6, was clear but unstable.

F. Determination of Antibody Activity

In preliminary studies to evaluate the retention of antibody activity in conjugates, we use radial immunodiffusion with a BSA-rabbit anti-BSA IgG system. Assay of antibody activity using the anti-BSA IgG system is based on the procedure of Mancini (100b). Two sets of agar plates (diam. 83 mm) are made by mixing 12.5 ml of 3% agar with an equal volume of BSA (30 μg/ml or 60 μg/ml) in 0.02 M PBS containing 0.01% merthiolate. The plates are left to set at 4°C, then holes (3 mm) are punched into the gel. Equal amounts of treated and untreated IgG (10 μl containing approximately 50 μg of IgG), are placed in wells in the same plate. The relative immunoactivity is calculated from the area of the ring of precipitation after 24 hr at 20°C.

G. Assay of Conjugates in Vitro

1. Procedure for Evaluating Conjugates by a Cell Proliferation Inhibition Assay

In this method, the effect of continuous exposure of target cells to test agents is studied. Initially the pattern of growth of the target cells in appropriate culture media is determined. Primary cultures from solid tumors are subcultured once to remove debris, leukocytes, macrophages, and fibroblasts. Five $\times 10^4$ cells in 1 ml of an appropriate medium in 35 $\times$ 10 mm petri dishes are incubated at 37°C in a 5% CO_2 atmosphere. When cells enter the logarithmic phase of proliferation, they are incubated with various concentrations of test agents. Every 24 hr cells are harvested from dishes (at least in triplicate for each concentration of the agents) and counted with an electronic cell counter. The IC_{50} for each of the agents (i.e., drug-linked antibody, drug alone, antibody alone, drug linked to nonspecific mouse IgG of the same subclass as the carrier antibody, and drug and antibody unlinked) is determined.

2. Procedure for Evaluating Conjugates by a Clonogenic Assay

In this method, we study the effect of a pulse exposure for 2 hr to various test agents on the survival and clonogenicity of target tumor cells. Our assay system is essentially that described by Lathan et al. (101). In brief, a stock agar solution is autoclaved and cooled to 50°C. Solutions containing 0.5% and 0.3% agar are prepared by diluting agar with prewarmed (50°C) media. Aliquots of 0.5% agar are dispensed into multiwell culture plates (96 wells–Falcon) and allowed to set under sterile conditions. Target cells (after exposure for 2 hr to appropriate concentrations of conjugates, free drug, antibody, a mixture of free drug and antibody, and drug linked to nonspecific mouse IgG) are diluted with 0.3% agar to give 10^3 cells/ml. One ml of the cell suspension is dispensed on top of the 0.5% agar layer and allowed to set for 2 hr. The culture plates are then transferred to a 5% CO_2/95% air incubator and colonies are counted after 14 days. For all in vitro assays, fetal calf sera are dialyzed against PBS to exclude interference with MTX activity by folic acid and its active derivatives in fetal calf sera. The IC_{50} of test agents (if tumor inhibiting) is determined.

H. Assay of MTX and Its Conjugates in Vivo

1. Models Based on Human Tumor Xenografts in Nude Mice

a. Choice of Models The choice of tumor models is determined by the tumor or tumors with which the carrier antibody reacts and the question on which the investigation is based. In our laboratory, we are at present investigating the potential of several panels of MAb against different histological types of human cancer (e.g., melanoma, renal cell carcinoma, chronic lymphocytic leukemia) for the production of optimally effective MTX-antibody conjugates.

The antitumor effect of conjugates is evaluated in appropriate human tumor xenografts in nude mice. Human tumor lines that are known to be able to grow in nude mice are mostly obtained from the Human Tumor Cell Bank through the American Type Culture Collection. Also, several human tumor lines in our laboratory were successfully adapted to grow in nude mice, e.g., the human chronic lymphocytic leukemia line EBV CLL-1 (102) and several melanoma lines (96).

b. Procedure for Assay of the Therapeutic Effect of Conjugates in Human Tumor Xenograft Models In all experiments for evaluating the antitumor effect of agents, tumor inocula contain the minimum number of cells that produce tumor in 100% of mice. Suspension of tumor cells are obtained from solid tumor after dissociation with 0.25% trypsin (GIBCO, Grand Island) and 20 μg/ml deoxyribonuclease I (Sigma, St. Louis, MD). Dead cells are separated from viable cells by a Ficoll-Isopaque density gradient (103). For MTX and conjugates, mice are usually given a total of 4 to 5 injections with an interval of 3 days in between injections (i.e., days 1, 4, 7, 10, and 13) (41,43). It should be pointed out that the systemic toxicity of MTX increases severalfold after linkage to macromolecular carriers (41). For example, the LD_{10} of free MTX for C57BL/6J mice is approximately 50 mg/kg but the LD_{10} dose for IgG-linked MTX is 5 mg/kg. The systemic toxicity of MTX further increases when the drug is linked to anti-TAA antibodies that cross-react with normal tissue components (especially kidney, vascular wall, splenic cells, etc.) even if equimolar amounts of unlinked antibody fail to show any gross toxic manifestation. In our laboratory, all mice treated with MTX or conjugates are given alkaline drinking water to prevent precipitation of MTX in the kidneys. In mice given subcutaneous tumor inoculation, the day of appearance of the tumor is noted, and tumors are measured at least 3 times a week.

c. Metastatic and Other Models to Answer Specific Questions MTX-antibody conjugates are likely to be most useful in the eradication of tumor cell emboli and micrometastases. Larger tumors can be effectively treated by surgery and/or radiation which, however, cannot remove hidden foci of tumor cells that are beyond the field of these two modalities of treatment. It is the progressive growth and lethality of micrometastases and tumor emboli that are not detectable that severely limits the usefulness of surgical excision and/or irradiation. We believe that antibody-linked MTX is ideal for the eradication of tumor micrometastases. The reasons for this include the following: (1) In contrast to large tumors that may have avascular and nectoric areas and also present other problems of accessibility to conjugates, cells in microfoci are likely to be easily accessible to systemically administered conjugates. (2) Most cells in a large tumor are usually not in cycle. On the other hand, cells in microfoci are more likely to be in cycle and thus be sensitive to phase specific agents such as MTX (7). (3) As cell kill by MTX follows second order kinetics, "cell cure" is more likely to be achievable with a small tumor burden. We have, therefore, developed several metastatic models of human tumor in addition to the metastatic mouse B16 melanoma and renal carcinoma models already described (7,104). For example, subcutaneous xenografts of our human chronic lymphocytic leukemia line EBV-CLL 1 (102) (the only human CLL line transplantable in nude mice), produces metastases in regional lymph nodes, spleen, liver, lungs, kidneys, adrenal, and other organs (102). After intrarenal inoculation or 10^6 cells of the human renal cell carcinoma line Caki-1 and removal of the tumor-inoculated kidney 20 days later, we observe tumor metastasis in lymph nodes, lungs, and liver in 100% of mice. The IC_{50} of MTX for EBV CLL (102) and the Caki-1 lines are, respectively, 88 mM and 300 mM. It should be pointed out that results from our laboratory and elsewhere (105,106) demonstrate that metastasis of human tumor xenografts in nude mice is more common than was thought to be the case. One of the reasons for the initial failure to detect metastases was the difficulty in keeping tumor-bearing nude mice alive (i.e., protecting them from lethal infections) for an adequate period to allow metastatic lesions to develop. The availability of metastatic human tumor models will facilitate studies on the effectiveness of MTX-antibody conjugates in the eradication of small secondary lesions after removal of the primary.

It may sometimes be necessary to develop tumor models that are appropriate to answer a specific question. For example, we evaluate the effect of MTX conjugates on human renal cancer lines using xenograft of renal cancer in the kidney of the host mouse. Such a model is more likely to resemble the clinical situation because the kidneys play an important role in the pharmacokinetics and excretion of MTX.

d. Advantages and Disadvantages of Human Tumor Xenograft Models
It should be stated that human tumor xenografts usually retain the metabolic characteristics and chemosensitivity profile of the tumor of origin (107). As all human tumors (even if of a given histiotype) do not respond equally to a given agent, a small battery of tumors of particular histiotype can adequately represent the heterogeneity of tumor cells observed clinically and thus provide a very useful preclinical screen (107). In our laboratory, we use xenografts of 3 to 5 different tumor lines of a given histiotype for evaluation of agents.

In the context of evaluation of MTX-antihuman tumor MAb conjugates in xenograft models, it should be realized that in this model the tumor cells (the target of the carrier antibody) are human in origin and those of the tumor host are murine. This model is therefore not suitable for evaluating the problems associated with cross-reactivity or nonspecific binding of the carrier antibody with one or more normal human tissues. Thus the specificity of the carrier antibody must be rigorously established by appropriate in vitro assays on a wide panel of normal tissues that should include kidney, lung, liver, bone marrow, blood vessels, leukocytes, etc. (96) before its clinical use.

2. The Murine EL4 Lymphoma Model

In our protocol for the evaluation of agents, we still include a rodent tumor model (the EL4 lymphoma in C57BL/6J mice), mainly as a reference point for comparison of antitumor activity of new conjugates. This is because in this model we have been successful in completely eradicating 10^4 to 10^5 tumor cells per animal using MTX conjugated to antitumor antibodies via a variety of linkages (41,108). Intraperitoneal inoculation of as few as 10^4 EL4 cells lead to progressive ascites tumor formation, extensive tumor infiltration of organs and tissues and subsequent death of 100% of tumor inoculated mice (8). Furthermore, the inverse correlation between the size of the tumor inoculum and survival provide rough estimates of the percentage of cell-kill based on prolongation of survival after a given therapeutic regimen (8). We realize that results obtained using polyclonal antibodies of rabbit origin cannot be readily extrapolated to MAb of mouse origin (even individual MAbs may differ in their sensitivity to conjugation procedures and their potential as therapeutic drug carriers), but the EL4 lymphoma model is useful for a rapid preliminary evaluation of new conjugates and for optimizing dosage and administration schedules.

ABBREVIATIONS

AELG	antiEL4 lymphoma IgG
BSA	bovine serum albumin
CLL	chronic lymphocytic leukemia
DCC	dicyclohexylcarbodiimide
DHFA	dihydrofolic acid
DHFR	dihydrofolate reductase
DMAPE	1,2-bis-(p-dimethylaminophenyl) ethane-1,2-diol
DMF	dimethylformamide
DMSO	dimethylsulfoxide
EDCI	1-ethyl-3-(3′-dimethylaminopropyl) carbodiimide
ELISA	enzyme-linked immunosorbant assay
HSA	human serum albumin
IC_{50}	concentration giving 50% inhibition
Ig	immunoglobulin
IgG	immunoglobulin G
INH	isonicotinic acid hydrazide
MAb	monoclonal antibody
MET	mercaptoethanol
MTX	methotrexate
MTX-AE	NHS-based active ester of MTX
MTX-gamma-ASP	gamma aspartate derivative of MTX
MTX-gamma-ASP-AE	NHS-based active ester of MTX-gamma-ASP
MTX-hyd	MTX hydrazide
NHS	N-hydroxysuccinimide
NRG	normal rabbit IgG
PBS	0.01 M sodium phosphate, pH 7.1., containing 0.145 M sodium chloride
PLL	polylysine
RCC	renal cell carcinoma
RT	room temperature
SDS-PAGE	polyacrylamide gel electrophoresis using sodium dodecylsulfate
THFA	tetrahydrofolic acid
TAA	tumor associated antigen

ACKNOWLEDGMENTS

The investigations reported in this chapter were supported by grants from the Medical Research Council of Canada and the Atlantic Institute of Biotechnology. We gratefully acknowledge the gift of MTX-gamma-ASP from Dr. J. R. Piper, Southern Research Institute, Birmingham, AL.

REFERENCES

1. Holland J. F. (1983) Karnofsky memorial lecture: breaking the cure barrier. *J. Clin. Oncol. 1*:75-90.
2. Baserga, R. (1981) The cell cycle. *N. Engl. J. Med. 304*:453-459.
3. Haynie, T. P., III, Hutchins, R.D., and McKelvey, E. M. (1984) Selected abstracts on radiolabeled antibodies in cancer. Oncology Overview U.S. Dept. of Health and Human Services. Natl. Technical Information Service, Springfield, Virginia.
4. Ghose, T., Blair, A. H., and Kulkarni, P. (1983) Preparation of antibody-linked cytotoxic agents. *Methods Enzymol. 93*:280–361.
5. Ghose, T., and Blair, A. H. (1987) The design of cytotoxic-agent-antibody conjugates. *CRC Critical Review of Therapeutic Drug Carrier Systems 3*: 263-361.
6. Blair, A. H., and Ghose, T. (1983) Linkage of cytotoxic agents to immunoglobulins. *J. Immunol. Methods 59*: 129–143.
7. Ghose, T., Blair, A. H., Vaughan, K., and Kulkarni, P. (1983). Antibody-directed drug targeting in cancer. In *Targeted Drugs* (Goldberg, E. P., ed.). John Wiley & Sons, New York, Vol. 2, p. 1-22.
8. Ghose, T., Guclu, A., Faulkner, J., and Tai, J. (1977) Suppression in vivo of the mouse EL4 lymphoma by rabbit antitumor sera. *J. Natl. Cancer Inst. 58*:693–700.
9. Ghose, T., Guclu, A., Tai, J., Mammen, M., and Norvell, S. T. (1977) Immunoprophylaxis and immunotherapy of EL4 lymphoma. *Eur. J. Cancer 13*:925-935.
10. Wright, P. W., and Bernstein, I. D. (1980) Serotherapy of malignant disease. *Prog. Exp. Tumor Res. 25*:140-162.
11. Young, W. W., and Hakomori, S.-I. (1981) Therapy of mouse lymphoma with monoclonal antibodies to glycolipid: Selection of low antigenic variants in vivo. *Science (Wash., D.C.) 211*:487–489.
12. Ritz, J., and Schlossman, S. F. (1982) Utilization of monoclonal antibodies in the treatment of leukemia and lymphoma. *Blood 59*:1-11.
13. Dillman, R. O., and Royston, I. (1984) Applications of monoclonal antibodies in cancer therapy. *Brit. Med. Bull. 40*:240-246.
14. Goodman, G. E., Beaumier, P., Hellstrom, I., Fernyhough, B., and Hellstrom, K.-E. (1985) Pilot trial of murine monoclonal antibodies in patients with advanced melanoma. *J. Clin. Oncol. 3*:340-352.
15. Houghton, A. N., Mintzer, D., Cordon-Cardo, C., Welt, S., Fliegel, B., Vadhan, S., Carswell, E., Melamed, M. R., Oettgen, H. F., and Old, L. J. (1985)

Mouse monoclonal IgG3 and antibody detecting GD3 ganglioside: a phase I trial in patients with malignant melanoma. *Proc. Natl. Acad. Sci. USA 82*: 1242-1246.

16. Miller, R. A., Maloney, D. G., Warnke, R., and Levy, R. (1982) Treatment of B cell lymphoma with monoclonal anti-idiotype antibody. *N. Engl. J. Med. 306*:517-522.
17. Drebin, J. A., Link, V. C., Weinberg, R. A., and Greene, M. I. (1986) Inhibition of tumor growth by a monoclonal antibody reactive with an oncogene-encoded tumor antigen. *Proc. Natl. Acad. Sci. USA 83*:9129-9133.
18. Ghose, T., Cerini, M., Carter, M., and Nairn, R. C. (1967) Immuno-radioactive agent against cancer. *Br. Med. J. 1*:90-93.
19. Ghose, T., and Guclu, A. (1974) Cure of a mouse lymphoma with radioiodinated antibody. *Eur. J. Cancer 10*:787-792.
20. Ghose, T., and Nigam, S. (1972) Antibody as carrier of chlorambucil. *Cancer 29*: 1398-1400.
21. Ghose, T., Norvell, S. T., Guclu, A., Cameron, D., Bodurtha, A., and MacDonald, A. S. (1972) Immunochemotherapy of cancer with chlorambucil-carrying antibody. *Br. Med. J. 1*:495-499.
22. Ghose, T., Tai, J., Aquino, J., Guclu, A., Norvell, S., and MacDonald, A. (1975) Tumor localization of ^{131}I-labeled antibodies by radionuclide imaging. *Radiol. 116*:445-448.
23. Ghose, T., Guclu, A., Tai, J., MacDonald, A. S., Norvell, S. T., and Aquino, J. (1975) Antibody as carrier ^{131}I in cancer diagnosis and treatment. *Cancer 36*:1646-1657.
24. Ghose, T., Norvell, S. T., Aquino, J., Belitsky, P., Tai, J., Guclu, A., and Blair, A. H. (1980) Localization of ^{131}I-labeled antibodies in human renal cell carcinomas and in a mouse hepatoma and correlation with tumor detection by photoscanning. *Cancer Res. 40*:3018-3031.
25. Ghose, T., Blair, A. H., Martin, R. H., Norvell, S. T., Ramakrishnan, S., Belitsky, P., and Ferrone, S. (1982) Tumor imaging by antitumor antibody linked radionuclides. *Tumor Imaging* (Bruchiel, S., Ed.). Masson Publishers, New York, pp. 167-178.
26. Ghose, T., Ferrone, S., Imai, K., Norvell, Jr., S. T., Luner, S. J., Martin, R. H., and Blair, A. H. (1982) Imaging of human melanoma xenografts in nude mice with a radiolabeled monoclonal antibody. *J. Natl. Cancer Inst. 69*:823-826.
27. Yamaizumi, M., Mekada, E., Uchida, T., and Okada, Y. (1978) One molecule of diphtheria toxin fragment A introduced into a cell can kill a cell. *Cell 15*:245-250.
28. Eiklid, K., Olsnes, S., and Pihl, A. (1980) Entry of lethal doses of abrin, ricin and modeccin into the cytosol of HeLa cells. *Exp. Cell Res. 126*: 321-326.
29. Baldwin, R. W., and Byers, V. S. (1986) Monoclonal antibodies in cancer treatment. *Lancet 1*:603-605.
30. Bale, W. F., Countreras, M. A., and Grady, E. D. (1980) Factors influencing localization of labeled antibodies in tumors. *Cancer Res. 40*:2965-2972.

31. Order, S. E. (1984) The use of radiolabeled antibody in cancer chemotherapy. *Dev. Oncol. 26*:257-261.
32. Ettinger, D. S., Order, S. E., Wharam, M. D., Parker, M. K., Klein, J. L., and Leichner, P. D. (1982) Phase I-II study of isotopic immunoglobulin therapy for primary liver cancer. *Cancer Treat. Rep. 66*:289-297.
33. Leichner, P. K., Klein, J. L., Siegelman, S. S., Ettinger, D. S., and Order, S. E. (1983) Dosimetry of ^{131}I-labeled antiferritin in hepatoma: specific activities in the tumor and liver. *Cancer Treat. Rep. 67*:647-658.
34. Johns, D. G., and Bertino, J. R. (1982) Folate antagonists. *Cancer Medicine* (Holland, J. F., and Frei, E., Eds.). Lea & Febiger, Philadelphia, pp. 775-790.
35. Jolivet, J., Cowan, K. H., Curt, G. A., Clendeninn, N. J., and Chabner, B. A. (1983) The pharmacology and clinical use of methotrexate. *N. Engl. J. Med. 309*: 1094-1104.
36. Uadia, P., Blair, A. H., Ghose, T., and Ferrone, S. (1985) Uptake of methotrexate linked to polyclonal and monoclonal antimelanoma antibodies by a human melanoma cell line. *J. Nat. Cancer Inst. 74*:29-35.
37. Uadia, P., Blair, A. H., and Ghose, T. (1984) Tumor and tissue distribution of a methotrexate-anti-EL4 immunoglobulin conjugate in EL4 lymphoma-bearing mice. *Cancer Res. 44*:4263-4266.
38. Uadia, P., Blair, A. H., and Ghose, T. (1983) Uptake of methotrexate linked to an anti-EL4-lymphoma antibody by EL4 cells. *Cancer Immunol. Immunother. 16*:127-129.
38a. Uadia, P. (1984) The uptake and mode of cytotoxic action of MTX-immunoglobulin conjugates. Ph.D. Thesis, Dalhousie University, pp. 87-121.
39. Ghose, T., and Blair, A. H. (1978) Antibody-linked cytotoxic agents in the treatment of cancer: current status and future prospects. *J. Natl. Cancer Inst. 61*:657-676.
40. Edwards, D. C. (1983) Targeting potential of antibody conjugates. *Pharmac. Ther. 23*:147-177.
41. Kulkarni, P. N., Blair, A. H., and Ghose, T. (1981) Covalent binding of methotrexate to immunoglobulins and the effect of antibody-linked drug on tumor growth in vivo. *Cancer Res. 41*:2700-2706.
42. Burstein, S., and Knapp, R. (1977) Chemotherapy of murine ovarian carcinoma by methotrexate-antibody conjugates. *J. Med. Chem. 20*:950-952.
43. Ghose, T., Blair, A. H., Uadia, P., Kulkarni, P. N., Goundalkar, A., Mezei, M., and Ferrone, S. (1985) Antibodies as carriers of cancer chemotherapeutic agents. *Ann. NY Acad. Sci. 446*:213-227.
44. Peterson, D. L., Gleisner, J. M., and Blakely, R. L. (1975) Bovine liver dihydrofolate reductase: purification and properties of the enzyme. *Biochemistry 14*:5261-5267.
45. Kulkarni, P. N., Blair, A. H., Ghose, T., and Mammen, M. (1985) Conjugation of methotrexate to IgG antibodies and their $F(ab')_2$ fragments and the effect of conjugated methotrexate on tumor growth in vivo. *Cancer Immunol. Immunother. 16*:127-129.

46. McCabe, R. P., Quaranta, V., Frugls, l., Ferrone, S., and Reisfeld, R. A. (1979). A radioimmunometric antibody-binding assay for evaluation of xenoantisera to melanoma-associated antigens. *J. Natl. Cancer Inst. 62*: 455-463.
47. Shimuzu, A., Kohler, C. P. M., Shinoda, T., and Putnam, F. W. (1971) Variation and homology in the mu and gamma heavy chains of human immunoglobulins. *Sci. 173*:629-631.
48. Beale, D., and Feinstein, A. (1976) Structure and function of the constant regions of immunoglobulins. *Q. Rev. Biophys. 9*:135-180.
49. Nezlin, R. S., Timofeev, V. P., Sykulev, Yu., K., and Zurabyan, S. E. (1978) Spin-labeling of immunoglobulin carbohydrates. *Immunochem. 15*:141-144.
50. Fanger, M. W., and Smyth, D. G. (1972) The oligosaccharide units of rabbit immunoglobulin G. Multiple carbohydrate attachment sites. *Biochem. J. 127*:757-765.
51. Fanger, M. W., and Smyth, D. G. (1972) The oligosaccharide units of rabbit immunoglobulin G. Asymmetric attachment of C2-oligosaccharide. *Biochem. J. 127*:767-774.
52. Hinrichs, W. A., and Smyth, D. G. (1970) Studies on the asymmetrically attached oligosaccharide of rabbit immunoglobulin G. I. Biosynthesis and stability of the C_2-oligosaccharide. *Immunol. 18*:757-759.
53. William, K. J., Golding, B., Givol, D., and Dwek, R. A. (1977) Specific spin labeling of the Fc region of immunoglobulins. *FEBS Letters 80*:133-136.
54. Spiro, R. G. (1971) Periodate oxidation of the glycoprotein Fetuin. *J. Biol. Chem. 239*:567-573.
55. Kornfeld, R., Keller, J. Baenziger, K., and Kornfeld, S. (1971) The structure of the glycopeptide of human gamma G myeloma proteins. *J. Biol. Chem. 246*:3259-3268.
56. Murayama, A., Shimeda, K., and Yamcinoto, T. (1978) Modification of immunoglobulin G using specific reactivity of sugar moiety. *Immunochem. 15*:523-528.
57. Taylor, J. E., Soldano, B., and Hall, G. A. (1985) A survey of the effects of changes in pH, solvent and salt concentration. *J. Am. Chem. Soc. 77*:2656-2657.
58. Crouthamel, C. E., Hayes, A. M., and Martin, D. S. (1951) Ionization and hydration equilibria of periodic acid. *J. Am. Chem. Soc. 73*:82-87.
59. Aminoff, D., and Morgan, W. T. J. (1951) Studies in immunochemistry, The oxidation of the human blood group A substance with the periodate ion. *Biochem. J. 48*:74-88.
60. Lee, C. Y., and Montgomery, R. (1961) The carbohydrate of ovalbumin. *Arch. Biochem. Biophys. 95*:263-270.
61. Rothfus, J. A., and Smith, E. L. (1963) Glycopeptides. IV. The periodate oxidation of glycopeptides from human gammaglobulin. *J. Biol. Chem. 238*:1402-1410.
62. Moe, O. A., Miller, S. E., and Buckley, M. I. (1951) Periodate oxidation of the formyl esters of starch. *J. Am. Chem. Soc. 73*:4185-4186.

63. Bobbit, J. M. (1956) Periodate oxidation of carbohydrates. *Advances in Carbohydrate Chemistry* (Wolfrom, M. L., Ed.). Academic Press Inc., New York, Vol. 11, pp. 1-41.
64. Dyer, R. J. (1956) Use of periodate oxidations in biochemical analysis. *Methods of Biochemical Analysis* (Glick, D., Ed.). Interscience, New York, Vol. 3, pp. 111-152.
65. Fleury, P., Courtois, J., and Grandchamp, M. (1949) Action of periodic acid on amine compounds. *Bull. Soc. Chim. Fr.*:88-94.
66. Nicolet, B. H., and Shinn, L. A. (1939) The action of periodic acid on aminoalcohols. *J. Am. Chem. Soc. 61*:1615.
67. Shinn, L. A., and Nicolet, B. M. (1941) The determination of threonine by the use of periodate. *J. Biol. Chem. 138*:91-96.
68. Carter, H. E., and Loo, Y. H. (1948) Oxidation of hydroxy-L-proline by periodate. *J. Biol. Chem. 174*:723-727.
69. Bragg, P. D., and Hough, L. (1958) The oxidation of proline, hydroxyproline and N-methylglycine with periodate. *J. Chem. Soc.*:4050-4056.
70. Eylar, E. H., and Jeanloz, R. W. (1962) Periodate oxidation of the acid glycoprotein of human plasma. *J. Biol. Chem. 237*:1021-1025.
71. Yamasaki, R. B., Osuga, D. T., and Feeney, R. E. (1982) Periodate oxidation of methionine in proteins. *Anal. Biochem. 126*:183-189.
72. Brot, N., and Wiessbach, H. (1983) Biochemistry and physiological role of methionine sulfoxide residues in proteins. *Arch. Biochem. Biophys. 223*: 271-281.
73. Fields, R., and Dixon, H. B. F. (1968) A spectrophotometric method for the microdetermination of periodate. *Biochem. J. 108*:883-887.
74. Bertoni, J. M. (1982) Inhibition of rat brain microsomal (Na^+ + K^+)-ATPase and K^+-p-nitrophenyl phosphatase by periodic acid. *Biochim. Biophys. Acta 688*:101-106.

74b. Chua, M. M., Fan, S. T., and Karash, F. (1984) Attachment of immunoglobulins to liposomal membrane via protein carbohydrate. *Biochim. Biophys. Acta 800*: 291-300.

75. Dopp, D., and Dopp, H. (1985) Carbonsaure-hydrazide. Methoden der organischen Chemie, Houben-Weyl (Falbe, J., Ed.). Georg Thieme, Stuttgart, Band E5, pp. 1154-1172.
76. Henecke, H. (1952) Methoden der Herstellung und Umwandlung von funktionellen N-Derivaten der Carboxylgruppe. *Methoden der organischen Chemie* (*Houben-Weyl*) (Muller, E., Ed.). Georg Thieme, Stuttgart, Band III, pp. 676-679 and 711.
77. Smith, P. A. S. (1946) The Curtius reaction. Preparation of hydrazides. *Organic Reactions* (Adams, E., Ed.). Wiley, New York, Vol. 11, pp. 366-369.
78. Rosowsky, A., Forsch, R., Uren, J., and Wick, M. (1981) Methotrexate analogues. 14. Synthesis of new gamma-substituted derivatives as dihydrofolate reductase inhibitors and potential anticancer agents. *J. Med. Chem. 24*:1450-1455.
79. Smith, R. F., Bates, A. C., Battisti, A. J., Byrnes, P. G., Mroz, C. T., Smearing, T. J., and Albrecht, F. X. (1968) Reactions of hydrazines with esters and carboxylic acids. *J. Org. Chem. 33*:851-855.

80. Baccolini, G., and Rosini, G. (1970) Phenyldichlorophosphite oxide as an activator in acylation reactions. Formation of amides and hydrazides. *Chim. Ind. (Milan) 52*:583-584.
81. Steglich, W., Schmidt, H., and Holitzer, O. (1978) Aktivierte carbonsaure-derivate; II. Eine einfache synthese von 2-oxo carbonsaure-hydraziden. *Synthesis*:622-624.
82. Wackerle, L. (1979) Racemisierungsfreie Aktivierung von Alpha-amino-sauren mittels Isocyaniden. *Synthesis*:197-198.
83. Jencks, W. P. (1959) Studies on the mechanism of oxime and semi-carbazone formation. *J. Am. Chem. Soc. 81*:475-481.
84. Anderson, B. M., and Jencks, W. P. (1960) The effect of structure on reactivity in semicarbazone formation. *J. Am. Chem. Soc. 82*:1773-1777.
85. Cordes, E. H., and Jencks, W. P. (1962) On the mechanism of Schiff base formation and hydrolysis. *J. Am. Chem. Soc. 84*:832-837.
86. Lindmo, T., Boven, E., Cuttitta, F., Fedorko, J., and Bunn, P. A., Jr. (1984) Determination of the immunoreactive fraction of radiolabeled monoclonal antibodies by linear extrapolation to binding at infinite antigen excess. *J. Immunol. Meth. 72*:77-89.
87. Kanellos, J., Pietersz, G. A., and McKenzie, I. F. C. (1985) Studies of methotrexate-monoclonal antibody conjugates for immunotherapy. *J. Natl. Cancer Inst. 75*:319-322.
88. Guclu, A., Tai, J., and Ghose, T. (1975) Endocytosis of chlorambucil-bound anti-tumor globulin following "capping" in EL4 lymphoma cells. *Immunol. Commun. 4*:229-242.
89. Ghose, T., Kulkarni, N., Ferrone, S., Giacomini, P., Norvell, S. T., Kulkarni, P., and Blair, A. H. (1983). Imaging human tumors in nude mice. *Radioimmunoimaging and Radioimmunotherapy* (Burchiel, S., and Rhodes, B. A., Eds.). Elsevier Science Publishing Co. Ltd., New York, pp. 255-263.
90. Embleton, M. J., Garnett, M.C., and Baldwin, R. W. (1984) Use of an anti-tumour monoclonal antibody for targeting MTX. *Protides Biol. Fluids 32*: 429-431.
91. Garnett, M. C., and Baldwin, R. W. (1986) An improved synthesis of a methotrexate-albumin-791T/36 monoclonal antibody conjugate cytotoxic to human osteogenic sarcoma cell lines. *Cancer Res. 46*:2407-2412.
92. Manabe, Y., Tsubota, T., Haruta, Y., Kataoka, K., Okazaki, M., Haisa, S., Nakamura, K., and Kimura, I. (1984) Production of a monoclonal antibody-methotrexate conjugate utilizing dextran-T40 and its biological activity. *J. Lab. Clin. Med. 104*:445-454.
93. Manabe, Y., Tsubota, T., Haruta, Y., Okazaki, M., Haisa, S., Nakamura, K., and Kimura, I. (1983) Production of a monoclonal antibody-bleomycin conjugate utilizing dextran-T40 and the antigen-targeting cytotoxicity of the conjugate. *Biochem. Biophys. Res. Commun. 115*:1009-1114.
94. Manabe, Y., Tsubota, T., Haruta, Y., Kataoka, K., Okazaki, M., Haisa, S., Nakamura, K., and Kimura, I. (1985) Production of a monoclonal antibody-mitomycin C conjugate utilizing dextran-T40, and its biological activity. *Biochem. Pharmacol. 34*:289-291.

95. Goding, J. W. (1978) Use of staphylococcal protein A as an immunological reagent. *J. Immunol. Methods 20*: 241-253.
96. Luner, S. J., Ghose, T., Chatterjee, S., Cruz, H. N., and Belitsky, P. (1986). Monoclonal antibodies to kidney and tumor-associated surface antigens of human renal cell carcinoma. *Cancer Res. 46*:5816-5820.
97. Lamoyi, E., and Nisonoff, A. (1983) Preparation of $F(ab')_2$ fragments from mouse IgG of various subclasses. *J. Immunol. Methods. 56*:235-243.
98. Futterman, S. (1957) Enzymatic reduction of folic acid and dihydrofolic acid to tetrahydrofolic acid. *J. Biol. Chem. 228*: 1031-1038.
99. Falk, L. C., Clark, D. R., Kalman, S. M., and Lng, T. F. (1976) Enzymatic assay for methotrexate in serum and cerebro spinal fluid. *Clin. Chem. 22*: 785-788.
100. Baccanari, D., Phillips, A., Smith, S., Sinski, D., and Burchell, J. (1975) Purification and properties of escherichia coli dihydrofolate reductase. *Biochemistry 14*: 5267-5273.
100b. Mancini, G., Carbonara, A. O., and Heremans, J. F. (1965) Immunochemical quantitation of antigens by single radial immunodiffusion. *Immunochemistry 2*: 235-254.
101. Lathan, B., von Hoff, D. D., and Elslager, E. (1984) Use of a human tumor cloning system to evaluate analogs of methotrexate and mitoxantrone. *Cancer Treat. Rep. 68*: 733-738.
102. Lee, C. L. Y., Uniyal, S., Fernandez, L. A., Lee, S. H. S., and Ghose, T. (1986) Growth and spread in nude mice of Epstein-Barr virus transformed B-cells from a chronic lymphocytic leukemia patients. *Cancer Res. 46*: 2497-2501.
103. Mavligit, G. M., Gutterman, J. U., and Hersh, E. M. (1973) Separation of viable from non-viable tumor cells using Ficoll-Hypaque density solution. *Immunol. Commun. 2*:463-472.
104. Tai, J., Guclu, A., Ghose, T., and Norvell, S. (1983) Inhibition of pulmonary metastases of B16 melanoma with irradiated tumor cells and BCG. *Cancer Immunol. Immunother. 15*:47-53.
105. Sordat, B. C., Ueyama, Y., and Fogh, J. (1982) Metastasis of tumor xenografts in the nude mouse. *The Nude Mouse in Experimental and Clinical Research* (Fogh, J., Giovanella, B. C., Eds.). Academic Press, New York, Vol. 2, pp. 95-147.
106. Lozzio, B. B., and Machado, E. N. (1982) Transplantation and dissemination of human hematopoietic malignant cells in nude and lasat mice. *The Nude Mouse in Experimental and Clinical Research* (Fogh, J., Giovanella, B. C., Eds.). Academic Press, New York, Vol. 2, pp. 521-567.
107. Poulsen, C. O. (1978) Status of chemotherapy, radiotherapy, endocrine therapy and immunotherapy. Studies of human cancer in the nude mouse. *The Nude Mouse in Experimental and Clinical Research* (Fogh, J., Giovanella, B. C., Eds.). Academic Press, New York, Vol. 1, pp. 437-456.
108. Ghose, T., Blair, A. H., Kulkarni, P., Vaughan, K., Norvell, S. T., and Belitsky, P. (1982) Targeting of radionuclides and drugs for the diagnosis and treatment of cancer. *Targeting of Drugs* (Gregoriadis, G., Ed.). Plenum Press, London, pp. 55-82.

5

Monoclonal Antibody-Mediated Targeting of Alkylating Agents for the Treatment of Cancer

MARK J. SMYTH, GEOFFREY A. PIETERSZ, and IAN FARQUHAR CAMPBELL McKENZIE

Research Centre for Cancer and Transplantation, University of Melbourne, Parkville, Victoria, Australia

I. INTRODUCTION

There are now many drugs available for the chemotherapy of cancer, and even though some of these are analogs, there are at least 20 different chemical entities capable of regressing cancer in man. Trends indicate that alkylating agents are broader in their effects against tumors than antimetabolites or hormonal agents, however, their action is not specific for neoplastic tissue. Several thousand derivatives of alkylating agents have been prepared, but generally they are unlikely to be of clinical value since they must inevitably affect many normal tissues. Even Chlorambucil (CBL) and Melphalan (MEL) (Fig. 1), two alkylating agents routinely used in the treatment of chronic lymphocytic leukemia, ovarian carcinoma, testicular carcinoma, and Hodgkin's disease, cause bone marrow depression and have other toxicities, especially with prolonged use.

Numerous attempts have been made to improve the selective cytotoxicity of many clinically used cytotoxic agents. The idea of targeting a cytotoxic drug to a tumor using a "tumor-specific" antibody has existed for many years, and the specific localization of drug-antibody complexes to a particular tumor enables the use of significantly lower doses of chemotherapeutic drugs. Various agents have been studied for their suitability when complexed with tumor-as-

CHLORAMBUCIL

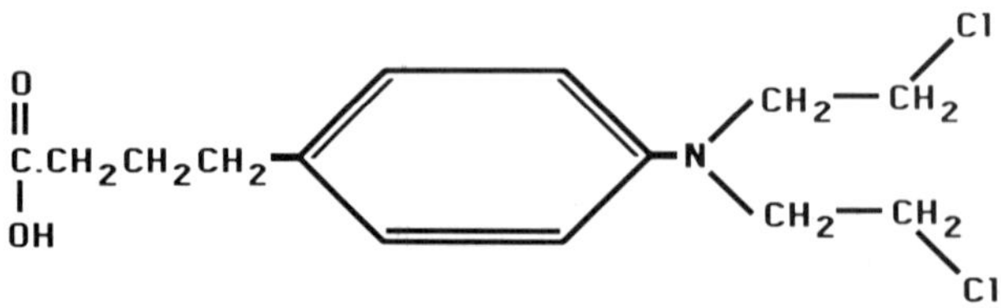

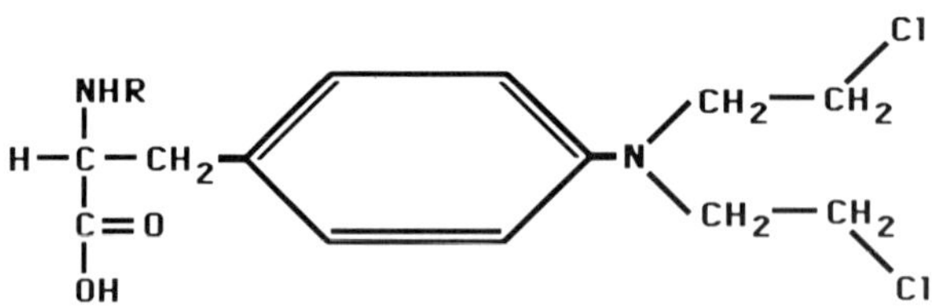

R = H MELPHALAN
R = CH_3CO N-ACETYL MELPHALAN

Figure 1 Structure of the alkylating agents.

sociated monoclonal antibodies (MAb). In many cases specific cytotoxicity towards antibody-reactive tumor cells was achieved in vitro, however, a significant loss of drug activity usually resulted upon coupling to antibodies (1-3). By contrast, *potentiation* of the cytotoxic action of some chemotherapeutic drugs was observed some years ago with studies demonstrating that mixing of antibody and the alkylating agent CBL led to a noncovalently bound complex that prevented the growth of transplanted tumors in conditions under which equivalent amounts of free CBL or antibody used alone were ineffective (4,5). These experiments were independently verified (6), and it was also observed that CBL and antibodies could act synergistically in inhibiting tumor growth when they were injected separately. The covalent coupling of CBL has involved water-soluble carbodiimides (7), but protein cross-linkage and polymerization have made these conjugates no more efficacious than noncovalently complexed CBL and antibody. Intermediaries and spacers, such as dextran (8) and polyglutamic acid (9), have been used, but these procedures were hindered by an inability to control the degree of coupling of CBL to antibodies. Despite these inadequacies, noncovalent and covalent CBL-antibody complexes have been used in the treatment of malignant melanoma (10) and neuroblastoma (11), but the success of these earlier trials was not clear due to the absence of suitable controls.

Our studies indicate that it is possible to covalently couple CBL to MAb using an active ester derivative of CBL to produce conjugates which have high drug:antibody ratios and greater in vitro and in vivo activity than free CBL (12). Although the antitumor effect of these CBL-MAb conjugates was reasonable, we considered that a greater efficacy could be achieved using a more potent alkylating agent, such as MEL. MEL is derived from phenylalanine and is taken into cells by an active carrier-mediated process using an amino acid transport system (13). We have used a novel approach to block this uptake by modifying the amino group of MEL to produce N-acetyl Melphalan (N-AcMEL). As MAb offer drugs an alternative route of entry into cells (14,15), N-AcMEL can gain entry into cells when coupled to MAb via an active ester derivative of N-AcMEL. It should be noted that it is difficult to directly couple MEL to MAb and that previous attempts to do this using a polyglutamic acid carrier produced an inactive conjugate (16). These N-AcMEL-MAb conjugates and conjugates of N-AcMEL and $F(ab')_2$ fragments were demonstrated to be specifically cytotoxic in vitro and in several different in vivo models (17,18). We now summarize the effects of coupling the two alkylating agents (CBL and MEL) to MAb and detail their in vitro and in vivo potency.

II. RESULTS

These studies were designed to assess the feasibility of coupling the alkylating agents CBL and MEL to MAb and to determine the specific cytotoxicity of the conjugates in vitro and in vivo in both ascites and solid tumor models. Initially it was necessary to establish conditions for the coupling of CBL to antibody and then to measure the residual drug and antibody activities in the conjugates. When a satisfactory coupling method was designed, in vitro and in vivo studies of the mode of action and activity of these conjugates could be examined. To couple MEL covalently to whole MAb or $F(ab')_2$ fragments, a less toxic derivative of MEL (N-AcMEL) was produced and coupled to MAb while maintaining drug and antibody activity. The specificity of action of these conjugates in vitro and in vivo was then determined and compared using different routes of administration.

A. Coupling to MAb and to Their F(ab')$_2$ Fragments

1. Chlorambucil

The anti-Ly-2.1 MAb (IgG2a), which reacts with the murine tumor ITT(1)75NS (E2), was reacted with different amounts of CBL active ester (Appendix) to produce conjugates that varied in the amount of drug coupled. It was found that an increasing amount of CBL could be covalently bound by increasing the amount of active ester of CBL present (Fig. 2) and up to 30 molecules of CBL could be bound without a great loss of protein, but when greater than 35 molecules were coupled, a substantial loss of protein solubility occurred. Thus a compromise had to be sought between higher CBL:MAb incorporation ratios and lower protein recoveries; CBL-anti-Ly-2.1 conjugates that were further tested in vitro and in vivo had between 20 and 35 molecules of CBL incorporated per molecule of anti-Ly-2.1. By extracting the noncovalently bound CBL from the CBL-anti-Ly-2.1 conjugate with ethyl acetate, it was found that 80% of the CBL was covalently bound. Only 10% of the physically bound CBL in noncovalent CBL-MAb complexes could not be extracted with ethyl acetate by the same procedure. Conjugates retained over 90% of their alkylating activity.

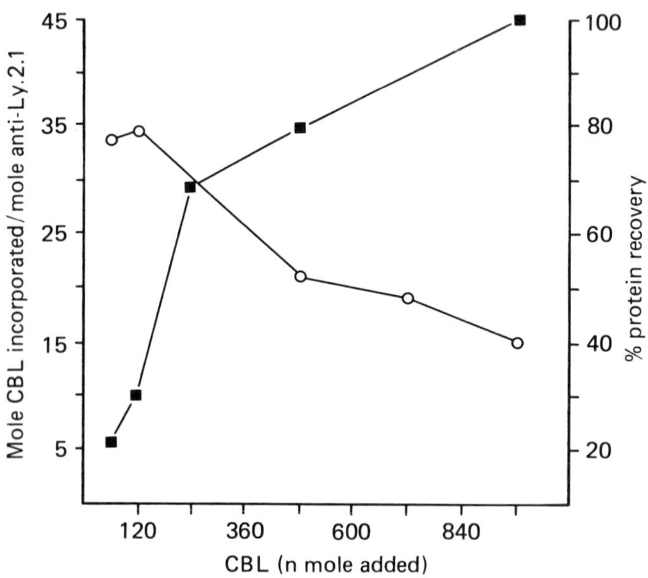

Figure 2 Coupling of CBL to anti-Ly-2.1 (0.5 mg). Moles of CBL incorporated per molecue anti-Ly-2.1 (■) and protein recovery (○) are shown as a function of the number of nmole CBL in the reaction mixture (abscissa).

2. N-acetyl Melphalan

The anti-Ly-2.1 MAb (IgG1) reactive with the same epitope of the Ly-2 molecule as the IgG2a MAb was added to different amounts of N-AcMEL active ester, and it was also found that up to 30 molecules of N-AcMEL could be covalently bound with good recovery of protein (data not shown). Again beyond these levels of incorporation, precipitation occurred due to loss of protein solubility, thus N-AcMEL-MAb conjugates that were tested further in vitro and in vivo had between 10 and 30 molecules of N-AcMEL incorporated per molecule of MAb. It was found that 90% of the N-AcMEL incorporated was covalently bound, and 90% of the alkylating activity was retained upon conjugation to the anti-Ly-2.1 MAb. In addition it was determined that from 20-25 molecules of N-AcMEL could be covalently coupled to the $F(ab')_2$ fragment of the anti-Ly-2.1 MAb (IgG1) with retention of good protein recovery (data not shown). $F(ab')_2$ conjugates that were further tested had between 10 and 25 molecules of N-AcMEL incorporated per molecule of $F(ab')_2$ MAb.

B. Antibody Activity of Drug-MAb Conjugates

Optimally 20-30 molecules of CBL or N-AcMEL could be covalently bound to MAb and their $F(ab')_2$ fragments with retention of alkylating activity and some loss of protein. For these drug-MAb conjugates to be specifically cytotoxic to tumor cells it was essential that their antibody activity be comparable to that of unmodified MAb, and so the antibody activity of the conjugates were measured.

1. Chlorambucil-MAb Conjugates

The titers (dilution at which 50% of the E2 target cells demonstrated rosettes) of anti-Ly-2.1 MAb (IgG2a) were measured before and after conjugation to CBL (Fig. 3). Anti-Ly-2.1 conjugates containing 25 and 35 molecules of CBL had titers of 1:15,000 and 1:10,000, respectively, while the unconjugated antibody titer was 1:50,000. There is clearly some loss of antibody activity following conjugation to CBL, however, the titers of these conjugates were sufficiently high to enable further experimentation. The CBL-MAb conjugates formed of CBL bound noncovalently to MAb (Appendix) had very similar titers to covalently bound CBL-MAb conjugates (data not shown).

2. N-acetyl Melphalan-MAb Conjugates

The titers of anti-Ly-2.1 MAb (IgG1) were measured before and after conjugation to N-AcMEL by the rosetting method; anti-Ly-2.1 conjugates containing 10 and 25 molecules of N-AcMEL had titers of 1:45,000 and 1:20,000, respectively, while the unmodified anti-Ly-2.1 titer was 1:75,000 (data not shown) (i.e., a similar loss of activity to that found with CBL).

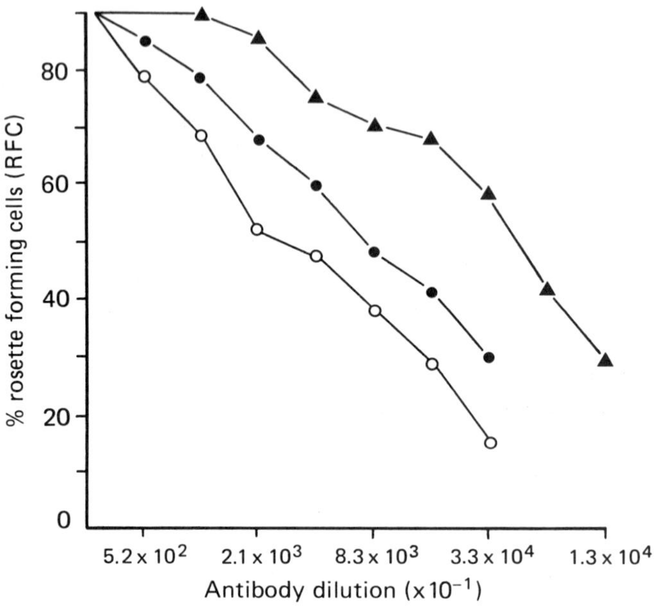

Figure 3 Antibody titer measured as the percentage of rosette-forming cells vs. antibody dilution of anti-Ly-2.1 conjugates on ITT(1)75NS target cells. Serial dilutions were performed on a 0.25 mg/ml solution of neat anti-Ly-2.1 (▲); or anti-Ly-2.1 with 25 (●) or 35 mol CBL/mol conjugate (○).

3. N-acetyl Melphalan-F(ab')$_2$ Conjugates

The titers of anti-Ly-2.1 MAb (IgG1) were measured before and after pepsin degradation and conjugation to N-AcMEL by a competitive radiolabel binding assay (Fig. 4) [in this case, titer = the dilution of cold antibody at which 35% (half the maximum binding) of the ^{125}I-anti-Ly-2.1 binding to E3 target cells was reduced]. F(ab')$_2$ conjugates containing 20 molecules of N-AcMEL had an antibody titers of 1:32, the unconjugated F(ab')$_2$ titer was 1:32, and the anti-Ly-2.1 titer was 1:100. There is some loss of antibody activity upon pepsin degradation of IgG to F(ab')$_2$ fragments, but no further loss occurred upon conjugation of up to 20 N-AcMEL molecules. However, when N-AcMEL incorporation ratios exceeded 20 molecules, a significant loss in antibody activity was observed (data not shown).

C. Cytotoxicity in Vitro

The cytotoxicity of all drug-MAb conjugates was initially assessed by measuring the percentage inhibition of [^{3}H]-thymidine uptake of tumor cells which

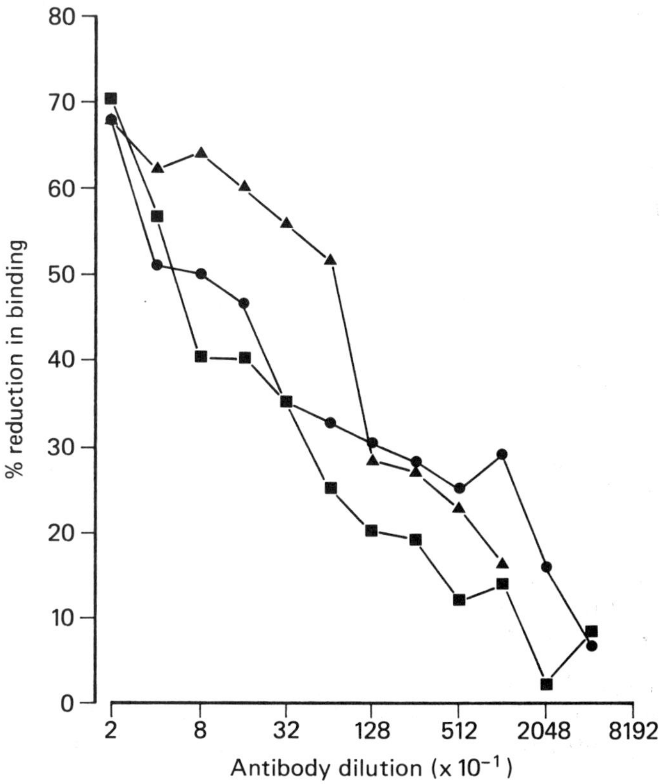

Figure 4 Titer measured as the percentage reduction in ^{125}I-anti-Ly-2.1 binding vs. antibody dilution of $F(ab')_2$ conjugate using 0.8 mg/ml solution of anti-Ly-2.1 (▲), anti-Ly-2.1 $F(ab')_2$ (■) or $F(ab')_2$ conjugate (●) 20 mol N-AcMEL/mol conjugate.

has been exposed to conjugate, free drug, or phosphate buffered saline (PBS) for 24 hr.

1. Chlorambucil-MAb Conjugates

The cytotoxicity of anti-Ly-2.1 conjugates was tested on Ly-2^+ E2 target cells and compared with that of free CBL or noncovalently bound CBL and anti-Ly-2.1 (Fig. 5). The activity of the bound drug was considerably increased over that of free CBL, with 50% inhibition in [^{3}H]-thymidine incorporation occurring at 2.6×10^{-6} M for the anti-Ly-2.1 conjugate compared to 1.7×10^{-5} M for free CBL (i.e., a fivefold increase). In addition CBL noncovalently bound to anti-Ly-2.1 was twice as cytotoxic toward E2 as free CBL alone. It should be

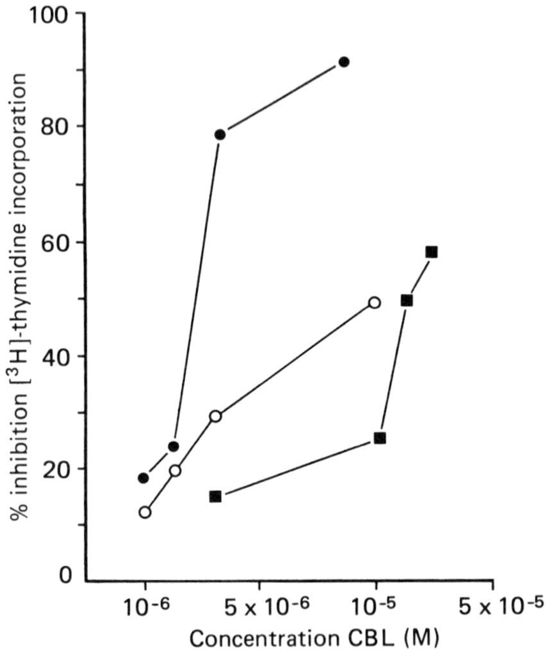

Figure 5 The inhibitory effect of CBL on E2 cells (see text) with the drug free (■), noncovalently bound to anti-Ly-2.1 MAb (30 mol CBL/mol conjugate) (○) or covalently bound to anti-Ly-2.1 MAb (30 mol/CBL mol conjugate) (●).

noted that the anti-Ly-2.1 MAb used in this study was found to have no cytotoxic action on target cells in vitro in the absence of complement.

2. N-acetyl Melphalan-MAb and N-acetyl Melphalan-F(ab$'$)$_2$ Conjugates

The cytotoxicity of the N-AcMEL-F(ab$'$)$_2$ conjugate was tested on Ly-2$^+$ E3 cells and compared with that of N-AcMEL covalently bound to intact anti-Ly-2.1 (IgG1) and N-AcMEL alone (Fig. 6). It was clear that the cytotoxic activity of the N-AcMEL-MAb and N-AcMEL-F(ab$'$)$_2$ conjugate was considerably greater than free N-AcMEL. For example, the 50% inhibition in [^{3}H]-thymidine incorporation occurred at a N-AcMEL concentration of 7.5×10^{-6} M for the F(ab$'$)$_2$ conjugate compared to 4.0×10^{-4} M for free N-AcMEL and 9.0×10^{-6} M for N-AcMEL-MAb (Fig. 6). Therefore, when the amino group of MEL was modified, an N-AcMEL derivative was produced which was 100-150 times *less* cytotoxic in vitro, however, upon coupling N-AcMEL to the anti-Ly-2.1 MAb or its F(ab$'$)$_2$ fragment, a 40-50-fold *increase* in cytotoxic activity was observed.

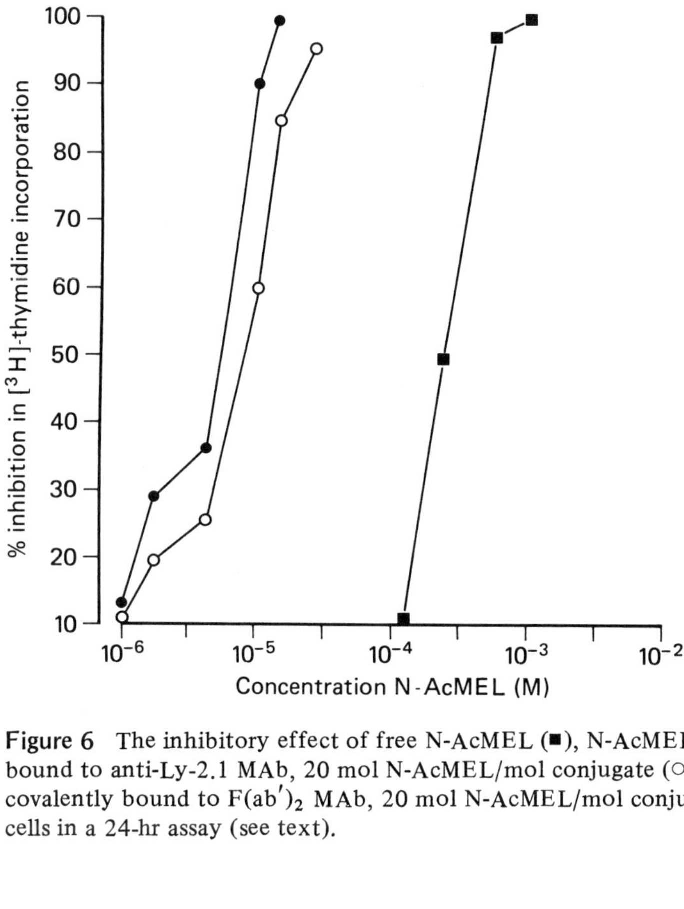

Figure 6 The inhibitory effect of free N-AcMEL (■), N-AcMEL covalently bound to anti-Ly-2.1 MAb, 20 mol N-AcMEL/mol conjugate (○) or N-AcMEL covalently bound to $F(ab')_2$ MAb, 20 mol N-AcMEL/mol conjugate (●) on E3 cells in a 24-hr assay (see text).

D. Specific Cytotoxicity in Vitro

After determining that both CBL-MAb and N-AcMEL-MAb conjugates were more cytotoxic than free CBL and N-AcMEL respectively, it was necessary to demonstrate that the inhibition observed was due to the specific binding to cells at the antibody-binding site. A number of different experiments were performed using the 30-min assay, including the testing of drug-MAb conjugates against Ly-2^+ and Ly-2^- cell lines; the testing of drug-MAb conjugates against Ly-2^{high} and Ly-2^{low} variants of the ITT(1)75NS cell line and the inhibition of drug-MAb cytotoxicity by competing free MAb.

1. Chlorambucil-MAb Conjugates

The CBL-anti-Ly-2.1 conjugate was shown to bind the Ly-2^+ E2 cell line and to exert its cytotoxicity on these cells after 30 min exposure, where 50% inhibition

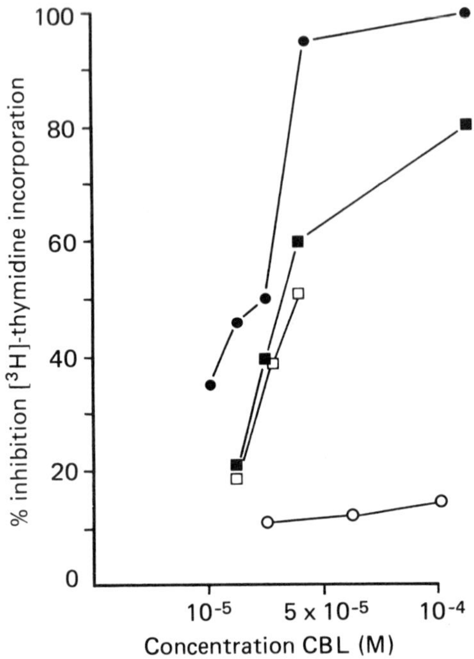

Figure 7 Inhibitory effect of free CBL (■) or CBL-anti-Ly-2.1 conjugate (20 mol CBL/mol conjugate) (●) on antibody-reactive cells (E2) and free CBL (□) or conjugate (○) on antibody-nonreactive cells (BW 5147) in the 30-min assay.

in [^{3}H]-thymidine incorporation occurred at 2.5×10^{-5} M compared with 3.0×10^{-5} M for free CBL (Fig. 7). It should be noted that the anti-Ly-2.1 conjugate demonstrated selectivity in its action by inhibiting the Ly-2$^+$ E2 cell line only; no inhibition of the Ly-2$^-$ BW5147 cell line was observed over the same molar concentration range.

To clarify that the cytotoxicity of the CBL-anti-Ly-2.1 conjugate was primarily dependent on the number of reactive antigen-binding sites on the target cells, Ly-2^{high} (E3) and Ly-2^{low} (D1) variants of the ITT(1)75NS cell line were used. Both the E3 and D1 tumors had an identical response to free CBL; however, the CBL-anti-Ly-2.1 conjugate was five times more cytotoxic toward E3 than D1 (Fig. 8). Clearly, therefore, cells with the highest antigen expression were more susceptible to the toxicity of CBL-MAb conjugates.

To ensure that the binding of CBL-MAb conjugate to target cells was specific and occurred at the antibody-binding site, inhibition studies of the binding of conjugate by free antibody were performed. At a CBL concentration of 10^{-4} M (50 μg anti-Ly-2.1), the cytotoxicity of the anti-Ly-2.1 conjugate on E2 target

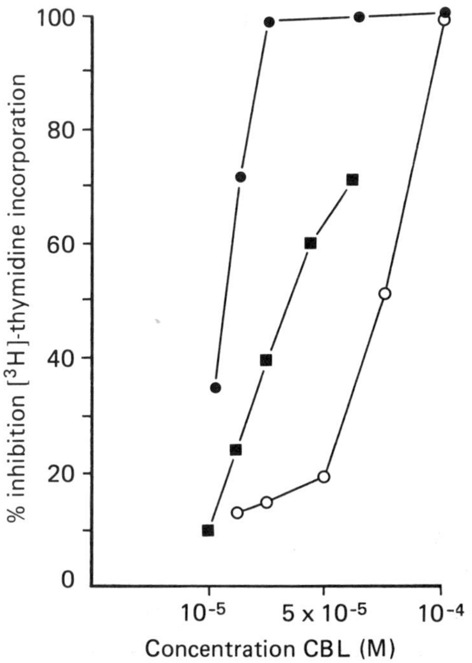

Figure 8 Inhibitory effect of free CBL (■) or CBL-anti-Ly-2.1 conjugate (30 mol CBL/mol conjugate) (●) on E3 cells and free CBL (■) or conjugate (○) on D1 cells in the 30-min assay.

cells was reduced by 70% in the presence of 100 μg of free anti-Ly-2.1 (Fig. 9), indicating that the cytotoxicity of the CBL-MAb conjugate was directly related to its antibody-binding ability.

2. N-acetyl Melphalan-MAb and N-acetyl Melphalan-F(ab′)$_2$ Conjugates

The N-AcMEL–anti-Ly-2.1 conjugate was demonstrated to bind the Ly-2$^+$ E3 cell line and to exert its cytotoxicity after 30 min exposure (Fig. 10): 50% inhibition of [^{3}H]-thymidine incorporation occurred at a N-AcMEL concentration of 3.2×10^{-5} M compared with 3.0×10^{-4} M for free N-AcMEL. By contrast, the Ly-2$^-$ cell line BW5147 OU$^-$ was three times more sensitive than E3 to free N-AcMEL, however, it was comparatively resistant to the cytotoxic effect of the anti-Ly-2.1 conjugate.

In addition, at a N-AcMEL concentration of 3×10^{-5} M (15 μg anti-Ly-2.1), the cytotoxicity of the anti-Ly-2.1 conjugate on E3 target cells was reduced by 80% by the addition of 100 μg of free anti-Ly-2.1 MAb (data not shown).

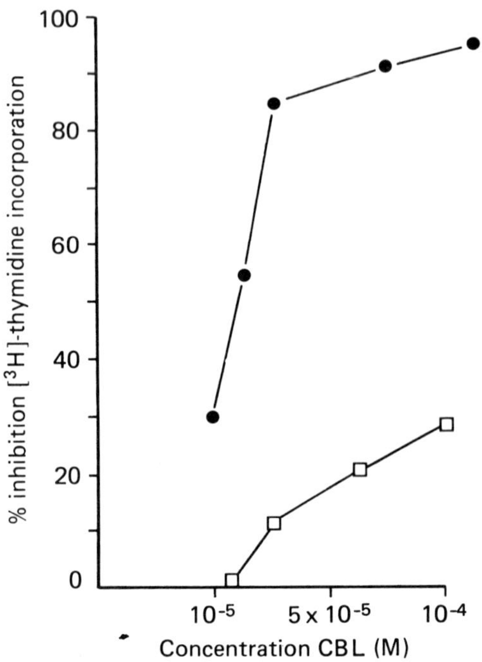

Figure 9 Inhibitory effect of CBL-anti-Ly-2.1 conjugate (30 mol CBL/mol conjugate) (●) and conjugate plus 100 μg neat anti-Ly-2.1 (□) on E2 target cells in the 30-min assay.

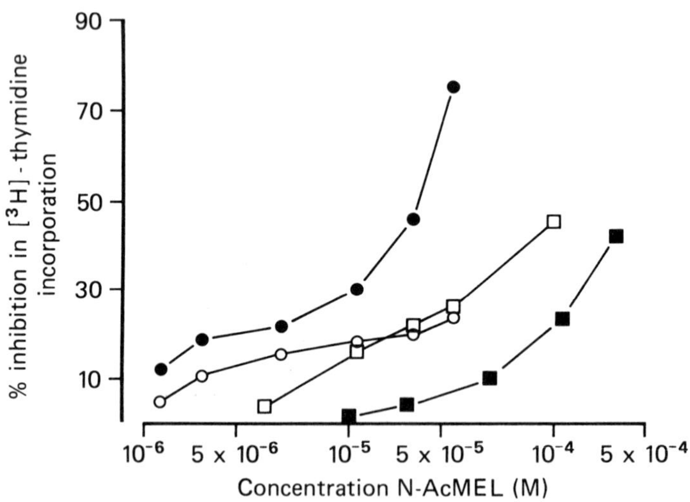

Figure 10 The inhibitory effect of free N-AcMEL (■) or N-AcMEL-anti-Ly-2.1 conjugate, 25 mol of N-AcMEL/mol of conjugate (●) on antibody reactive cells (E3) and free N-AcMEL (□) or conjugate (○) on antibody-nonreactive cells ($BW5147OU^-$) in the 30-min assay.

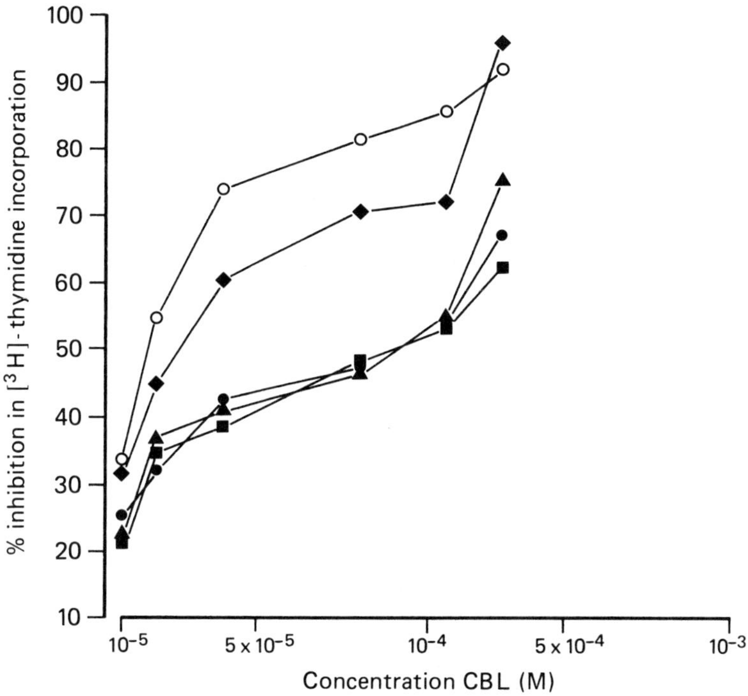

Figure 11 The inhibitory effect of free CBL (■) or CBL in the presence of 500 μg/ml of anti-Ly-2.1 IgG2a (○), IgM (♦), IgG3 (▲), and IgG1 (●) on E3 cells in a 24-hr assay.

The N-AcMEL-F(ab′)$_2$ conjugate demonstrated a 50% inhibition in [^{3}H]-thymidine incorporation into E3 cells at a N-AcMEL concentration of 1.5×10^{-5} M compared with 1.5×10^{-4} M for free N-AcMEL (data not shown). By contrast EL4 (Ly-2$^-$), which was 10 times more sensitive than E3 to free N-AcMEL, was relatively resistant to the cytotoxic effect of the F(ab′)$_2$ (Ly-2$^+$) conjugate over the molar concentration range tested. Therefore, both the N-AcMEL-anti-Ly-2.1 and N-AcMEL-F(ab′)$_2$ conjugates were specifically cytotoxic for Ly-2$^+$ cell lines.

E. The Synergy of Chlorambucil and MAb

It had previously been shown, using polyclonal antibodies, that CBL and antibody did not have to be covalently bound to antibody to selectively inhibit tumor cell growth. Our studies examined this phenomenon using MAb and have sought to determine how antibody may serve to focus and increase the

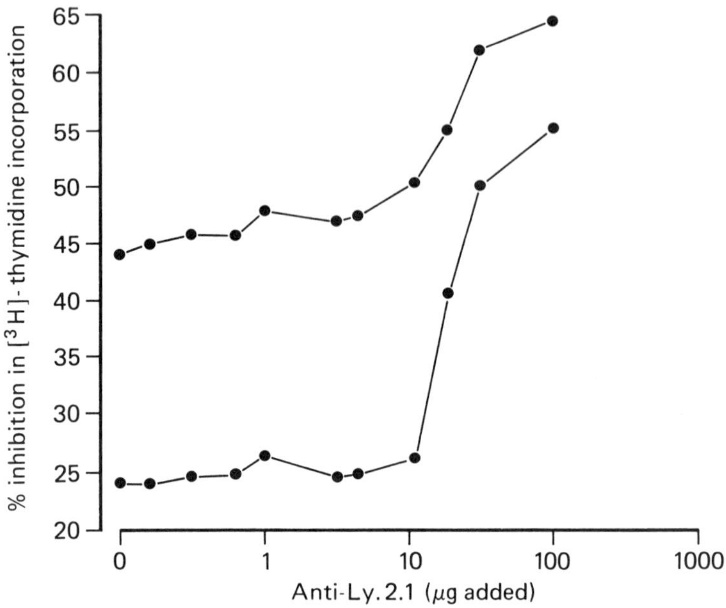

Figure 12 The inhibitory effect of free CBL (6×10^{-6} M or 10^{-5} M) in the presence of different amounts of anti-Ly-2.1 (IgG2a) on E3 cell in a 24-hr assay.

cytotoxic effect of CBL. In vitro, it was demonstrated that the MAb has to be reactive with and bind to tumor target cells for CBL to have an enhanced cytotoxicity (19). Furthermore, not all MAb are effective—the synergistic action of CBL and four different classes of anti-Ly-2.1 MAb on the Ly-2.1$^+$ E3 cell line varied considerably. CBL was 3-5 times more cytotoxic to E3 cells in the presence of either an IgM or IgG2a MAb. By contrast, the IgG1 or IgG3 MAb did not enhance the cytotoxicity of CBL (Fig. 11). In addition, the F(ab$'$)$_2$ fragment of the IgG2a MAb did enhance the cytotoxicity of CBL, demonstrating that this synergistic action is not F_c mediated. In all of the studies of CBL-antibody synergism to date (5,6,20), a saturating amount of antibody has been used, and it was critical to vary the amount of MAb to determine the limiting amount of MAb required for its synergistic action with CBL in preventing tumor growth in vitro. At least 25-50 μg/ml of anti-Ly-2.1 is required for a synergistic action with CBL, and this corresponds to a minimum saturating concentration of anti-Ly-2.1 MAb on 10^5 E3 cells (50 μg/ml) (Fig. 12).

In other studies (19) it was found that specific binding of the MAb to the cell was essential for the synergistic action of CBL and MAb and that the MAb did not have to be internalized for noncovalent CBL-MAb conjugates to exert their cytotoxic action (19), thus the synergy of CBL and MAb at 4°C—a temperature at which endocytosis is prevented was examined. The reduction in temperature did not prevent the synergistic action of CBL and anti-Ly-2.1 (250 or 500 μg/ml) or the cytotoxicity of free CBL (Fig. 13), suggesting that internalization of the anti-Ly-2.1 MAb was not a prerequisite for its synergistic action with CBL.

F. Mode of Action of Drug-MAb Conjugates

1. Chlorambucil-MAb Conjugates

It was clear that the cytotoxic action of CBL-MAb conjugates involved specific binding of antibody, internalization, and lysosomal degradation (21). These studies involved inhibition of conjugate cytotoxicity using free MAb, inhibi-

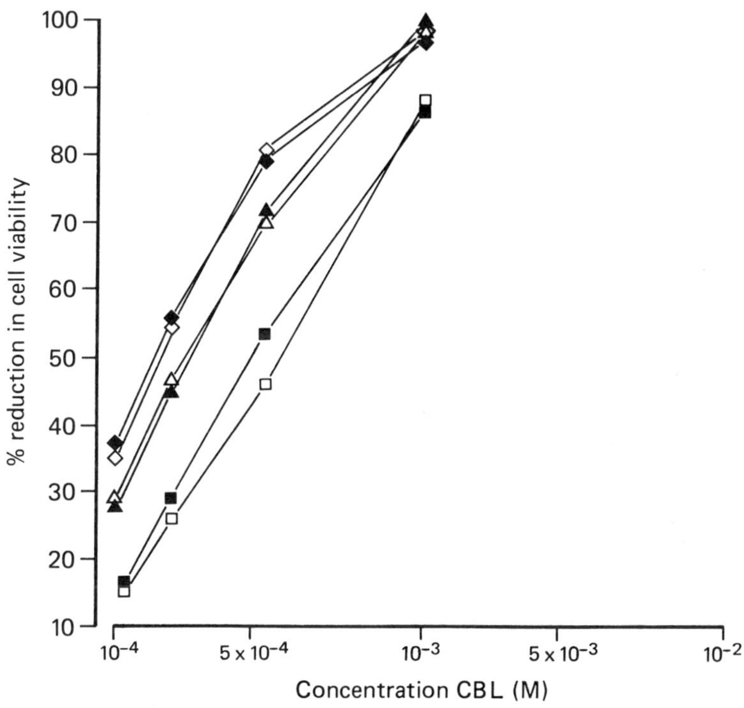

Figure 13 The percentage reduction in tumor cell viability using the temperature dependence assay for CBL at 4°C (□) and 37°C (■), CBL plus 50 μg anti-Ly-2.1 (IgG2a) at 4°C (△) and 37°C (▲), and CBL plus 100 μg anti-Ly-2.1 (IgG2a) at 4°C (◇) and 37°C (◆).

tion of lysosomal degradation and cytotoxicity using NH_4Cl and chloroquine, and inhibition of endocytosis and cytotoxicity using 2-deoxyglucose (2-dG) and sodium azide.

2. N-acetyl Melphalan-MAb Conjugates

Detailed study of the mode of cytotoxic action of N-AcMEL-MAb conjugates has yet to be performed, however, it was clear that free MAb was capable of inhibiting the cytotoxicity of the N-AcMEL-MAb conjugate while L-leucine, a competitive inhibitor of MEL active carrier-mediated uptake was unable to reduce the conjugate's cytotoxic effect. When MEL was incubated with 1 mM L-leucine a 25-40% reduction in cytotoxic activity on CEM (transferrin receptor $(TFR)^+$) cells was observed over the MEL concentration range (10^{-5} to 10^{-4} M) (Fig. 14). However, the same concentration of L-leucine was unable to reduce the cytotoxic action of N-AcMEL and N-AcMEL-anti-TFR upon CEM cells, suggesting that both N-AcMEL and N-AcMEL-anti-TFR enter cells by a different mechanism to MEL, the former probably by passive diffusion, and the latter via the TFR receptor.

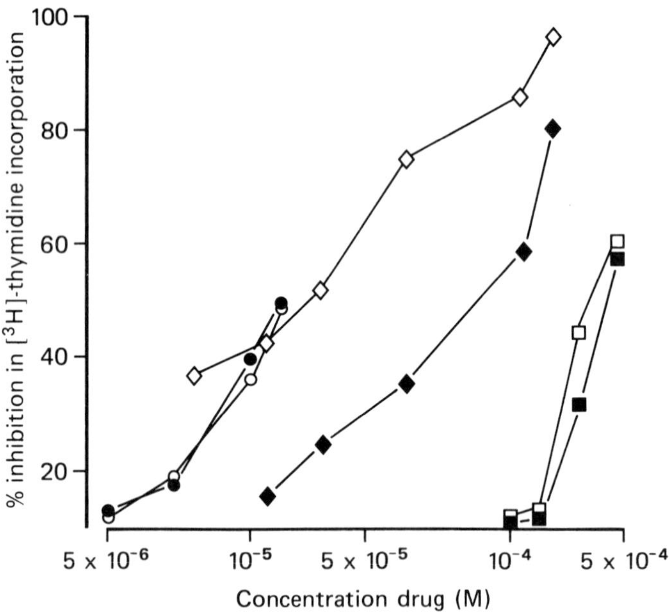

Figure 14 Effect of L-leucine on the sensitivity of CEM cells to MEL (◇), N-AcMEL (□), or N-AcMEL-anti-Ly-2.1 conjugate, 30 mol N-AcMEL/mol of conjugate (○). 1 mM L-leucine not present during exposure (open symbols); 1 mM L-leucine present (closed symbols).

G. In Vivo Efficacy of Drug-MAb Conjugates

As the specificity and cytotoxicity of these drug-MAb conjugates had been fully characterized, an investigation of their antitumor effect in vivo was undertaken. All in vivo experiments were performed with the E3 variant of the murine thymoma ITT(1)75NS, which in vivo is a rapidly proliferating tumor with a doubling time of less than 24 hr; the tumor is Ly-2.1$^+$ but grows rapidly in B6CF$_1$ mice which are Ly-2.2, i.e., the anti-Ly-2.1 MAb reacts only with the tumor.

1. Chlorambucil-MAb Conjugates

In order to demonstrate the in vivo efficacy of CBL-MAb conjugates against peritoneal tumors, groups of 10 B6CF$_1$ mice were given i.p. injections of 10^5 tumor cells. Six hr later the mice were given (i.p.) either PBS, anti-Ly-2.1, CBL, CBL-anti-Ly-2.1 conjugate, or a noncovalent mixture of anti-Ly-2.1 and CBL on days 0, 1, 2, 3, 7, and 13 after tumor inoculation. The average amount of CBL and antibody received per injection was 4 μg and 40 μg, respectively. The PBS-treated mice had a survival time of 20 days, whereas the group that received CBL died after 22 days (Fig. 15). By contrast, 100% of mice treated with covalently linked CBL-anti-Ly-2.1 conjugate (and 80% of mice treated with

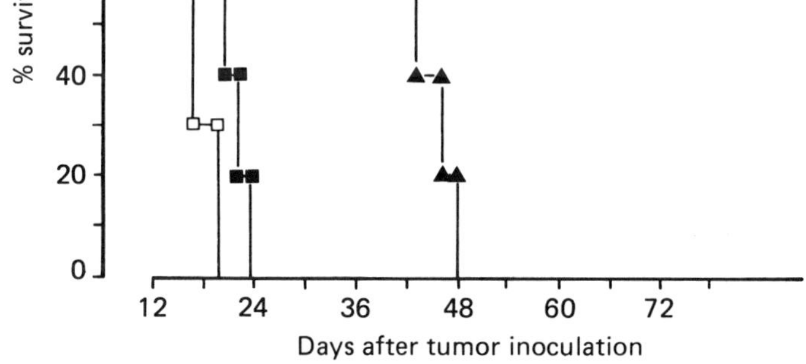

Figure 15 Survivial of B6CF$_1$ mice bearing the ITT(1)75NS E3 tumor. Groups of 10 mice were inoculated (i.p.) with 10^5 cells/mouse; 6 hr later, mice received i.p. PBS (□), free CBL (■), neat anti-Ly-2.1 (▲), noncovalent anti-Ly-2.1 and CBL (○), or CBL-anti-Ly-2.1 conjugate (●).

the noncovalent conjugate) survived tumor-free for more than 200 days—compared to the 48-day survival observed with mice receiving anti-Ly-2.1 MAb alone. In the tumor growth study, groups of 10 B6CF$_1$ mice given a s.c. injection of 2 × 10^6 tumor cells developed a solid tumor 0.3 cm^2 in size, 6 days after inoculation. These mice with established tumors were then given an injection of one of the five treatments listed above. The amount of CBL and anti-Ly-2.1 MAb received per injection was 2 and 20 μg, respectively, on days 6 and 7 after tumor inoculation; on days 8, 9, 12, and 13 this dosage was doubled to 4 μg CBL and 40 μg antibody. Tumor growth was inhibited in mice that had received antibody in their treatments, while tumor growth was unaffected in mice that had been given PBS or CBL alone. By day 15, the mean tumor size of the group receiving CBL-anti-Ly-2.1 conjugate was 60% that of PBS-treated control mice, the conjugate group having significantly smaller tumors than those receiving noncovalently bound CBL-anti-Ly-2.1 or anti-Ly-2.1 alone (Fig. 16).

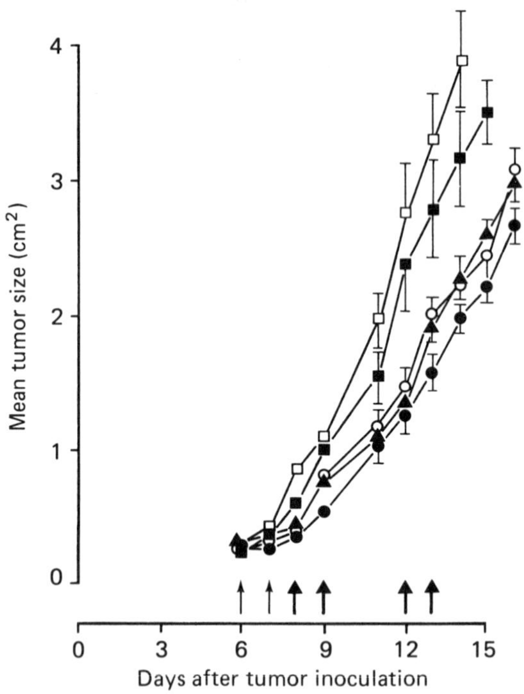

Figure 16 Growth of the thymoma ITT(1)75NS E3 in B6CF$_1$ mice given a s.c. injection of 2 × 10^6 cells [6 days later (tumor size = 0.3 cm^2)]. Groups of 10 mice were given treatments i.p., denoted (↑); PBS (□), free CBL (■), CBL-anti-Ly-2.1 conjugate (●), noncovalently conjugated CBL-anti-Ly-2.1 (○), and anti-Ly-2.1 (▲). Error bars represent ± standard error of the mean.

Thus the CBL-anti-Ly-2.1 conjugate had some effect on tumor growth in the group with solid tumors, however, this was disappointing considering the 100% survival of mice with tumor in the ascites form.

2. N-acetyl Melphalan-MAb and N-acetyl Melphalan-F(ab')$_2$ Conjugates

Groups of 10 B6CF$_1$ mice were given i.p. injections of 3 × 10^5 E3 cells and 4 hr later were given either PBS, MEL, N-AcMEL, a noncovalent conjugate of anti-Ly-2.1 and N-AcMEL, or N-AcMEL-anti-Ly-2.1 conjugate. Each reagent was further administered on day 1 after tumor inoculation: The amount of drug and MAb received per injection was 15 and 150 μg, respectively, with one group of N-AcMEL-anti-Ly-2.1 conjugate mice receiving only 7.5 and 75 μg, respectively. The PBS-treated mice had a survival time of 25 days, while the group receiving N-AcMEL survived 30 days (Fig. 17). By contrast, 90% of the mice treated with a total of 30 μg of N-AcMEL-anti-Ly-2.1 and 30% of the mice treated with 15 μg of conjugate or 30 μg of MEL survived tumor-free for more than 200 days.

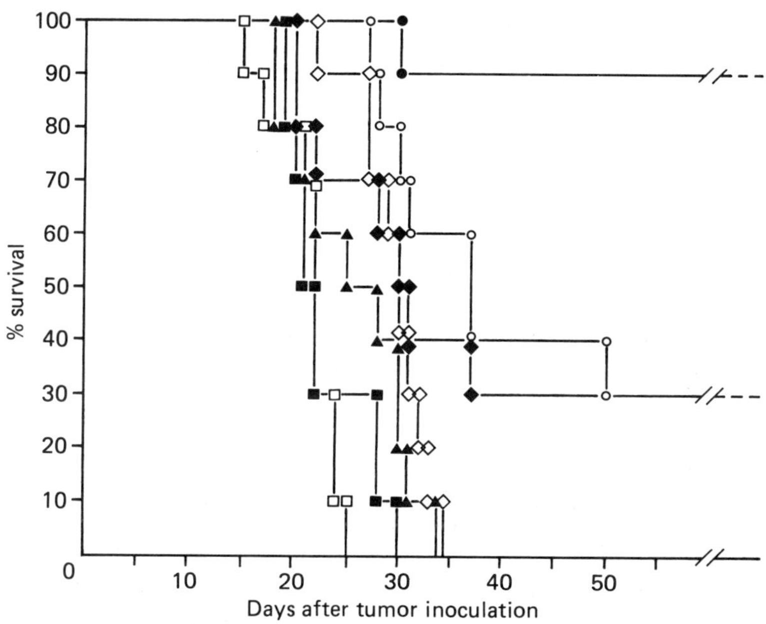

Figure 17 Survival of B6CF$_1$ mice bearing the ITT(1)75NS E3 tumor. Groups of 10 mice were inoculated with 3 × 10^5 cells/mouse; 4 hr later mice received i.p. either PBS (□), free MEL, 30 μg (♦), free N-AcMEL, 30 μg (■), neat anti-Ly-2.1, 300 μg (▲), noncovalently bound anti-Ly-2.1 and N-AcMEL, 30 μg (◇) and N-AcMEL-anti-Ly-2.1 conjugate, 15 μg (○) and 30 μg (●).

These groups survived significantly longer than mice receiving either noncovalently bound N-AcMEL-anti-Ly-2.1 or anti-Ly-2.1 alone, their survival time being only 35 days. Thus N-AcMEL-MAb (covalently bound) and CBL-MAb conjugates (covalently and noncovalently bound) were effective in eradicating peritoneal tumors, thereby prolonging the survival time of the mice. After finding that doses as large as 100 μg of N-AcMEL-anti-Ly-2.1 were required to produce a significant decrease in tumor growth when treatments were administered i.p.(17), we attempted to evaluate the effectiveness of three different sites of delivery (i.p., i.v., and intratumor). Mice carrying a solid E3 tumor (growing s.c.) received injections either i.p. or i.v. on days 4 and 6, or directly into the tumor on days 8 and 9 after tumor inoculation, with either PBS, anti-Ly-2.1, a noncovalent N-AcMEL-anti-Ly-2.1 conjugate, or the covalent N-AcMEL-anti-Ly-2.1 conjugate. The amount of N-AcMEL and anti-Ly-2.1 received per injection was 10 and 100 μg, respectively. As noted previously, those mice receiving antibody in their treatments had smaller tumors than those receiving PBS alone, regardless of the route of administration (Fig. 18). The administration of 20 μg of N-AcMEL demonstrated that the efficacy of i.p. conjugate treatment was limited to high dose therapy, as the mice that received N-AcMEL-anti-Ly-2.1 conjugate did not at any stage have significantly smaller tumors than those receiving either noncovalent N-AcMEL-anti-Ly-2.1 or anti-Ly-2.1 alone (Fig. 18A). However, when treatments were administered i.v., the N-AcMEL-anti-Ly-2.1 conjugate-treated mice had a 70% slower rate of tumor growth (days 8 to 15) than PBS-treated mice, while mice receiving anti-Ly-2.1 alone or noncovalently bound N-AcMEL-anti-Ly-2.1 had tumor growth rates similar to PBS-treated mice (Fig. 18B). Mice receiving N-AcMEL-anti-Ly-2.1 conjugate directly into the tumor had smaller tumors than those given intratumor injections of the other reagents (Fig. 18C).

Considering the promising results and greater utility of i.v. delivery, higher doses of N-AcMEL-anti-Ly-2.1 conjugate were tested to assess the limitations of N-AcMEL-MAb conjugates in this model; N-AcMEL-F(ab′)$_2$ were also tested. Mice with solid E3 tumors growing s.c. received (on days 3, 5, and 6 after tumor inoculation) either PBS, anti-Ly-2.1, MEL, N-AcMEL-anti-TFR (as a negative control), N-AcMEL-anti-Ly-2.1-F(ab′)$_2$, or N-AcMEL-anti-Ly-2.1. The amount of drug administered was 8 μg on day 3, 15 μg on day 5, and 7 μg on day 6 (i.e., a total of 30 μg). As previously noted, those mice receiving N-AcMEL and anti-Ly-2.1 in their treatments had smaller tumors than those receiving PBS, MEL, or antibody alone (Fig. 19). By day 11 the mean tumor size of F(ab′)$_2$ conjugate-treated mice was 15% that of PBS-treated mice and 20% that of N-AcMEL-anti-TFR-treated mice. The individual tumor growth curves of F(ab′)$_2$ conjugate-treated mice revealed that 9/10 of the mice demonstrated a reduction in tumor size during the treatment period (day 5 to 6), and five of these tumor completely regressed and did not redevelop (Fig. 20). At

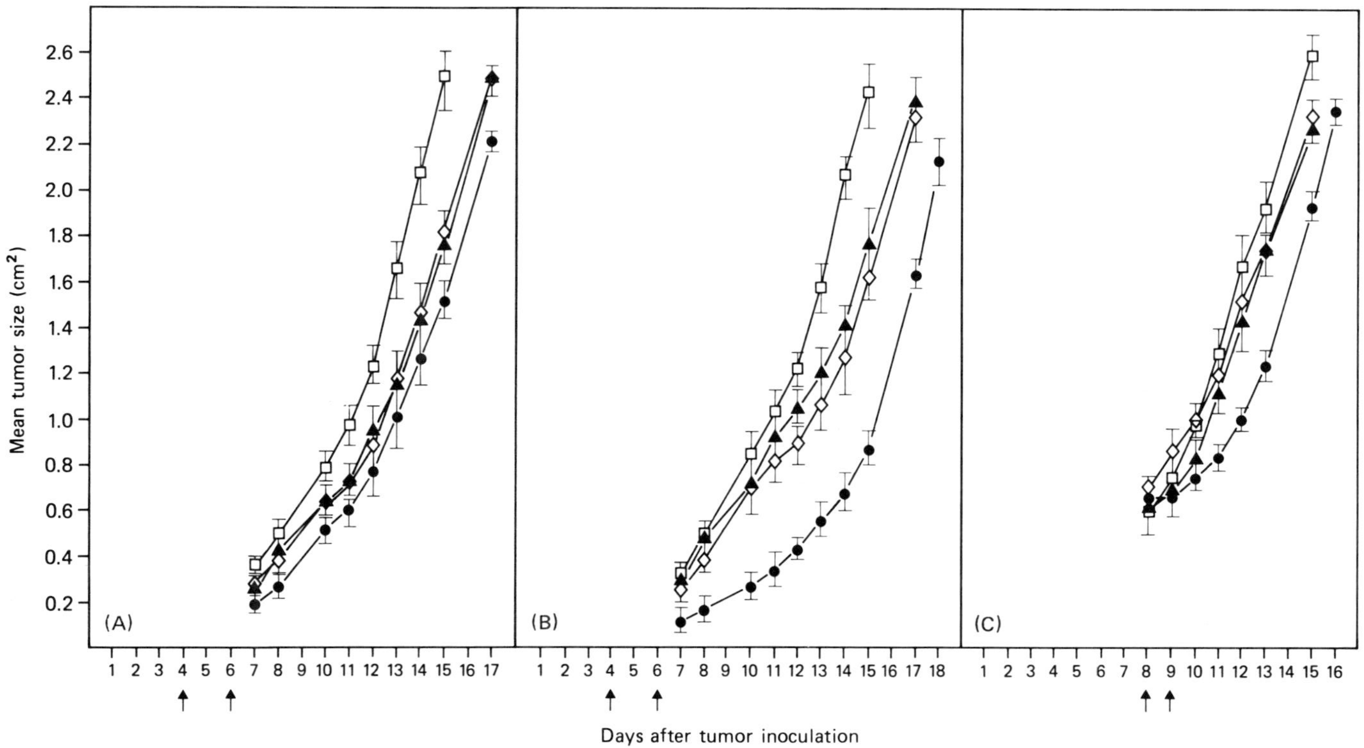

Figure 18 Growth of the thymoma ITT(1)75NS E3 in $B6CF_1$ mice given injections s.c. of 2×10^6 cells. Groups of 10 mice were given the following treatments, denoted (↑): PBS (□), anti-Ly-2.1 (▲), N-AcMEL-anti-Ly-2.1 conjugate (●) and noncovalently conjugated N-AcMEL-anti-Ly-2.1 (◇) either i.p. (A), i.v. (B), or into the tumor (C). Points, mean tumor diameter, bars, SE.

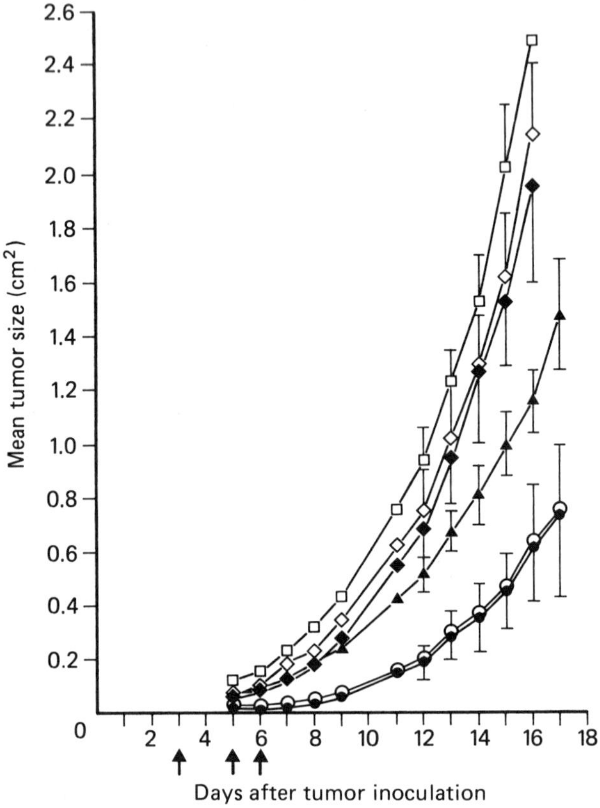

Figure 19 Growth of the thymoma ITT(1)75NS E3 in CBF_1 mice injected s.c. with 2×10^6 cells. Groups of 10 mice were given the following treatments i.v., denoted (↑): PBS (□), free MEL (♦), N-AcMEL-F(ab')$_2$ conjugate (●), N-AcMEL-anti-Ly-2.1 IgG conjugate (○), N-AcMEL-anti-TFR conjugate (◇), and anti-Ly-2.1 (▲). Error bars represent ± standard error of the mean tumor size.

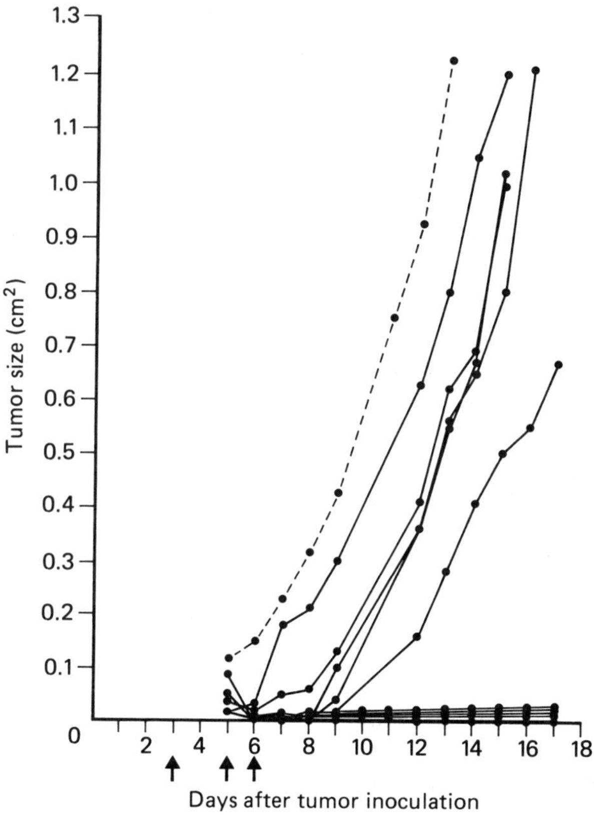

Figure 20 Individual tumor growth curves of B6CF$_1$ mice injected s.c. with 2×10^6 ITT(1)75NS E3 tumor cells and treated i.v. (↑) on days 3, 5, and 6 with N-AcMEL-F(ab′)$_2$ conjugate. The broken line represents the mean tumor size of PBS-treated mice.

the termination of F(ab′)$_2$ conjugate treatment the remaining four tumors began to increase in size, growing at variable rates, all slower than the mean growth rate of PBS-treated mice. In the group treated with N-AcMEL-IgG (anti-Ly-2.1) conjugate, 4/10 of the tumors were completely eradicated (data not shown). By varying the tumor cell number and treatment schedule in several other experiments, we were unable to demonstrate a major difference in the in vivo efficacy of the N-AcMEL-IgG conjugate and the F(ab′)$_2$ conjugate.

III. DISCUSSION

The specificity, monoclonality, and unlimited source of MAb makes them ideal vehicles for carrying toxins and drugs to tumor cells. However, a number of limitations exist which hinder the use of drug-MAb conjugates, such as modification of drug and MAb activity following the coupling procedure and an inability to deliver large amounts of drug to the tumor due to chemical and physical barriers.

With the production of MAb with high tumor reactivity, toxic agents such as isotopes, antibiotics, plant toxins, and antimetabolites have been coupled and targeted both in vitro and in vivo (22). Considerable research has been performed with ricin-antibody conjugates, which appear valuable for the in vitro treatment of bone marrow cells, but because of their broad reactivity cannot be used safely in vivo unless they are chemically modified (23). By contrast, fewer studies have researched the use of drug-MAb conjugates because most drugs are complex organic molecules that are coupled to antibodies with difficulty (2,3, 24). For example, we have recently coupled Doxorubicin (2) and Methotrexate (1) to MAb, and although the drug-MAb conjugates were specific, they only had one-tenth of the activity of the free drug. By contrast, CBL-MAb conjugates were highly specific and had greater in vitro and in vivo antitumor activity than *free drug* or MAb alone. The major difference between CBL and the other drugs was the ability to couple large amounts of CBL (up to 30 molecules CBL/molecule MAb) to the MAb to produce a conjugate with greater potency and specificity than free CBL. The reason why CBL and N-AcMEL are more readily coupled to MAb than other antineoplastic drugs is not clear, but it may be that these alkylating agents are smaller and less hydrophobic than the majority of chemotherapeutic agents.

Using N-hydroxysuccinimide (NHS) to produce an active ester derivative of CBL, 15-30 molecules of CBL could be incorporated per molecule of MAb with good retention of antibody activity and protein recovery. The CBL-anti-Ly-2.1 conjugate was shown to retain the cytotoxic effect of CBL, increasing the 24-hr antitumor activity of bound CBL to five times that of an equimolar amount of free CBL (Fig. 5). With the specific in vitro (and in vivo) binding of CBL-MAb to target cells, the conjugate exhibited cytotoxicity only to Ly-2^+ cells (Fig. 7), which could be inhibited by a competing anti-Ly-2.1 MAb (Fig. 9). The cytotoxicity was partially dependent on the antigen density on the target cells; and the Ly-2^{high} E3 cell line was found to be five times more susceptible to the cytotoxic activity of the CBL-anti-Ly-2.1 conjugate than was the Ly-2^{low} D1 cell line (Fig. 8). In vivo the survival times of mice inoculated with the murine E3 tumor clearly demonstrated that CBL, covalently or noncovalently bound to MAb, was a more effective tumor inhibitor than free CBL or antibody alone (Fig. 15)—indeed these conjugates were able to cure mice bearing tumors in the ascites form. This however is somewhat analogous to the in vitro treatment of tumor cells, and more stringent tests against established solid tumors demonstrated that the efficacy of these conjugates was far from satisfactory. No difference was observed in the in vivo efficacy of noncovalently and covalently bound CBL-anti-Ly-2.1 conjugates, and it appears from other studies (6) that even separately administered CBL and antibody can be equally effective. It would appear therefore that a strong affinity exists between CBL and antibody which prevents rapid dissociation in vivo and results in noncovalently bound CBL-MAb having a marked antitumor effect.

On the basis of our study and others (20,25), we envisage two possible explanations for the synergy of CBL and antibody. The first proposes that the specific binding of the MAb at saturating levels triggers an increased cell membrane permeability to CBL, however, the uptake of [^{3}H]-CBL by immune serum-treated cells was not different from that of control serum-treated cells (20). The second involves a protein-drug interaction, whereby the reactive MAb concentrates the CBL on the surface of the target cell, enabling it to structurally damage the cell membrane by alkylation; however, the exact nature of this CBL-MAb interaction remains doubtful.

Considering the favorable aspects of CBL-MAb conjugates (i.e., high drug: MAb coupling ratios and increased cytotoxicity over free drug), we reasoned that a greater effectiveness against solid tumors could be achieved by using more potent alkylating agents, such as MEL. In this case the studies are of interest and differ from previous studies of the coupling of alkylating agents to antibodies in several ways. To reduce the nonspecific toxicity of MEL, the MEL was initially rendered 100 times less toxic by blocking its normal mode of entry into cells. This was done by modifying the amino group of MEL to form an N-acetyl derivative of the drug (i.e., to produce a prodrug). This N-AcMEL derivative has two advantages compared with MEL: it is nontoxic and its active ester can easily be coupled to MAb. The N-AcMEL is conveyed to tumor cells by the MAb and probably enters the cell by endocytosis of the conjugate; the N-AcMEL-MAb conjugate therefore has little systemic toxicity simply because N-AcMEL has a reduced cytotoxicity, and only upon entry into the cell and cleavage from the MAb does N-AcMEL become as active as MEL itself.

As with CBL, the N-AcMEL active ester was successfully coupled to MAb and conjugates of up to 30 molecules of N-AcMEL per molecule of MAb were obtained which retained 50-80% of the MAb activity. The N-AcMEL-anti-Ly-2.1 (IgG1) conjugate was demonstrated to increase the antitumor activity of bound N-AcMEL to 40-50 times that of an equimolar amount of free N-AcMEL (Fig. 6). The antibody-binding activity of these N-AcMEL-MAb conjugates clearly resulted in their selective cytotoxicity (Fig. 10) in which the N-AcMEL-anti-Ly-2.1 conjugate displayed cytotoxicity only to Ly-2$^+$ cells. In addition, the cytotoxic effect the N-AcMEL-anti-Ly-2.1 conjugate had on E3 target cells was reduced by 80% on addition of anti-Ly-2.1, and L-leucine, a competitive inhibitor of MEL uptake, was unable to protect E3 cells from the cytotoxic action of N-AcMEL-anti-Ly-2.1 conjugate (Fig. 14). Thus it appears feasible that the internalized N-AcMEL of N-AcMEL-MAb conjugates is broken down by the lysosomes to release the more active MEL molecule.

The in vivo efficacy of the N-AcMEL-anti-Ly-2.1 conjugate was investigated in several tumor models using different modes of administration. The survival times of mice inoculated i.p. with murine E3 tumor clearly demonstrate that N-AcMEL covalently bound to anti-Ly-2.1 is a more effective tumor inhibitor than free N-AcMEL, N-AcMEL noncovalently bound to anti-Ly-2.1, or anti-Ly-2.1 alone (Fig. 17). Although MEL alone enabled 30% of the mice to survive tumor-free for >200 days, its use would be hindered by its narrow therapeutic range (>100 μg is toxic to a mouse), and therefore N-AcMEL-anti-Ly-2.1 conjugate treatment is comparatively safer and more efficacious. More critical tumor growth models using subcutaneously growing established tumors demonstrated that N-AcMEL-anti-Ly-2.1 was the most effective tumor inhibitor (Fig. 18A-C) and that intravenous delivery was the best route of administration, however, further experiments in which treatments are administered at an earlier stage are required to accurately assess the value of intratumor treatment. Intratumor therapy is a limited technique, applicable to tumors which cannot be resected; intravenous therapy is more applicable and consequently additional experiments were undertaken in which greater doses of N-AcMEL-anti-Ly-2.1 conjugate were administered i.v. and their in vivo efficacy compared to that of N-AcMEL-anti-Ly-2.1 $F(ab')_2$ conjugates.

In vitro the N-AcMEL-$F(ab')_2$ conjugate was demonstrated to be equally cytotoxic and specific for Ly-2^+ target cells as the N-AcMEL-anti-Ly-2.1 IgG conjugate. In vivo, however, $F(ab')_2$ fragments would have several advantages as carriers of N-AcMEL. An important feature of $F(ab')_2$ fragments is their inability to bind Fc receptors on macrophages and Kupffer cells, which should therefore limit conjugate accumulation in the liver and the reticuloendothelial system. Also, due to their smaller size, $F(ab')_2$ conjugates should more easily penetrate the capillary network of a tumor. Surprisingly, by varying the tumor cell number and treatment schedule in several tumor growth experiments, we were unable to demonstrate a major difference in the in vivo efficacy of the N-AcMEL-IgG conjugate and the $F(ab')_2$ conjugate. It was shown that *small* established subcutaneous tumors could be eradicated using multiple doses (total = 30 μg) of N-AcMEL-anti-Ly-2.1 IgG or N-AcMEL-$F(ab')_2$ conjugate (Fig. 19). Individual tumor growth curves demonstrated that 9/10 of the tumors treated with $F(ab')_2$ conjugate (Fig. 20) were reduced in size, and five of these tumors were completely eradicated. Similar individual profiles were observed for N-AcMEL-anti-Ly-2.1 IgG-treated mice (data not shown). This suggests, therefore, that the shorter half-life (faster clearance) may balance the advantage of the $F(ab')_2$ conjugate treatment (less nonspecific binding) such that neither conjugate is more effective than the other. It is not clear which of these properties of MAb is the most important when delivering cytotoxic drugs to tumors, however the lower immunogenicity of $F(ab')_2$ fragments compared with whole IgG and the similar cytotoxicity of their conjugates suggests that the $F(ab')_2$ conjugates may have greater potential for clinical use.

It appears that the in vitro and in vivo properties of CBL and N-AcMEL were similar when covalently coupled to MAb, and both have greater in vitro and in vivo antitumor activity than free drug. Further, it is likely that both of these conjugates are endocytosed and degraded within the lysosomes of the tumor cell. In relation to other reported drug-MAb conjugates (1-3,23), CBL-MAb and N-AcMEL-MAb conjugates compare favorably. Unlike toxin-MAb conjugates (e.g., whole Ricin (26)), the intravenous use of which is hampered by the nonspecific interaction of the B chain with normal cells (via mannose receptors), CBL-MAb and N-AcMEL-MAb conjugates have demonstrated no sign of nonspecific toxicity (for doses of up to 16 mg/kg), and they are not subject to rapid reticuloendothelial clearance. In addition, the production, purification, and cost of CBL-MAb and N-AcMEL-MAb conjugates are minimal compared to those involved in synthesizing Ricin-MAb or Daunomycin-MAb conjugates—and because a large number of molecules can be incorporated there is no need for the use of intermediary carriers or spacers (22). Problems with CBL-MAb and N-AcMEL-MAb conjugates do exist, however, which are either unique to alkylating agents or common to all drug-MAb conjugates. In contrast to toxins (one molecule is sufficient to kill a cell), alkylating agents do not offer the greatest chance of killing tumor cell populations that have a low density of cell surface antigens. In addition, a definitive study of the stability of these conjugates in plasma is necessary considering the potential hydrolysis of the chloroethyl (alkylating) groups of the drug. This may be a major limitation in the intravenous use of these drug-MAb conjugates, and, consequently, continuous infusion may be required to improve this type of immunochemotherapy.

Generally, tumor accessibility, heterogeneity, and the development of an immune response to drug-MAb conjugates are problems which still must be surmounted. The use of "cocktails" of drug-MAb conjugates recognizing different antigens on target cells, or combination therapy of nontoxic doses of another antineoplastic agent in conjunction with these drug-MAb conjugates may overcome the problem of heterogeneity. Also, the production of human MAb, while still in its earliest stages, has had a measure of success (27) and improvements in fusion techniques should increase the availability of such reagents in the future. With the current appraisal of drug-MAb conjugates for the treatment of cancer, there is a need for studies to determine the causes of poor tumor accessibility and to uncover methods of improving tumor localization by MAb.

This is readily apparent when one considers that N-AcMEL-MAb conjugates represent an advance in drug-MAb conjugate development by virtue of their ability to completely eradicate small (0.20 cm^2) subcutaneous solid tumors, yet the removal of larger tumors remains beyond the limit of current immunochemotherapy.

IV. APPENDIX

A. Tumor Cells

EL4 (28) BW5147, BW5147 OU^- (oubain resistant) (29), E2, E3, and D1 clonal variants of the murine thymoma ITT(1)75NS (12) and the human T cell leukemia CEM (30) were used. The murine cell lines were maintained in vitro in DME or RPMI (CEM), supplemented with 10% heat-activated newborn calf serum (Flow Laboratories, Sydney, Australia), 2 mM glutamine (Commonwealth Serum Laboratories, Melbourne, Australia), 100 IU penicillin/ml (Commonwealth Serum Laboratories), and 100 μg/ml streptomycin (Glaxo Laboratories, Melbourne). For in vivo experiments E3 was maintained by serial passage in the ascites form in (C57BL/6 $\times$ BALB/c) F_1 ($B6CF_1$) mice; cells from the ascites fluid were washed and centrifuged (400 $\times$ *g*, 5 min) twice in DME in PBS (pH 7.3), resuspended in PBS and injected s.c. or i.p. into $B6CF_1$ mice.

B. Mice

$B6CF_1$ mice were produced in the Department of Pathology, University of Melbourne.

C. MAb

MAb used in this study were (a) anti-Ly-2.1, reactive with murine Ly-2.1 specificity (murine IgG2a unless specified) (31) and (b) A3C6 (anti-TFR), reactive with the human transferrin receptor (murine IgG1) (17). The MAb were isolated from ascitic fluid by precipitation with 40% ammonium sulfate, dissolution in PBS, and dialysis with the same buffer. These crude preparations were either adsorbed onto Protein A-Sepharose (Pharmacia Inc., Piscataway, NJ), washed extensively in PBS (pH 7.3), and eluted with 0.2 M glycine-HC1 (pH 2.8); or passed through an Affigel blue column (Bio-Rad Laboratories, Sydney, Australia) and eluted with PBS. Following neutralization, MAb were dialyzed against PBS, aliquoted, and stored.

D. Preparation of $F(ab')_2$ by Pepsin Degradation

The optimal conditions for the degradation of IgG1 for the preparation of $F(ab')_2$ fragments of the anti-Ly-2.1 MAb (IgG1) were 0.1 M citrate, pH 3.8 at

37°C for 6-8 hr using IgG concentrations of 1 to 2 mg/ml and pepsin concentrations of 25 μg/ml (32). Intact IgG was removed using Protein A-Sepharose (Pharmacia), and each preparation was calculated for yield (>80%) and characterized by polyacrylamide gel electrophoresis under reducing and nonreducing conditions.

E. Preparation of N-acetyl Melphalan

A suspension of MEL (200 mg) in dry DMF (1.5 ml) was treated with acetic anhydride (68 μl) and stirred for 1 hr and then a further aliquot of acetic anhydride (68 μl) was added and stirred for 3 hr when a clear solution was obtained. The reaction mixture was then poured into water and extracted with dichloromethane, and the extract was washed with water and dried over anhydrous sodium sulfate. Evaporation of the dichloromethane yielded an oil which was triturated with ether, and the resulting solid (62% yield) was recrystallized using dichloromethane ether. Thin layer chromatography on silica gel plates (DC-Plastik-tolien Kieselgel 60F 287; Merck) using chloroform:methanol (2:1) indicated only one spot ($R_f = 0.35$), indicating that a pure sample of N-AcMEL had been produced.

F. Preparation and Quantitation of Conjugates

An active ester of CBL or N-AcMEL was prepared by dissolving 5.0 mg of CBL or N-AcMEL in 100 μl of DMF and NHS (2.2 mg in 200 μl of DMF) added, followed by N, N-dicyclohexylcarbodiimide (3.9 mg in 200 μl of DMF). The reaction mixture was left at room temperature for 1 hr and for 18 hr at 4°C (it was discarded after 4 weeks if unused). A solution (10 to 50 μl) of CBL or N-AcMEL active ester (1.5 to 7.0 mmol) in DMF was added to 0.5 to 1.0 ml solution containing 0.5 to 2.0 mg of affinity purified MAb or its $F(ab')_2$ fragment, the mixture was reacted for 1 hr at room temperature and any precipitated protein was removed by centrifugation. Free drug and other unreacted starting materials were removed by gel filtration (Sephadex G-25, PD-10 Pharmacia). The amount of drug incorporated in the drug-MAb conjugate was determined by absorbance spectrophotometry at 258 nm (E_{258} N-AcMEL = $1 \times 10^4\ M^{-1}\ cm^{-1}$) after subtracting the protein contribution following its estimation by the Bradford dye-binding assay (33). The alkylating activity of the conjugate was determined by a modification of the Epstein Method (34). For noncovalent conjugates a 10 to 50 μl solution of CBL or N-AcMEL in DMF was mixed with MAb producing a noncovalently associated drug-MAb complex, which was also purified by gel filtration on a PD-10 column. Free drug was prepared by dissolution in 0.5 M $NaHCO_3$.

G. Antibody Activity

A rosetting assay (35) was used to determine the antibody activity of the drug-antibody conjugates and this was compared to the activity of free antibody that had undergone the same procedures used in the coupling method. In addition the antibody activity of N-AcMEL-$F(ab')_2$ conjugates was compared with whole IgG1 and $F(ab')_2$ fragments in a competitive binding assay using radiolabeled whole IgG1 MAb. In this assay doubling dilutions were performed using 25 μl of anti-Ly-2.1, 25 μl of $F(ab')_2$ conjugate, or 25 μl $F(ab')_2$ anti-Ly-2.1 in a 96-well round-bottom plate, and to these 25 μl of ^{125}I-anti-Ly-2.1 was added; 50 μl of E3 target cells (1 -5 $\times$ 10^6/ml) were then added and incubated for 30 min before washing (x3) in PBS and counting individual samples in a gamma counter. It should be noted that control wells did not include 25 μl of "cold" antibody or conjugate and results were counted as the percentage reduction in ^{125}I-anti-Ly-2.1 binding of control samples.

H. Drug Activity

Two assays were performed to assess drug activity. They differed in the time the drug-MAb conjugate was in contact with the cells (24 hr or 30 min).

1. 24-hr Assay

This assay was designed to determine whether drugs had an increased, similar, or reduced cytotoxicity when coupled to MAb. One hundred μl of cells (1-5 $\times$ 10^6/ml) was added to a 96-well flat-bottom microtiter plate and incubated for 2-3 hr at 37°C. Antibody, free drug, and drug-antibody conjugates were filtered through a 0.2 μm Millipore filter to ensure sterility, and dilutions were performed in sterile PBS; 50 μl of antibody, free drug, or conjugate was added to the cells with the use of duplicate wells per sample; control wells received 50 μl of medium or PBS, and the cells were cultured at 37°C in 7% CO_2 atmosphere for 24 hr. As a variation of this procedure, to assess the synergy of CBL and anti-Ly-2.1 MAb, different amounts and different subclasses of the anti-Ly-2.1 MAb (50 μl) were added after 50 μl of CBL had been added to the E3 target cells. Similarly, inhibition by L-leucine was performed as in the 24-hr assay (above), except that cells were incubated in the presence or absence of 1 mM L-leucine over the 24-hr period.

2. 30-min Assay

This assay was designed to determine the specificity of drug-MAb conjugates after a brief exposure to tumor cells. Two hundred μl of cells (1-5 $\times$ 10^6/ml) was collected in sterile plastic centrifuge tubes, resuspended in sterile drug, antibody, or conjugate and mixed for 30 min at 37°C. The cells were centrifuged (400 *g* $\times$ 5 min) and then resuspended in growth medium; cells (100 μl) were then seeded into a microtiter plate using duplicate wells for each sample and incubated for 16-24 hr. To assess the inhibition of conjugate cytotoxicity by "cold" antibody, cells were preincubated with 100 μg of free MAb before following the 30-min assay procedure.

After the incubation period in the above assays, 50 μl of medium containing 1 μCi of [^{3}H]-thymidine (sp act = 15 Ci/mmol; Amersham International Ltd., Amersham, England) was added, and the plates were incubated for 3-6 hr. Cells were then harvested onto a glass fiber filter paper with the use of a cell harvester and dried for 10 min at 80°C, and individual samples were separated and counted on a beta counter (Tri Carb 460C; Packard Instrument Co., La Grange, IL). Incorporation of [^{3}H]-thymidine was expressed as a percentage inhibition in incorporation of controls (growth inhibition was similar to cell cytotoxicity as measured by the in vitro uptake of trypan blue). The standard error for any given point was generated by multiple determinations and did not exceed 5% for any point.

3. Temperature Dependence Assay

To investigate the entry of drugs and MAb into cells their cytotoxicity was examined at 4°C, a temperature at which the endocytotic mechanisms of the cell are prevented. Five hundred μl of cells (1-5 $\times$ 10^6/ml) were added to a 24-well flat-bottom plate and incubated for 2 hr at 4°C or 37°C. Five hundred μl of CBL or CBL and MAb (250-500 μg/ml) were added to the cells using duplicate wells/sample; control wells received 500 μl medium ± MAb. Cells were left at 4°C or 37°C for 6 hr, 25 μl of each sample was removed and added to an equal volume of aniline blue solution. The number of viable cells was counted in a Neubauer hemocytometer and the result expressed as a percentage reduction in the viability relative to the control samples.

I. In Vivo Experiments

1. Survival Study

This experiment was principally designed to determine the drug-MAb conjugates' ability to eradicate ascites tumor cells in vivo. Tumor cells were injected i.p. into mice, and 4 or 6 hr later a series of i.p. treatments were begun. The percentage of mice in each group which survived was recorded.

2. Tumor Growth

Tumor cells were injected s.c. into the abdominal wall and were allowed to develop into palpable tumors before commencing treatment. Mice were then subjected to a series of i.p. treatments, and the size of the tumors was measured daily with a caliper square measuring along the perpendicular axes of the tumors; the data were recorded as a mean tumor size (products of two diameters ± SE).

Experimental groups of 8 to 10 mice, all of the same sex and age, were used in each experiment; and individual mice could be monitored for the size of their tumors.

ABBREVIATIONS

MAb	Monoclonal antibody(ies)
CBL	Chlorambucil
MEL	Melphalan
N-AcMEL	N-Acetyl Melphalan
PBS	Phosphate Buffered Saline
2-dG	2-Deoxyglucose
DME	Dulbecco's Modified Eagles Medium
NHS	N-Hydroxysuccinimide
i.p.	Intraperitoneal(ly)
i.v.	Intravenous(ly)
s.c.	Subcutaneous(ly)

ACKNOWLEDGMENTS

The authors wish to thank Mimi Morgan, Ruth Godding, and Antoinette Gentile for their secretarial assistance. We also thank: Journal of the National Cancer Institute for Figures 2, 3, 5, 7, 8, 9, 15, and 16; British Journal of Cancer for Figures 4, 6, 19, and 20; Cancer Research for Figures 10, 14, 17, and 18, and the Journal of Immunology for Figures 11, 12, and 13.

REFERENCES

1. Kanellos, J., Pietersz, G. A., and McKenzie, I. F. C. (1985) Studies of Methotrexate-monoclonal antibody conjugates for immunotherapy. *J. Natl. Cancer Inst. 75*:319-332.
2. Pietersz, G. A., Zalcberg, J. R., and McKenzie, I.F. C. The use of adriamycin-monoclonal antibody complexes for specific anti-tumor activity. Unpublished data.
3. Hurwitz, E., Levy, R., Maron, R., et al. (1975) The covalent binding of daunomycin and adriamycin to antibodies with retention of both drug and antibody activities. *Cancer Res. 35*:1175-1178.
4. Ghose, T., and Blair, A. H. (1978) Antibody-linked cytotoxic agents in the treatment of cancer. *J. Natl. Cancer Inst. 61*:657-676.
5. Ghose, T., and Nigam, S. P. (1972) Antibody as carrier of chlorambucil. *Cancer 29*:1398-1400.
6. Davies, D. A. L., and O'Neill, G. J. (1973) In vivo and in vitro effects of tumor specific antibodies with chlorambucil. *Br. J. Cancer 28*:285-298.

7. Ross, W. C. J. (1975) The conjugation of chlorambucil with human γ-globulin. *Chem. Biol. Interactions 10*:169-172.
8. Rowland, G. F. (1977) Effective anti-tumor conjugates of alkylating drug and antibody using dextran as the intermediate carrier. *Eur. J. Cancer 13*: 593-596.
9. Rowland, G. F., O'Neill, G. J., and Davies, D. A. L. (1975) Suppression of tumor growth in mice by a drug-antibody conjugate using a novel approach to linkage. *Nature 255*:487-488.
10. Ghose, T., Norvell, S. T., Guclu, A., Cameron, D., Bodurtha, A., Tai, J., and McDonald, A. S. (1977) Immunochemotherapy of malignant melanoma with chlorambucil-bound antimelanoma globulins: Preliminary results in patients with disseminated disease. *J. Natl. Cancer Inst. 58*:845-852.
11. Melino, G., Forrest, D. M., and Castello, M. A. (1984) 32nd Annual Colloquium, Protides of the Biological Fluids, Brussels.
12. Smyth, M. J., Pietersz, G. A., Classon, B. J., and McKenzie, I. F. C. (1986) Specific targeting of chlorambucil to tumors with the use of monoclonal antibodies. *J. Natl. Cancer Inst. 76*:503-510.
13. Vistica, D. T., Rabon, A., and Rabinovitz, M. (1979) Amino acid conferred protection against melphalan: interference with melphalan therapy by L-leucine, a competitive substrate for transport. *Cancer Lett. 6*:7-13.
14. Garnett, M. C., Jacobs, E., Embleton, M. J., and Baldwin, R. W. (1984) Studies on the mechanism of action of a drug-carrier-antibody conjugate. *Biochem. Soc. Trans. 12*:1035-1036.
15. Smyth, M. J., Pietersz, G. A., and McKenzie, I. F. C. (1987) The mode of action of methotrexate-monoclonal antibody conjugates. *Immunol. Cell Biol. 65*:189-200.
16. Brent, L., Horsburgh, T., Rowland, G., and Wood, P. (1980) Failure to increase the in vivo immunosuppressive activity of anti-lymphocyte globulin by conjugation with melphalan. *Transplantation 29*:280-282.
17. Smyth, M. J., Pietersz, G. A., and McKenzie, I. F. C. (1987) Selective enhancement of antitumor activity of N-acetyl melphalan upon conjugation to monoclonal antibodies. *Cancer Res. 47*:62-69.
18. Smyth, M. J., Pietersz, G. A., and McKenzie, I. F. C. (1987) The in vitro and in vivo antitumor activity of N-AcMEL-F$(ab')_2$ conjugates. *Br. J. Cancer 55*:7-11.
19. Smyth, M. J., Pietersz, G. A., and McKenzie, I. F. C. (1986) Potentiation of the in vitro cytotoxicity of chlorambucil by monoclonal antibodies. *J. Immunol. 137*:3361-3366.
20. Rubens, R. D., and Dulbecco, R. (1974) Augmentation of cytotoxic drug action by antibodies directed at cell surface. *Nature 248*:81-82.
21. Smyth, M. J., Pietersz, G. A., and McKenzie, I. F. C. (1987) The cellular uptake and cytotoxicity of chlorambucil-monoclonal antibody conjugates. *Immunol. Cell Biol. 65*: 315-321.
22. Ghose, T., Blair, A. H., and Kulkarni, P, (1983) Preparation of antibody linked cytotoxic agents. *Methods Enzymol. 93*:280-333.

23. Vitetta, E. S., Krolick, K. A., Miyama-Inaba, M., et al. (1983) Immunotoxins: A new approach to cancer therapy. *Science 219*:644-650.
24. Embleton, M. J., Rowland, G. F., Simmonds, R. G., et al. (1983) Selective cytotoxicity against human tumor cells by a vindesine-monoclonal antibody conjugate. *Br. J. Cancer 47*:43-49.
25. Tung, E., Goust, J. M., Chen, W. Y., Kang, S. S., Wang, I. Y., and Wang, A. C. (1983) Cytotoxic effect of anti-idiotype antibody-chlorambucil conjugates against human lymphoblastoid cells. *Immunology 50*:57-64.
26. Pietersz, G. A., Kanellos, J., and McKenzie, I. F. C. (1986) The use of whole ricin-antibody conjugates for the treatment of tumors in mice. In: Membrane Mediated Cytotoxicity. UCLA Symposia on Molecular and Cellular Biology. New Series. Vol. 45. (B. Bonavida and R. J. Collier, Eds.). A. R. Liss Inc., New York.
27. Cote, R. J., Morrissey, D. M., Houghton, A. N., Beattie, E. J., Jr., Oettgen, H. F., and Old, L. J. (1983) Generation of human monoclonal antibodies reactive with cellular antigens. *Proc. Natl. Acad. Sci. USA 80*:2026-2030.
28. Horowitz, B., Madras, B. K., Meister, A., Old, L. S., Boyse, E. A., and Stockert, E. (1968) Asparagine synthetase activity of mouse leukemias. *Science 160*:533-535.
29. Hyman, R., and Stallings, V. (1974) Complementation patterns of Thy-1 variants and evidence that antigen loss variants "pre exist" in the parental population. *J. Natl. Cancer Inst. 52*:429-436.
30. Foley, G. E., Lazarus, H., Farber, S., Geren Uzman, B., Boone, B. A., and McCarthy, R. E, (1965) Continuous culture of human lymphoblasts from peripheral blood of a child with acute leukemia. *Cancer 18*:522-529.
31. Hogarth, P. M., Edwards, J., McKenzie, I. F. C., Goding, J. W., and Liew, F. Y. (1982) Monoclonal antibodies to murine Ly-2.1 cell surface antigen. *Immunology 46*:135-144.
32. Parham, P. (1983) On the fragmentation of monoclonal IgG1, IgG2a and IgG2b from BALB/C mice. *J. Immunology 131*:2895-2902.
33. Bradford, M. M. (1976) A rapid and sensitive method of quantitation of microgram quantities of protein utilizing the principle of protein-dye binding. *Anal. Biochem. 72*:248-253.
34. Epstein, J., Rosenthal, R. W., and Ess, R. J. (1955) The use of α-(4-nitro benzyl) pyridine as analytical reagent for ethylene imines and alkylating agents. *Anal. Chem. 27*:1435-1439.
35. Parish, C. R., and McKenzie, I. F. C. (1978) A sensitive rosetting method for detecting subpopulations of lymphocytes which react with alloantisera. *J. Immunol. Methods 20*:173-183.

6

Suppressor Deletion Therapy

Selective Elimination of T Suppressor Cells Using a Hematoporphyrin-Conjugated Monoclonal Antibody

J. KEVIN STEELE*
University of British Columbia, Vancouver, British Columbia, Canada

DANIEL LIU
Quadralogic Technologies, Inc., Vancouver, British Columbia, Canada

ANTHEA TENCH STAMMERS, HEATHER DEAL, STEPHEN WHITNEY,† and JULIA G. LEVY
University of British Columbia, Vancouver, British Columbia, Canada

I. INTRODUCTION

The concept that specific antibodies, conjugated to toxic or isotopically labeled materials, could be used to deliver a killing signal or a means of localization to tumors, is not new. Even though this concept has been with us for many decades, it was not until the development of hybridoma technology that many investigators felt that targeted immunotherapy and immunoimaging had the potential of developing into standard procedures. Even though a substantial amount of research has been carried out during the past ten years on these subjects, development of appropriate reagents for use in targeting and diagnosis have proved to be quite elusive. As work in these areas progresses, some of the more obvious problems in the development of such reagents become clear.

The approach we have used in this study to effect targeted immunotherapy is distinct from more traditional methods, in that targets for our immunotoxins are T suppressor cells and the goal of the treatment is immune modulation such

**Current affiliation*: Harvard Medical School, Boston, Massachusetts
†*Current affiliation*: Quadralogic Technologies, Inc., Vancouver, British Columbia, Canada

that tumor-bearing animals are able to reject their own tumors. The results reported here indicate that this may be a feasible approach.

II. INHERENT PROBLEMS

A. Conjugation Procedures

The preparation of suitable reagents to be used as either immunotoxins or diagnostic probes must involve procedures which rapidly yield reproducible and stable conjugates. The procedure must permit suitable loading of the toxin or isotope onto the antibody with minimal loss of biological reactivity of both participants. Also, protocols must be developed to minimize situations in which the monoclonal antibody (MAb) involved will either lose solubility or undergo some degree of aggregation. Because each monoclonal antibody used in the development of diagnostic or therapeutic conjugates will be unique owing to their monoclonality, a procedure which works very well for one MAb may completely denature another. Selection of appropriate MAbs is of primary importance. Ideally, the MAb of choice should exhibit both high affinity and avidity for the targeted antigen, should show no tendency to aggregate, and should be shown to be stable under the conjugation procedures to be used. Aggregation appears to be one of the major problems in this area both in terms of rendering immunotoxins more immunogenic in the patient, and because aggregates are thought to accumulate more readily in organs such as the liver due to the readiness with which Fc receptor-bearing (FcR) cells bind aggregated Ig. In attempts to minimize these effects, some investigators have attempted to use Fab or $(Fab')_2$ fragments. This approach also carries with it a set of problems in that many MAbs are less stable after peptic or papain digestion, and because the molecule is smaller, less efficient loading may result.

B. Biodistribution

While immunotoxins of various types may be highly efficient in vitro in specifically targeting tumor cells, the ability of such reagents in vivo to locate and destroy or facilitate imaging of tumor cells represents requirements of much greater complexity. Not only are immunotoxins concentrated, immediately after administration, in organs such as liver, lung, and kidney, but in vivo degradation of the reagents may lead to accumulation of antibody and targeting agent differentially in different tissues and organs. As mentioned above, one of the major causes of organ accumulation of administered antibody conjugates is the presence of FcR-containing cells, such as alveolar macrophages, dendritic cells, Kupffer cells, etc. It is known that these cells bind not only the Fc portion of antibodies but that they have a greater propensity for binding aggregated reagents than monomeric forms. Thus, as mentioned above, preparation of MAb conjugates using monomeric reagents or enzyme-degraded fragments may be an essential step in the preparation of suitable materials. The problem of degradation in vivo of conjugates is one of some complexity, since mechanisms for such degradation are no doubt many and varied. In this regard, the stability of the conjugation procedure is one of considerable importance, and the formation of covalent bonds is desirable where possible. Of equal importance is the maintenance of preparations with minimal levels of denatured protein, since there will be a greater likelihood of this being degraded over native protein, which could lead to incorrect estimates when biodistribution is being assessed.

C. Immunogenicity of Conjugates

The use of human monoclonal reagents for imaging and immunotherapeutic purposes is obviously desirable, since these would be less immunogenic than MAbs of murine origin. However, there are two distinct problems associated with this as yet largely hypothetical situation. Despite enormous efforts over the past few years on the development of suitable partners for human fusions and of novel immortalizing procedures for the development of human monoclonal cell lines, problems of stability and secretion are still considerable. Thus, most human B cell fusion products to date, even if they are stable, have been low antibody secretors, so that their value as reagents have been limited. Also, while human MAbs may be less immunogenic than murine products, it is still likely that patients receiving them would develop anti-idiotypic antibodies. Also, it is probable that conjugated drugs would constitute immunogenic haptens in association with the carrier antibody. Both of these problems are obviously also inherent in the use of murine MAbs as immunotherapeutic or imaging agents. There is now some data available indicating that an immune response to administered MAbs lessens the therapeutic effect observed on earlier administration (1-3). There are, however, two points that should be raised regarding these potential problems. First, it is possible to tolerize individuals to subsequent injections of xenogeneic proteins (conjugated or unconjugated) by a relatively simple procedure developed by Sehon and associates (4). These investigators have shown that conjugation of a variety of antigens, including monoclonal antibodies to polyethylene glycol (PEG) renders them tolerogenic. A single injection of PEG-conjugated materials will rapidly render recipients immunologically tolerant to subsequent administration of the unconjugated material. This result has been shown to be mediated through the development of T suppressor cells (5). Second, it is not at all clear that the development of anti-idiotypic antibodies in the recipient will have an adverse effect on the immunotherapy. Since it is postulated (and there is evidence that support this (6-8)) that anti-idiotypic antibodies represent the internal image of the antigen, then anti-idiotypic antibodies resembling tumor-associated antigens could constitute useful, immunogenic signals to the T-cell repertoire. There is some circumstantial evidence supporting this in observations made by Koprowski and colleagues (9) that, of patients treated with MAbs for recurrent gastrointestinal adenocarcinoma, those developing anti-idiotypic antibodies in fact did better than similarly treated patients who did not. It would appear, however, that for immunotherapeutic regimens using MAbs, control and understanding of the intrinsic response to the reagents is of critical importance.

D. Tumor Markers

It now appears clear that, with the exception of a few notable examples, most tumors do not expess tumor-unique gene products. By and large, tumor-associated antigens constitute those components of tumor cells which represent inappropriately expressed gene products in comparison to the normal counterpart or overtly displayed cellular constituents which are normally cryptic. These classes of tumor-associated antigen may represent differentiation or fetal antigens, growth factor, or other receptors or cryptic cell surface carbohydrates, such as the Thomsen-Freidenrich or T antigen (10). In order to represent a suitable tumor marker for imaging and/or immunotherapy, a number of criteria have to be met. While not being necessarily tumor unique, the desirable marker must be present on tumor cells at significantly higher concentrations than on normal cells. It should also be present on tumor cell surfaces and not be shed or liberated from the cell surface in its intact form, since its presence in blood would lead to the formation of soluble immune complexes, also readily picked up by FcR-containing cells or simply by phagocytic cells. These two requirements are important in the selection of a marker for imaging purposes. Additional properties are desirable if a marker is to be used as a target for immunotherapy. Cancerous cells are thought to be the products of self-renewing stem cells, which possess a defect of which the end result is a blockade in terminal differentation of the non-self-renewing progeny of that stem cell. It is, therefore, essential to recognize that a tumor consists of a small population of self-renewing defective stem cells and their partially differentiated progeny. If the purpose of immunotherapy is to diminish tumor load without eliminating the disease or to locate tumor masses with imaging, then markers displayed on the partially differentiated progeny can be used as targets. If, however, the purpose of the therapy is to eliminate the disease, it is essential to use a marker known to be present on the malignant stem cell. Unfortunately, this area of tumor biology is at this time so poorly understood, as is the nature of the self-renewing population, that this problem is extraordinarily difficult to deal with. The necessity for targeting stem cells becomes less critical for immunotherapy if the toxic agent can act over a distance greater than a single cell diameter, such as isotopes like ^{67}Cu or ^{131}I and reagents which induce singlet oxygen formation, such as hematoporphyrin. A second property of tumor markers suitable as targets for immunotherapy is that they do not undergo rapid antigenic modulation. It has been found that a number of markers on lymphoid cells which might be appropriate targets for immunotherapy of some leukemias undergo marked modulation in the presence of antibody (11). While this is a consideration for immunotherapy, the extent of its significance in the overall picture of tumor markers is not yet known. Some of the most promising results regarding tumor markers are in the area of cell surface carbohydrate antigens. Many classes of tumors bear the Thomsen-Friedenrich (TF) antigen (beta-gal (1 → 3)-alpha-ga1NA$_c$), usually cryptic on normal cells. Monoclonal antibodies to the TF antigen could conceivably be used as broad-based imaging agents or immunotoxins. The feasibility of this type of approach has already been demonstrated using both monoclonal antibodies and peanut agglutinin, a lectin with selective affinity for TF antigen (12,13).

In the experimental approach and results to be presented here, we have used a monoclonal antibody with specificity not for a tumor antigen, but for a population of T suppressor cells. The antibody has been conjugated to the photoactivable molecule, hematoporphyrin. The hypothesis on which we based this work was that tumor-bearing animals have the potential for mounting an immune response to their tumors, but in nature the response is down-regulated by T suppressor cells. By selectively eliminating this T cell subset in vivo using targeted immunotherapy, immune modulation should permit immune rejection of tumors. The results obtained indicate that this approach to immunotherapy may have some potential.

III. BACKGROUND

There is a considerable body of literature covering the use of photoactivable chemicals as chemotherapeutic agents in the treatment of tumors (14). Hematoporphyrin (Hp) and Hpd have been found, in a number of studies, to have a greater affinity for malignant cells than for normal cells (reviewed in Refs. 14 and 15). Photoactivation of Hp and Hpd in the range of 600 nm results in the release of singlet oxygen, which is thought to be the major component of the activation process delivering the cytotoxic signal in association with cell membranes. Hp and particularly Hpd have been used to treat a number of human cancers, including breast, lung, and bladder (16-18). Currently, a commercially available form of Hpd, photophrin, is being used in a number of centers for the treatment of locally recurring breast tumors and lung cancer. There are some problems associated with these treatments. While Hpd appears to have an enhanced affinity for malignant cells over normal, it still accumulates in normal tissues and is retained in the body for considerable time periods. At dose levels of 2.0-2.5 mg/kg body weight, it has been observed that severe photosensitivity can persist for 8-10 weeks following treatments. Side effects are unpleasant, taking the form of ulcerating skin lesions and necrosis.

Some years ago in this laboratory, we undertook a study to determine whether Hp-MAb conjugates could be used as immunotoxins for the treatment of an experimental murine tumor. It was felt that such conjugates might have advantages over other immunotoxins because of their lack of toxicity in the absence of light activation. Provided animals are maintained in the dark following administration of the conjugate up to a time when its tumor:nontumor ratio was optimal, maximum toxicity upon activation with light would occur at the tumor sight. Also, the enhanced tumor concentration of Hp resulting from the specificity donated by the MAb, might permit the use of lower doses of Hp. The studies using a murine myosarcoma system and a MAb raised to it in this laboratory resulted in some interesting observations (19). We showed that in this system, MAb-Hp conjugates administered intravenously (i.v.) were capable of homing to tumors implanted on the backs of DBA/2 mice (syngenic for the tumor system used), that exposure of animals to light following treatment could result in partial or complete regression of tumors, and that the effect was specific for those animals receiving specific MAb-Hp conjugate. We found further that the dose level of Hp required to have this effect was considerably below (<10%) dose levels recommended for therapy using Hp alone and, perhaps most surprising, that the optimal time following treatment for light activation was in the range of 6-9 days. This last observation implied that the time required for maximum accumulation of MAb-Hp into tumor tissue was considerably longer than one would anticipate, although there are other reported results using MAb-isotope conjugates that imply that accumulation of these reagents in tumors may increase over a fairly protracted time course (this of course would occur while levels in other tissues would be declining).

In further studies using different MAb-Hp conjugates, we showed that we could specifically kill cells producing a human leukemia-associated antigen (20) in vitro and that again the effects of the specific conjugate over appropriate controls was about an order of magnitude more effective. Thus, these studies showed that Hp could be effectively linked to MAbs while retaining the specificity of the MAb and the biological activity of Hp and that these conjugates could exert an effect on specific targets both in vivo and in vitro.

As mentioned above, treatment of cancer with immunotoxins targeted to TAA have had only limited success, owing possibly to any of a number of factors already commented on. We, therefore, have undertaken a somewhat different approach in the studies reported here. For many years, work in this laboratory has been directed to a study of immune regulation during tumor growth. In the P815 mastocytoma system of DBA/2 mice we demonstrated that, while mice injected with P815 cells mounted a transient positive immune response to the tumor as assessed by the measurement of tumor-specific cytotoxic T lymphocytes (CTL) in tumor-bearers' spleens, this response was swiftly overridden by the development of T suppressor cells (TsC) specific for the P815 tumor (21,22). The T suppressor cells in this system were further shown to secrete an antigen-specific factor (TsF) which could replace TsC in the down-regulation of the development of T killer cells, capable of specifically killing P815 in a syngeneic system (23). Subsequently, a MAb (B16G) was developed to the P815-specific TsF that was shown to bind to an invariant portion of the TsF molecule. Thus, B16G was found to bind to essentially all TsFs secreted by TsC in DBA/2 mice (24). Early work with the B16G MAb demonstrated that i.v. administration of B16G enhanced immune function in mice, including resistance to a variety of tumors, presumably by binding to and inactivating TsC in treated animals (24). Because of these earlier findings, we have undertaken the present study to determine whether B16G-Hp conjugates could act as better immunotoxins in the elimination of TsC in tumor-bearing animals. The hypothesis to be tested was that tumor-bearing mice will have significant levels of TsC circulating in the blood and that treatment with B16G-Hp followed by exposure to light should eliminate them, thus allowing the immune system of the tumor-bearing animal to effectively destroy tumor cells. This type of treatment, if successful, could have application in a broad variety of systems, and we have termed it suppressor deletion therapy.

IV. RESULTS

A. Loading Experiments and Biological Activity

The procedures described in the Appendix for the conjugation of Hp to MAbs is so efficient that the ratio of Hp:MAb conjugated can basically be dictated by the relative concentrations of the two reactants. During the development of this technology it became clear that excessive loading of Hp onto the B16G MAb resulted in loss of antibody-binding capacity. By and large, experiments regarding loading have indicated that molar ratios of Hp:MAb of 100:1 or greater almost invariably result in loss of antibody specificity. Further experiments have shown that, at least with a number of MAbs tested under these conditions, when loading ratios get beyond 50:1, the probability of antibody inactivation is high. For these reasons, ratios between Hp and B16G during conjugation were set up such that loading ratios of about 50:1 would be achieved.

Similar observations were made when experiments were carried out using affinity purified rabbit anti-mouse Ig (RαMIg) as antibody for Hp labeling. Control experiments showed that all procedures involved in the EDCl coupling (dialysis against distilled water, lyophilization, treatment with DMSO) did not reduce the activity of this conventional antibody—only excessive loading did this. Thus, recognizing that carbodiimide coupling involves random reactions of activated Hp with free amino groups on either MAbs or conventional antibody, the probability that amino groups involved in either the actual antigen-binding site of the antibody or those amino groups indirectly involved with tertiary structure will be increased if loading ratios are increased beyond 50:1. For this reason, standard procedures were set up such that loading would not exceed this ratio.

In these studies, two Hp-labeled antibodies were used. The MAb, B16G, was used in a series of experiments and was labeled with Hp a number of times, but ratios in all instances were in the range of 50:1. Similarly, Hp-RαMIg ratios were also in this range.

Another advantage of the rapid coupling method described here is that the possibility of the formation of noncovalent stable associations between Hp and MAb was minimized. The method described here resulted in essentially no noncovalent association, as shown by TLC of conjugates. This point is of significance when precise measurement of loading efficiency is required. This is exemplified by the following: We carried out an experiment in which Hp was mixed with B16G in aqueous conditions and left at room temperature for 2 hours. The mixture was then extensively dialyzed, following which remaining Hp was determined spectrophotometrically. We found that approximately 50% of the added Hp was still associated with the MAb (initial mixes contained 60 μg Hp/mg B16G) after 24 hours and 2 changes of dialysate.

The association constant between Hp and B16G was determined with fluorescence depolarization. The results (Fig. 1) show that in an aqueous environment association between Hp and B16G is quite rapid, with an association constant of $Ka = 7.6 \times 10^{-6}$ (M^{-1}). This kind of noncovalent association on immunotoxins to be used in vivo could lead to significant calculation errors. It is assumed that our procedures, using nonaqueous solvents and rapid coupling procedures, would minimize such difficulties.

B. Specificity of Hp:Antibody Conjugates in Targeting Cells in Vitro

The purpose of the experiments reported here was to determine whether a monoclonal antibody with specificity for a T suppressor factor (TsF), when conjugated to Hp, could eliminate subpopulations of T cells (T suppressor cells (TsC) and thereby modulate immune responsiveness. The MAb, B16G, was used in these experiments, since we had shown previously that it binds to a "constant" epitope of TsF and is expressed on the surface of TsC of DBA/2 mice (21). In order to determine whether B16G-Hp conjugates could kill TsC, experiments were undertaken using a T-cell hybridoma, A10, shown to secrete a TsF to which B16G binds. Initially, experiments were carried out in which B16G-Hp was titrated over a range of 20-150 ng/ml of Hp in determining its ability to specifically kill A10 cells in comparison to the cell lines P815 and L1210 (a syngeneic mastocytoma and thymoma, respectively, of DBA/2 mice). The results (Fig. 2)

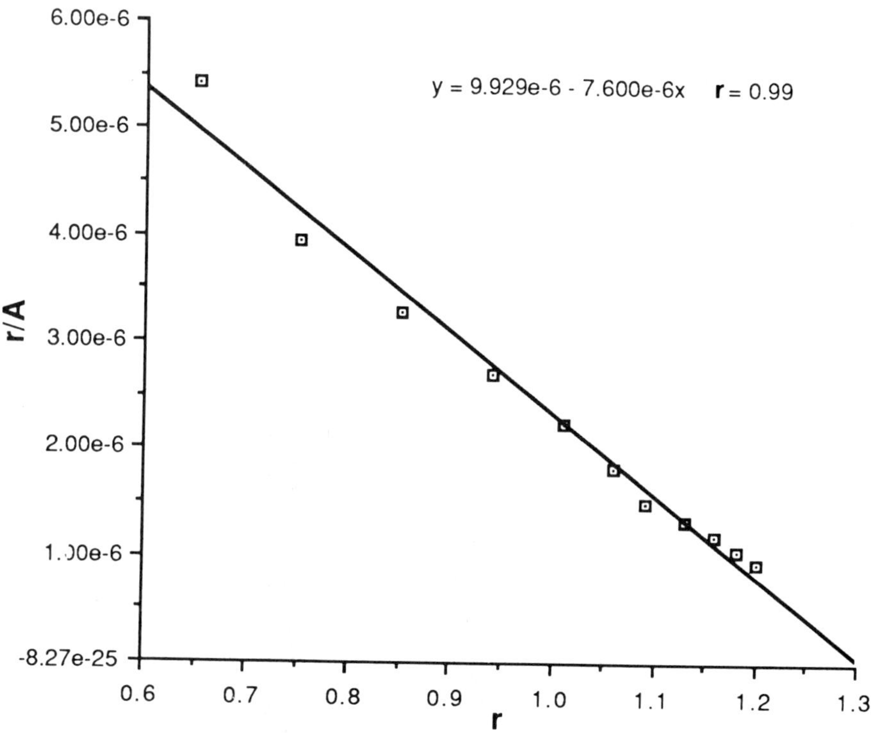

Figure 1 Scatchard plot showing the noncovalent binding of Hp with B16G in PBS. Results are plotted according to the method of Scatchard (45) using the expression $r/A = nKa - rka$, where r is the number of Hp molecules bound per mole of protein, n the number of binding sites, Ka the association constant, and A the concentration of free Hp. The plot of r/A against r is a straight line and Ka is 7.8×10^{-6}

show that under the experimental conditions described the conjugate appears to preferentially kill A10 cells. These results were based on [^{3}H]-thymidine uptake of cells following 30 minutes of exposure sequentially to both B16G-Hp and light. In another study, direct counting of P815 and A10 cells were carried out using eosin Y exclusion. B16G-Hp-treated cells were washed, resuspended and exposed to light for 1-4 hours. Cell counts were made at hourly intervals. Results for two different experiments are shown in Figures 3 and 4. It can be seen that assessment of cell killing by direct count yields results analogous to those found with [^{3}H]-thymidine uptake. The differential killing of A10 was shown not to be attributable to a greater sensitivity of A10 to Hp than control cells, since when an equivalent experiment was carried out using both B16G-Hp

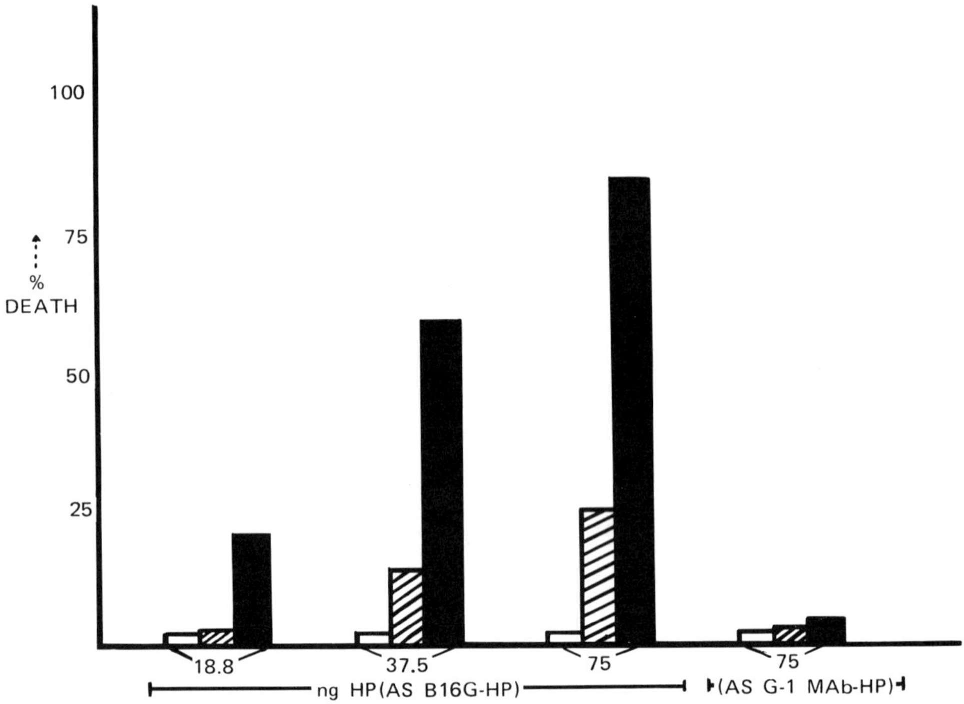

Figure 2 The effect of B16G-Hp in comparison to that of C-MAb-Hp on A10 (■), L1210 (▨), or P815 (□). Percent death was calculated from the level of inhibition of [^{3}H]-thymidine incorporation of treated cells in comparison to control samples of cultures taken at time zero and maintained in the dark during culture.

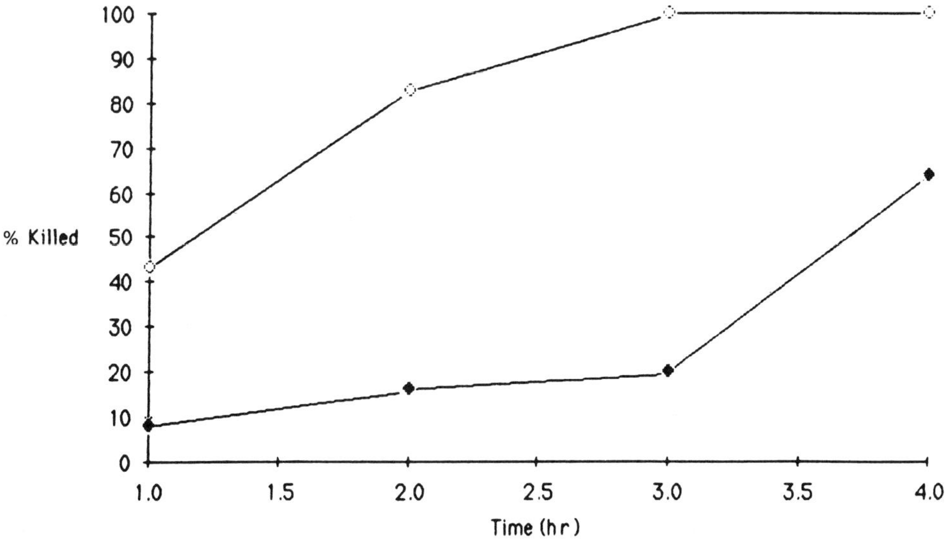

Figure 3 The effect of B16G-Hp at a concentration of 80 ng Hp/ml on viability of A10 cells (◇—◇) and P815 (◆—◆). Cells were exposed to B16G-Hp in the dark, washed, and maintained under light conditions throughout the experiment. Aliquots were removed at hourly intervals and counted for viability.

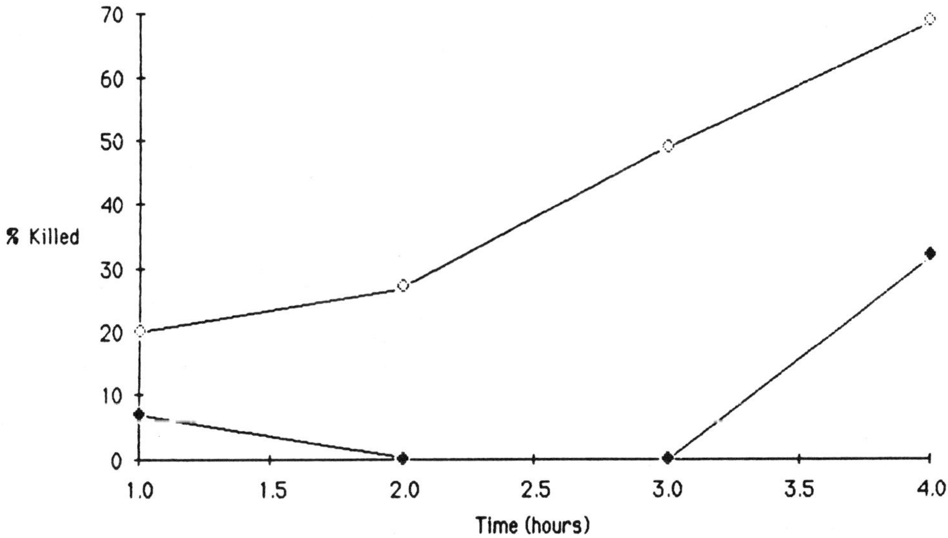

Figure 4 The effect of B16G-Hp at a concentration of 40 ng Hp/ml on the viability of A10 cells (◇—◇) and P815 cells (◆—◆). Cells were exposed to B16G-Hp in the dark, washed, and maintained under light conditions throughout the experiment. Aliquots were removed at hourly intervals and counted for viability.

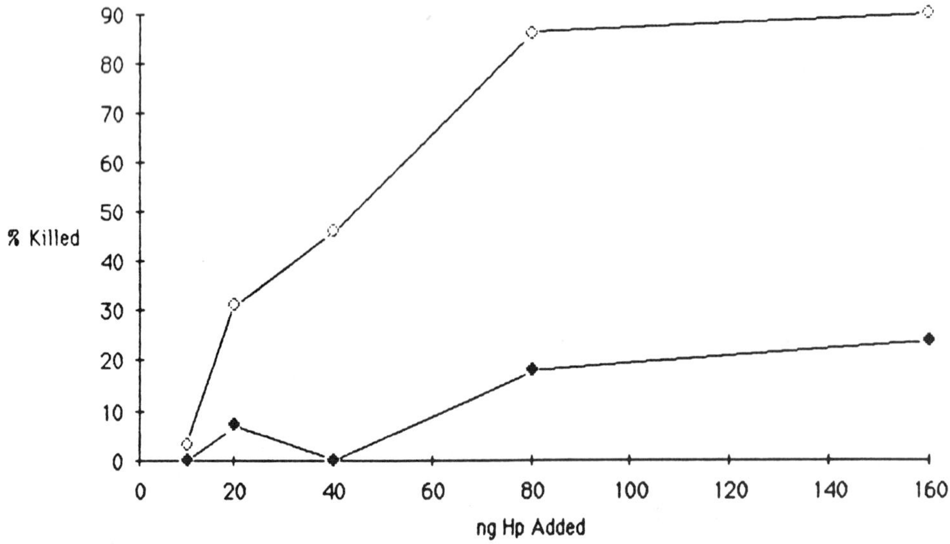

Figure 5 The effect of B16G-Hp (◇—◇) and C-MAb-Hp (◆—◆) on the A10 cell line. Conjugates were added to 10^6 A10 cells at various concentrations in the dark for 30 minutes. Cells were washed under dark conditions, resuspended in DME and exposed to light for an additional 30 minutes. Cells were washed again and set up in microtiter wells for 24-hour culture with [^{3}H]-thymidine. Percent killing was calculated from control cultures, which had been treated in an identical manner but in the absence of Hp conjugates.

and an irrelevant MAb-Hp conjugate on A10 cells in the [^{3}H]-thymidine uptake assay, selective killing of A10 with B16G-Hp was observed (Fig. 5). In a similar manner, experiments were carried out using RαMIg.Hp as the immunotoxin. A10 cells were exposed to either B16G or an irrelevant MAb. They were washed and exposed to RαMIg-Hp at various concentrations, washed again, and exposed to light for 30 minutes. Again, selective killing of A10 cells coated with B16G was observed (Fig. 6).

C. Effect of MAb-Hp Conjugates in Vivo

Further experiments involved in vivo testing of B16G-Hp conjugates. DBA/2 mice were injected in the right flank subcutaneously with 10^4 P815 cells. On day 8, when tumors were palpable, animals were randomly sorted into groups and injected i.v. with 200 μl of PBS containing nothing, Hp, B16G-Hp, B16G

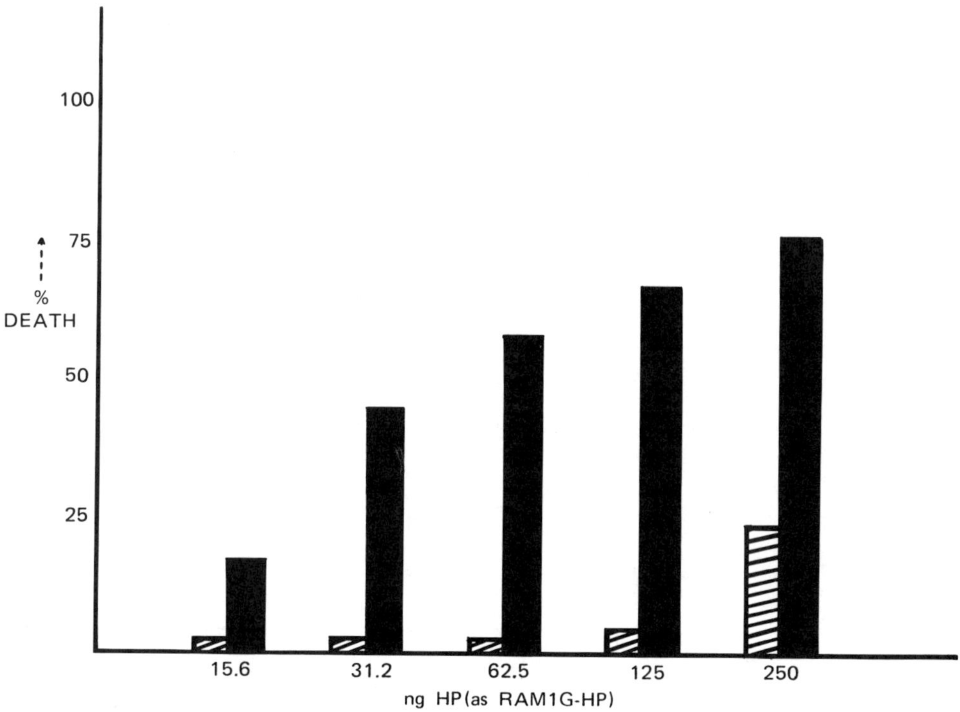

Figure 6 The effect of RαMIg-Hp on A10 cells previously labeled with either B16G (■) or C-MAb (▨). Percent killing was calculated as described in Fig. 5.

plus Hp (mixed immediately before injection to minimize effects of noncovalent association), B16G, or a control MAb-Hp conjugate (C-MAb-Hp), all at equivalent levels of both Hp (10 μg per animal) and MAb (100 μg). They were maintained in the dark for 2 hours, after which they were exposed to strong light for 5 hours and then treated normally. Animals were monitored daily, their tumor size was measured, and the time of death was recorded. In five separate experiments done using these reagents (and two different preparations of B16G-Hp), essentially the same results were observed, in that a significant number of B16G-Hp-treated animals underwent tumor regression (some permanent), while all other experimental groups demonstrated the expected pattern of tumor growth and death. The results of one such experiment are shown in Figure 7, in which the slowing of tumor growth in B16G-Hp-treated animals is apparent. A summary of survival patterns in all experiments done is given in Table 1. In all experiments, the treatments other than B16G-Hp resulted in 100% death and survival times not significantly different from PBS-treated controls. It would,

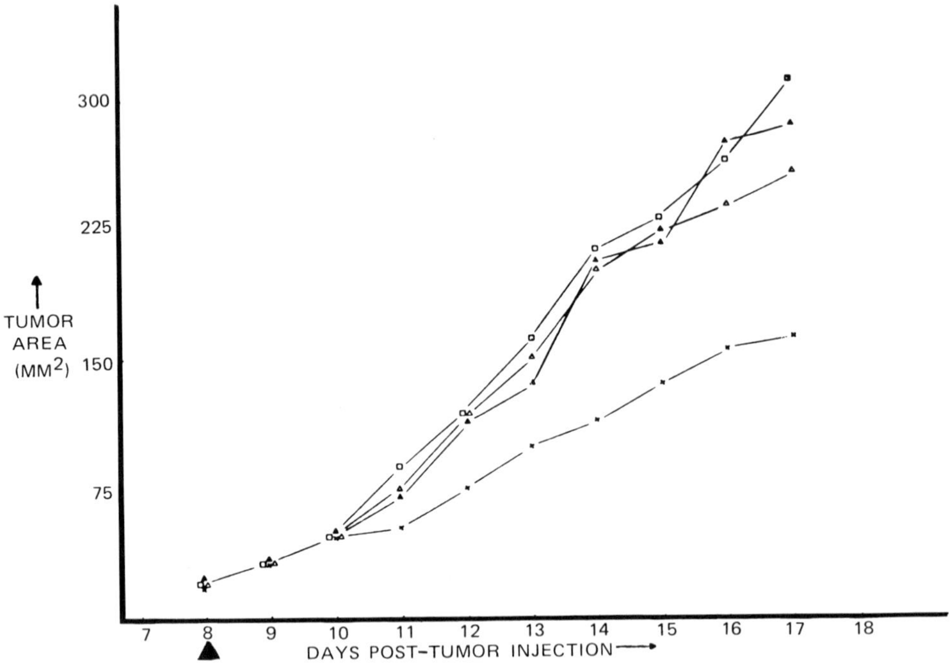

Figure 7 Growth of P815 tumor in mice receiving 10^4 P815 cells 8 days prior to receiving PBS (△–△), Hp (□–□), B16G plus Hp (▲–▲), or B16G-Hp (x–x). Tumor size was assessed in individual mice by two cross-sectional measurements using calipers. Differences in tumor area between B16G-Hp-treated animals and all other experimental groups became significant at day 14 at the level of $p < 0.05$ as determined by Student's t-test. Each group contained 8 animals.

therefore, appear that Hp alone under these conditions was having no direct effect on tumor growth. In each experiment, some animals treated with B16G-Hp underwent complete tumor regression and were tumor-free 100 days following initiation of the experiment. In only two experiments (experiments 2 or 6) was there no significant increase in survival time in B16G-Hp-treated animals. However, in both of these groups 3/8 of treated animals underwent complete tumor regression, and these animals could not be included in averaged survival times. In experiment 6, a lower level of conjugate was administered (5 μg Hp), but the rate of tumor regression was the same as that seen with higher levels.

A further experiment was undertaken to determine whether noncovalently associated Hp with B16G could influence the outcome of these kinds of experi-

Table 1 Survival Data on All B16G-Hp Experiments

Experiment	Treatment	Mean survival time (days ± SEM)	p^a	Number of cures	Percent tumor free after 100 days
1	PBS	25 ± 1.1		0/7	0
	B16G-Hp	41.3 ± 6.4[b]	<0.001	3/9	33
2	PBS	23.5 ± 2.4		0/6	0
	Hp	21.0 ± 2.3	NS	0/8	0
	B16G-Hp	24.2 ± 3.8	NS	3/8	37.5
3	PBS	24.1 ± 2.0		0/7	0
	Hp	23.4 ± 2.1	NS	0/7	0
	B16 + Hp	23.5 ± 3.2	NS	0/6	0
	B16-Hp[c]	29.2 ± 4.6	<0.05	2/7	29
4	PBS	25.2 ± 2.8		0/8	0
	B16G	28.3 ± 4.6	NS	0/8	0
	Hp	24.2 ± 1.9	NS	0/8	0
	B16G + Hp	24.6 ± 2.1	NS	0/7	0
	B16G-Hp	36.7 ± 2.5	<0.01	3/7	43
5	PBS	23.8 ± 2.1		0/8	0
	Hp	27.0 ± 3.8	NS	0/8	0
	C-MAb-Hp	20.3 ± 2.1	NS	0/8	0
	B16G-Hp	34.0 ± 3.5	<0.05	1/8	12.5
6	PBS	23.1 ± 2.9		0/8	0
	Hp	27.2 ± 4.0	NS	0/9	0
	B16G	26.3 ± 4.6	NS	0/8	0
	C-MAb-Hp	26.5 ± 4.1	NS	0/8	0
	B16G-Hp[c]	28.0 ± 3.5	NS	3/8	37.5

All animals received 10^4 P815 cells on day 0 and various intravenous injections on day 8. In all but experiments 3 and 6, mice received a total dose of 10 μg Hp and 100 μg MAb.

[a]*p* values are based on Student's *t*-test, in which survival times in individual groups were compared to values for PBS controls.

[b]Averaged survival times on B16G-Hp-treated animals utilizes data taken only from animals that died from their tumors (i.e., long-term survivors are not included).

[c]In experiment 3, animals received 23.4 μg Hp and 100 μg MAb. In experiment 6 animals received 5.4 μg Hp and 100 μg MAb.

ments. Preparations of B16G, Hp, and B16G plus Hp were made up in PBS and left at room temperature for 2 hours, after which they were injected i.v. into DBA/2 mice which had received 10^4 P815 cells 8 days earlier. Tumor growth and survival were followed. The results (Table 2) show unequivocally that noncovalent associations in vitro can certainly exhibit an effect in vivo, in that mice receiving the B16G plus Hp mixture demonstrated a remarkable regression rate with 3/8 apparent cures. It is probable that when longer-term effects, such as immunotoxins homing on localized tumor masses, as opposed to almost immediate interaction of immunotoxins with circulating cells (as in this model), are being studied, this effect may not be so dramatic. These results, however, clearly show the importance of precise quantifiable procedures for effecting covalent bonds between antibodies and ligands.

These results are compatible with the concept that B16G-Hp is successfully binding to circulating TsC and essentially eliminating them during the period that experimental animals are being exposed to strong light (2-6 hours after administration of conjugates). Animals were not shaved, so it is likely that sufficient light penetration took place through the ears and the tail to permit activation of the Hp. The P815 system has been studied extensively in this laboratory during the past decade. It has been established by us, as well as others (21,22,25), that P815-bearing animals develop tumor-specific TsC fairly early in tumor growth. We have not been able to establish, however, whether the development of these TsCs actually affects the course of tumor growth in this experimental model. The data presented here are consistent with the possibility that the elimination of these TsCs permits the immune mechanisms involved (probably CTL) to bring about rejection of tumors in at least some animals.

Table 2 Survival Data on P815-Bearing Mice Receiving B16G, Hp, or a Mixture of the Two

Treatment	Mean survival time (days ± SEM)	Number of cures	Percent cure
PBS	24 ± 4.1	0/8	0
Hp	28.1 ± 6.3	0/8	0
B16G	25.6 ± 3.3	0/8	0
B16G + Hp	27.8 ± 3.1	3/8	37.5

All mice received 10^4 P815 cells on day 0 and other treatments i.v. on day 8. Mice received 100 μg B16G and 10 μg Hp. The mixture of B16G and Hp was allowed to react for 120 minutes at 29°C prior to injection.

As can be seen in Table 1, in all of the separate experiments carried out with B16G-Hp, some treated animals underwent complete tumor rejection (between 12.5 and 43%, depending on te e experiment), whereas others went on to die of their tumors. It was thought that the difference in response to B16G-Hp treatment on the part of individuals in the group might be attributable to differences in initial tumor growth (i.e., tumor size) early in the course of the experiment. In order to examine this possibility, data from all individuals treated with B16G-Hp were pooled, and tumor measurements from those animals that underwent regression were compared with those of animals that went on to die of their tumors. The results (Fig. 8) show that while tumor size in mice that underwent

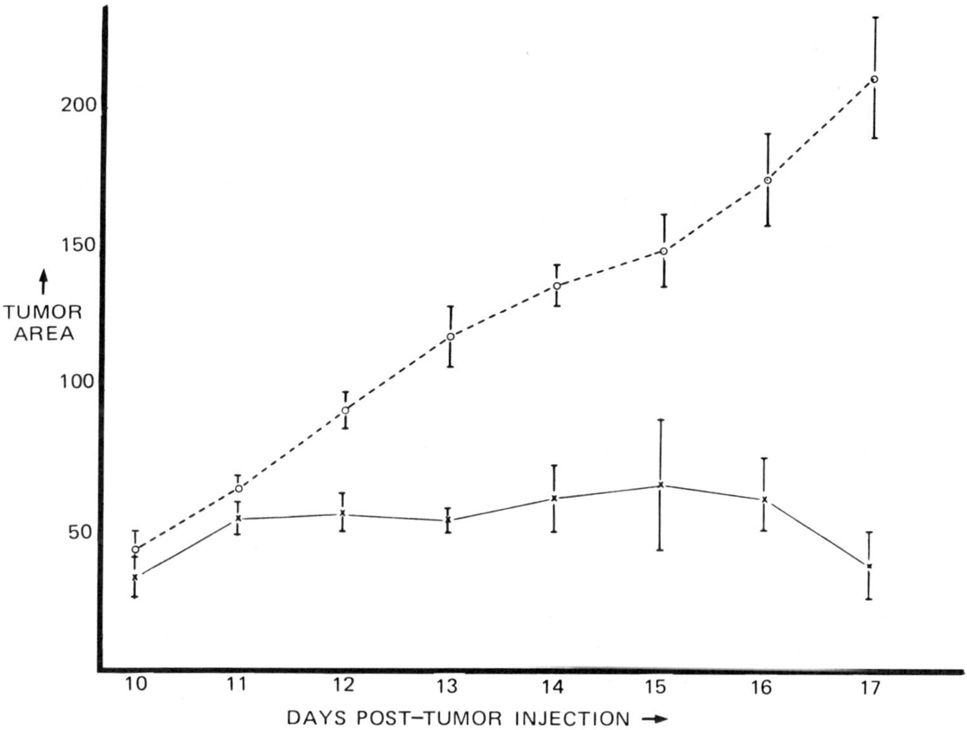

Figure 8 Comparison of P815 tumor growth curve in progressor (unresponsive to conjugate treatment) and regressor mice (ultimately cured of tumor) receiving B16G-Hp conjugate. Data are pooled from 5 different experiments and include a total of 38 mice. Porgressors (○–○) are defined as those mice that died of their tumors and regressors (x–x) as those that underwent permanent regression (>100 days). Error bars indicate the magnitude of standard error of the mean for each point.

regresson on days 10 and 11 was not significantly less than that of progressor animals at that time, by day 13 the differences are highly significant ($p <$ 0.005). By day 18, approximately one-third of the regressor mice had completely rejected their tumors, whereas the remainder showed scabbing at the tumor site. Thus, any obvious distinction between regressor and progressor mice is not evident, at least on the basis of tumor size at the time that treatment was initiated.

A second MAb, EA2, has been characterized in our laboratory and was shown to have almost identical properties to B16G. It was used in conjugation with Hp in an experiment in which the L1210 tumor was used instead of P815. DBA/2 mice were injected s.c. with 5×10^3 L1210 cells. On day 7, when tumors were palpable, animals were randomly sorted into groups and given intravenous injections of 0.2 ml PBS, control MAb-Hp conjugate, Hp, or EA2-Hp. Ratio of Hp:MAb on a molar basis in each case was 30:1, and animals received a total dose of 10 μg Hp. Animals were maintained in the dark for two hours, following which they were exposed to light as discussed above. Tumor growth curves and survival curves are shown in Figures 9 and 10. In this experiment, it can be seen that the EA2-Hp conjugate had a dramatic effect on both the rate of tumor growth and survival, in that all treated animals successfully rejected measurable tumors completely and remained tumor-free, whereas in control groups only 15-30% of the animals showed tumor rejection. Thus, this mode of treatment does not appear to be restricted to a single tumor model or to a single species of monoclonal, although B16G and EA2 both react with the same protein molecule(s).

D. Effect of B16G-Hp on the Generation of P815-specific CTL

A number of experiments have been carried out to determine whether treatment of experimental animals with B16G according to the protocols described above lead to the development of enhanced P815-reactive CTL activity in tumor-bearing mice. Results of a series of experiments are shown in Figure 11.

In this series, DBA/2 mice were injected on day 0 with P815 (10^4 cells s.c.) and on day 8 they received either B16G-Hp or a control MAb-Hp conjugate (C-MAb-Hp). Intravenous Hp levels in all instances were 10.0 μg and MAb concentrations 100 μg. On days 9, 10, 12, and 16, 4 animals from each group were sacrificed and their spleens used to assess CTL activity against P815. The results (Fig. 11) show a rapid effect of B16G-Hp, in that on day 9 there is a significant increase in CTL activity in the spleens of mice receiving B16G-Hp. Somewhat surprising is the apparent transience of this increased activity, since by days 10-12 it is no longer present, and by day 16 control animals show significantly higher levels of CTL activity than the experimental group. These observations were easily reproducible and were independent of Hp levels be-

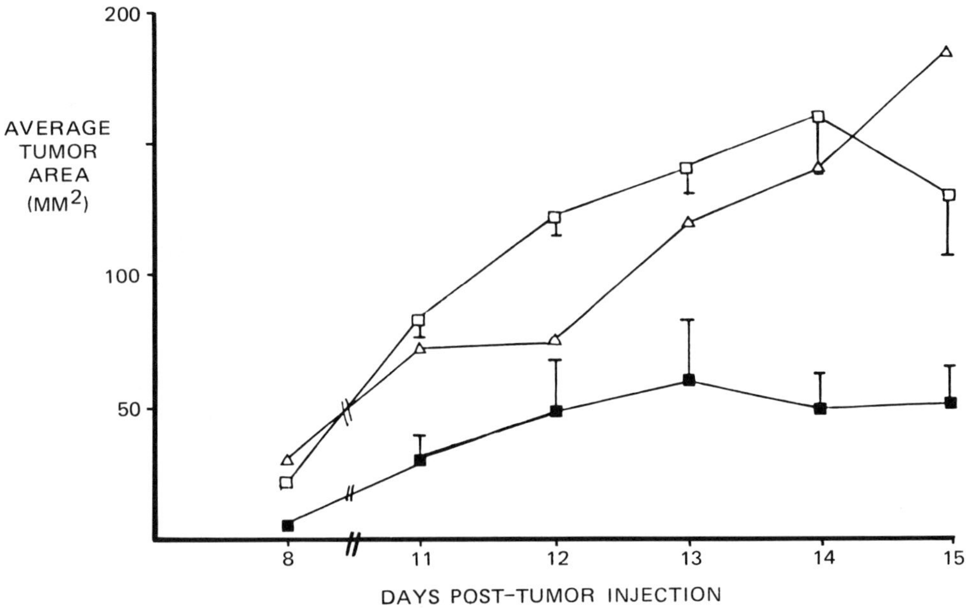

Figure 9 Growth of the L1210 tumor in mice receiving 5 X 10^3 L1210 7 days prior to receiving intravenous injections of Hp (△—△), C-MAb-Hp (□—□), or EA2-Hp (■—■). Tumor size was assessed in individual mice by two cross-sec-sectional measurements. Error bars indicate standard error of the mean and are shown where the differences between C-MAb-Hp (the most appropriate control) and EA2-Hp are significantly ($p < 0.02$) different by Student's t-test.

tween 5-15 μg/animal. It is impossible at this time, to explain the cellular kinetics of what we observe in the spleen of treated mice. The treatment used in these experiments serves to affect tumor rejection in this tumor system in about 30% of treated animals. Fluctuations in splenic CTL activity under the conditions described here may reflect differences in lymphocyte traffic from the spleen, and we do not have sufficient information to even speculate on these events.

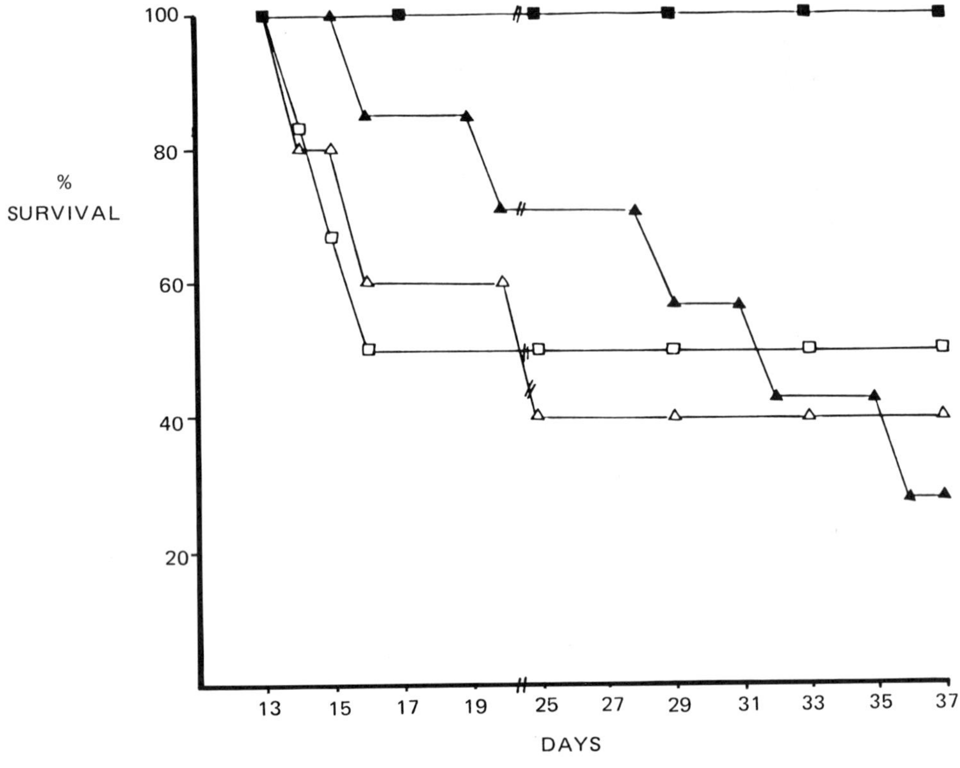

Figure 10 Survival of DBA/2 mice injected with 5×10^3 L1210 cells 7 days prior to receiving intravenous injections of Hp (△—△), C-MAb-Hp (□—□), PBS (▲—▲), or EA2-Hp (■—■).

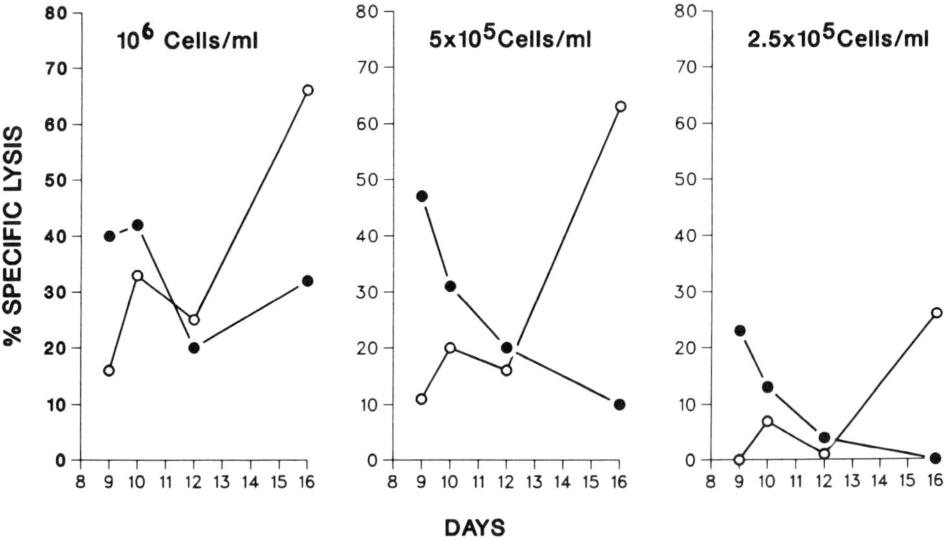

Figure 11 CTL activity of splenocytes of DBA/2 mice against P815 tumor cells at various time intervals after injection of P815 tumor cells. Mice received i.v. injections of either C-MAb-Hp (○–○) or B16G-Hp (●–●). Each data point represents average of octuplicate samples from 4 individual animals. At each cell concentration, the differences between the experimental and control animals was significant at least $p < 0.05$ on days 9 and 16. On other days there was no significant difference between data points.

V. DISCUSSION

The approach to targeted therapy suggested in the foregoing is novel and may have some advantages over more than the potential application of traditional immunotoxins. As mentioned earlier, there are many problems in the use of monoclonal antibodies to tumor-associated markers in conjugation with isotopes or cytotoxic reagents as targeting agents. Attesting to these problems is the fact that a decade after the introduction of hybridoma technology, the use of MAbs in this fashion is still essentially at the experimental level, and their unequivocal success in this application remains to be established.

Over the past few years, attitudes toward TAA have also changed. It is generally assumed that, by and large, tumor cells do not differ antigenically in any radical sense from their normal counterparts, with the possible exception of expression of cryptic carbohydrate antigens and oncofetal antigens. That they may express differing ratios of certain markers or carbohydrates of modified configuration is not questioned. If this then is the status of tumor "antigenicity," a major unanswered question pertains to the overwhelming evidence in the literature that in animal models, the tumor-bearing animal almost always mounts a detectable (if transient) response to its own tumor (26-33). There are also many references to detection of antitumor immunity (both T-cell- and B-cell-mediated) and antigen-specific suppression in patients with cancers of one type or another (34-38). Given that there appear to be few, if any, tumor-specific antigens associated with human cancers, one must then assume that specific antitumor responses seen in cancer patients are, in fact, a form of autoimmunity. There is some evidence in some cancers that the presence of such immune responsiveness may have prognostic significance (39,40).

Research in this laboratory has been directed to understanding immune regulation, particularly as it pertains to the interactions between TsC subpopulations. Some time ago, we demonstrated that the transience of the immune response in syngeneic DBA/2 mice to the P815 mastocytoma correlated with the development of tumor-specific TsC. If one looks at this transient tumor immunity as a form of autoimmunity, it is not surprising that the response is modulated by regulatory T, cells whose role it may be to maintain self-tolerance.

Later developments in this laboratory lead to the isolation of a B-cell hybridoma which secretes a MAb with specificity for a population of TsC and apparently the "constant" region of a TsF secreted by them (24). This MAb, B16G, was used subsequently to screen for T-cell hybridomas which secreted B16G-reactive molecules. A number of T-cell hybridomas have been isolated in this way (41,42). The one of particular interest here, A10, secretes a molecule which is bound by B16G and binds to an as yet uncharacterized antigen associated with the membrane of P815 cells. We have argued that the A10 hybridoma represents the prototype of a Ts1 population and secretes a first-order TsF which triggers the suppressor cell cascade and binds nominal antigen. It is further suggested that A10 represents a cell population present in normal animals that aids in the maintenance of self-tolerance.

In a number of experiments, we have used A10 and its soluble factor in attempts to modulate the immune response of DBA/2 mice to the P815 tumor. We have shown that active immunization of mice with A10 or its soluble factor results in enhanced resistance to challenge with P815 tumor cells (43). The studies reported in depth here were undertaken to determine whether selective removal of first-order TsC with B16G conjugated to Hp would also enhance tumor immunity. The results are self-evident in showing that immune modulation can be effected in this way.

It is assumed that treatment of animals with B16G-Hp followed by light results in the elimination of a significant number of circulating TsC. This event presumably destroys the balance of the suppressor cell circuitry and permits the ongoing immune response to P815 to continue without modulation, with the result that a finite number of tumor-bearing animals are capable of completely rejecting their tumors. It is predicted that this kind of treatment is applicable to any situation in which an "auto" response is possible (probably a high percentage of tumors), and preliminary experiments with the L1210 tumor system imply this. Ongoing studies are underway in which other tumor systems are being investigated. Also, animals treated with B16G-Hp are being examined for autoimmune responses of various kinds. It is predicted that this type of treatment could have a number of side effects, enhanced autoimmunity being the most likely possibility. Nevertheless, its potential application in human therapy is of interest. We have shown that B16G appears to react with an epitope present on human TsC and TsF as well as murine cells (44), and studies are being done to characterize the subpopulation of human cells with which it reacts.

V. METHODOLOGY

A. Carbodiimide as a Coupling Agent

Carbodiimide is a much used and important reagent, which effectively serves as a condensing agent, bringing about the formation of a peptide bond between ligands according to the scheme shown in Figure 12 (45). Initial protonation of carbodiimide is considered to yield the intermediate (1) which is attached by a carboxylate anion to produce the O-acylurea (2) (46). This O-acyluria participates in conjugation with amino groups on carrier protein molecules to form the stable peptide bond.

Traditional conjugations utilizing carbodiimide with antibodies have been done in aqueous buffer. These conditions tend to lower the efficiency of bond formation because of the destabilization of O-acylurea, and individual systems have to be worked out for optima of pH, timing, and other conditions as shown in Figure 13.

The approach taken originally for the coupling of porphyrins to monoclonal antibodies also involved in aqueous environment for the reaction (19). Coupling was prolonged and loading of porphyrins to MAbs varied unpredictably from one batch to another. Also, recovery of biological activity of the MAb was unpredictable owing no doubt to random location of hematoporphyrin molecules on antibody molecules.

More recently, we have carried out carbodiimide reactions in a variety of organic solvents. We find that a number of solvents can be used in which a variety of MAbs can be successfully coupled while retaining their biological activity. Carbodiimide coupling under these kinds of conditions can be very carefully controlled and loading is so efficient that assessment of the kind of ratios required can be made prior to reaction and appropriate mixtures set up.

R : CH_3CH_2-

R' : $(CH_3)_2NCH_2CH_2CH_2$-

Ab : Antibody

R' : Hematoporphyrin

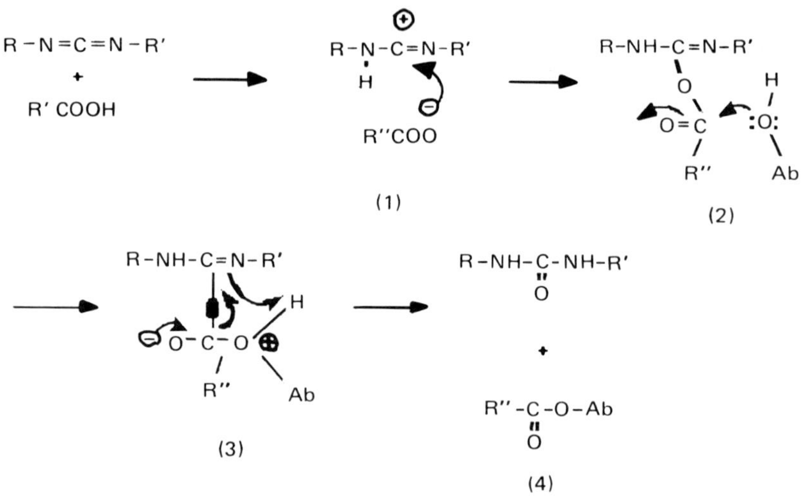

Figure 12 Mechanism of carbodiimide conjugation. Initial protonation of carbodiimide yields intermediate (1), which is attacked by a carboxylate anion to produce the O-acylurea (2), which participates in the conjugation of Hp with monoclonal antibodies.

B. Experimental Conditions

Fresh 1-ethyl-3-(3-dimethylaminopropyl) carbodiimide · HCl (EDCl, 20 mg from Sigma) was mixed with hematoporphyrin (1.0 mg, from Aldrich) in 1.0 ml of DMSO (spectro grade) at room temperature under N_2 for 30 minutes. Then lyophilized B16G (previously purified on DEAE-Sephadex and dialyzed against distilled H_2O prior to lyophilization) was dissolved in the reaction mixture for 1 minute. Molar ratios of Hp to MAb were modified from one coupling to another to test the loading capacity of this particular MAb. The reaction mixture was diluted with 3.0 ml of phosphate buffered saline (PBS), pH 7.5, containing 50 μl of monoethanolamine to quench the reaction. The resulting mixture was stirred for an additional 2 minutes and then dialyzed exhaustively against PBS at 4°C.

R : CH_3CH_2-

R' : $(CH_3)_2NCH_2CH_2CH_2$-

Ab : Antibody

R'' : Hematoporphyrin

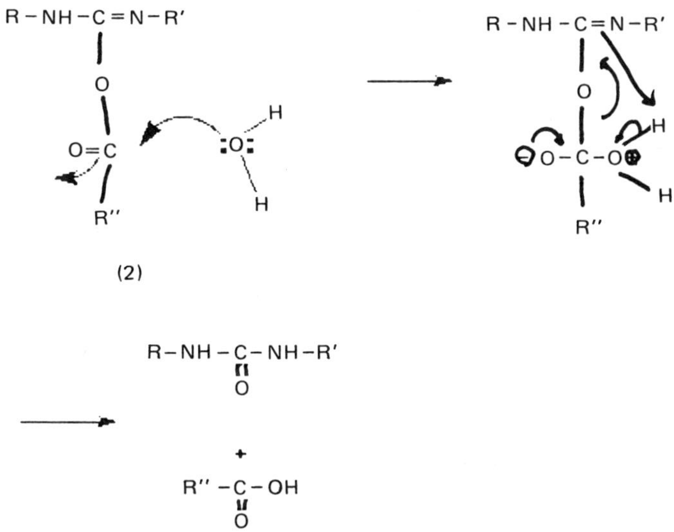

Figure 13 Mechanism by which water molecules can destabilize O-acylurea so that optimal coupling cannot be effected.

As stated above, a number of couplings of B16G to Hp were carried out with varying levels of Hp attached. We determined that when heavy loading was effected (>100 molecules Hp per molecule of MAb), significant inactivation of the MAb occurred. In most experiments, loading of between 40-50 molecules of Hp permitted maintenance of antibody activity and was therefore used as the range for loading.

The ratio of Hp:MAb was calculated spectrophotometrically by taking the absorbance at 505 nm of 0.644 for 80 μg Hp per ml. Protein concentration was determined by 280 nm absorbance (1.4 = 1.0 mg B16G per ml) prior to conjugation. Protein concentration following conjugation was determined by biorad assay.

C. Measurement of Noncovalent Association of Hp with B16G

Hp, and more specifically, Hpd, are reported to associate with cell membranes, particularly those of malignant cells. The nature of the association is not understood. We had some concern that Hp might associate in a noncovalent manner with MAb molecules, so that estimates of loading efficiency might not be accurate. This would have particular significance in situations where coupling reactions were taking place over a prolonged period of time. Noncovalent associations of Hp molecules can be demonstrated by running conjugates on TLC plates under circumstances where uncoupled Hp molecules will migrate away from the protein and can be detected under a chromatoviewer. However, this approach, while demonstrating the problem, does not yield quantified results. In order to examine the potential magnitude of the problem, the following experiment was carried out.

Hp and B16G were mixed in PBS at a ratio of 60 μg Hp/mg B16G. Actual concentrations were Hp at 30 μg/ml and B16G at 500 μg/ml. The mixture was maintained at room temperature in the dark for 2 hours, after which it was dialyzed against 2 liters of PBS with two buffer changes over 24 hours at 4°C in the dark. After this, relative concentrations of B16G and Hp inside the dialysis tube were assessed spectrophotometrically. It was found that approximately 50% of the Hp was still associated with the B16G molecule. Subsequent studies of this nature confirmed that even after a relatively short time (45-60 min), considerable association between Hp and various test MAbs took place. The association of Hp with B16G was quantified in the following manner.

Using a Perkin-Elmer 650-10 S fluorescence spectrophotometer, fluorescence depolarization was used to determine the association of Hp with B16G. The excitation wavelength was 400 nm, the emission wavelength 610 nm. Sensitivity range was 1.0 and slit width 5.0 nm. Two procedures were followed. A solution containing 285 ng Hp in 1.0 ml PBS was added to the cuvette. Aliquots of 100

μl of B16G (510 μg/ml) in PBS were added to the Hp solution, and fluorescence of this was also measured for comparison with test samples. Similarly, a 1.0 ml solution of B16G (510 μg) was titrated in reverse with 100 μl aliquots of Hp at a concentration of 2.85 μg/ml. The amount of free vs. bound Hp was determined using the following equation:

$$Hp_b = F_0/F_b * 285 \text{ ng}$$

where Hp_b is bound Hp, F_0 is the fluorescence difference (mixture – control), and F_b the fluorescence of Hp which is completely bound. The amount of free Hp was then calculated by subtracting bound Hp from the total. Results were plotted according to the method of Scatchard (47) using the expression:

$$R/A = nka - rKa$$

where r is the number of moles of Hp bound per mole of protein, n is the number of binding sites, Ka the association constant, and A the concentration of free Hp. The results are shown in Figure 1.

D. Cell Lines and Cell Products

The MAb B16G was used as the major targeting antibody throughout this study. It was produced in our laboratory and has been described extensively elsewhere (24). Antibody purified from ascites fluid, along with an appropriate negative control MAb (CMAb) of the same Ig subclass as B16G, was labeled with Hp as described above. The material was tested for specific activity by a standard ELISA reaction carried out under dark conditions. Plates, subsequent to addition of Hp-labeled MAb, were wrapped in foil throughout the reaction time. They were washed and treated with secondary antibody under conditions of dim light. A second MAb, EA2, shown to have similar properties to B16G, was also used in a number of experiments. It was handled in essentially the same manner as B16G.

The T-cell hybridoma, A10, was also used in these experiments, and has been described in detail elsewhere (41). Briefly, this hybridoma is a fusion product of the T-cell fusion partner BW5147 and thymocytes from P815 membrane extract-primed DBA/2 mice. The A10 hybridoma secretes a TsF molecule which specifically enhances the growth of P815 tumor in DBA/2 mice. The factor released is bound by B16G. The A10 cell is considered to be a prototype of Ts1 cells controlling the immune response to the P815 tumor in this mouse strain.

The tumor cell lines P815 and L1210 were used in these experiments. Both are syngeneic for DBA/2 mice and have been maintained in this laboratory for the past 10 years.

E. Direct Cytotoxicity of Hp Conjugates

In order to determine whether B16G-Hp conjugates were capable of specifically killing subpopulations of murine T lymphocytes, the A10 hybridoma described above was used. Experiments were done as follows. A10 or control cells (P815 or L1210) were grown in vitro in DME plus 10% FCS at 37°C and 10% CO_2. Cells in log phase of growth and >90% viable were washed and resuspended in serum-free DME. In direct killing experiments, MAb-Hp conjugates or appropriate control materials were added to aliquots of cells under dark conditions. Cells were incubated for 30 minutes at 37°C and washed three times by centrifugation through serum-free DME, all under dim light conditions. They were then exposed to light for 30 minutes, washed again 3 times and resuspended in DME plus 10% FCS. Cells were suspended at a concentration of 1.0×10^6 in 1.0 ml of DME for light exposure. The light source was a bank of four fluorescent tubes (General Electric F20T12-cool white). The spectrum of light generated ranged from 300-750 nm. The intensity of the light was measured by a YS1-Kettering Model 65 RAdiometer and was 1.5 milliwatts per cm^2. Cells were exposed at a distance of 11.0 cm where temperatures never exceeded 25°C. Treated cells were assessed for viability immediately after treatment using Eosin Y dye exclusion, or were dispensed into microtiter wells (triplicate or quandruplicates of 200 μl each) and [^{3}H]-thymidine (2 μCi in 50 μl medium) added to each well. Cultures were incubated overnight, at which time they were harvested on a MASH harvester, and cells were assessed for relative viability by comparison of [^{3}H]-thymidine incorporation of experimental samples to cell samples which had been treated identically but had not been exposed to Hp or Hp-MAb conjugates. (See Figs. 2-5.)

In another series of experiments, rabbit anti-mouse Ig (RαMIg) was affinity purified and labeled with Hp by standard procedures described here. It was similarly assessed for biological activity following labeling. Cell killing experiments utilizing RαMIg-Hp allowed for another level of control in these experiments, since all cell samples treated received identical Hp conjugate while receiving different MAbs as primary antibodies. In these experiments, cells to be tested were treated first with unlabeled MAbs (B16G or control) for 30 minutes at 37°C. Following washing, all samples (except untreated controls) were treated with RαMIg-Hp under dark conditions for a further 30 minutes at 37°C, washed three times, resuspended in serum-free medium, and exposed to light for 30 minutes. They were then washed, resuspended in medium plus FCS, and treated as described above. In this way, we were able to assess the specificity of B16G-Hp conjugates for the A10 T-cell hybridoma. (See Fig. 6.)

F. Experimental Design

In vivo experiments on DBA/2 mice bearing the P815 mastocytoma were carried out to determine whether B16G-Hp could effectively kill TsC in these animals and whether such treatment would alter the course of tumor growth. Mice were injected subcutaneously in the left flank with 10^4 P815 cells in 0.2 ml. They were rested for 8 days, at which time tumors were just palpable (approximately 25 mm^2 in area). Animals were randomized into experimental groups and injected intravenously with B16G-Hp, B16G plus Hp, control MAb-Hp, Hp alone, or PBS in 0.2 ml. All levels of Hp and MAb were the same in all groups. Animals were left in the dark for 2 hours, exposed to light (the same as that described for cells) for 4 hours, and thereafter were maintained under normal conditions. Animals were monitored daily for tumor growth and survival. The area of growing tumors was estimated my multiplying values for two cross-sectional tumor measurements using callipers. All measurements were made blind. (See Figs. 7-10.)

G. Measurement of Cytotoxic T Lymphocytes in B16G-Hp-treated Animals

Because we noted an effect on tumor growth in mice treated with B16G-Hp, we undertook experiments to determine whether the enhanced tumor resistance seen in these animals was associated with increased immunological activity, such as the generation of P815-reactive CTL. Animals were treated with B16G-Hp or control materials described earlier. At various time intervals after treatment, groups were sacrificed and their spleens removed and tested for CTL to P815 as described previously (43). Briefly, DBA/2 spleen cells were plated in doubling dilutions in V-bottom plates (Linbro #76-023-05) from 10^6 to 1.2×10^5 cells in 100-μl aliquots per well in replicates of 8. P815 cells were obtained from ascites fluid of DBA/2 mice, washed 3 times and incubated at 2-6 $\times 10^6$ cells/ml in 50 μg/ml of mitomycin C in complete RPMI (RPMI, 10 mM Hepes, 5×10^{-5} M 2-mercaptoethanol, 10% fetal calf serum, penicillin, streptomycin) at 37°C and 5% CO_2 for 1 hour. P815 cells were washed 3 times, resuspended in complete RPMI, and 100 μl containing 2.5×10^4 cells was added to all wells containing spleen cells. Five days later, cells were resuspended and 100 μl from all wells was transferred to U-bottom plates (Linbro #76-24-205). Fresh P815 cells were labeled for 1½ hours with ^{51}Cr at 0.2 mCi/2 $\times 10^6$ cells. The cells were washed, then incubated at 37°C and 5% CO_2 in complete RPMI for 3 to 4 hours. The labeled P815 cells were then washed 3 times, resuspended in complete RPMI, and 100 μl containing 10^4 cells was added to all wells, including 2 rows of 8 replicates of labeled P815 cells alone for calculation of spontaneous and maximum ^{51}Cr release. The plates were centrifuged at 100 rpm for 5 minutes and then incubated at 37°C and 5% CO_2. After 18 hours, plates were again centrifuged and 100 μl of supernatant was removed from all wells except for rows of P815 cells alone, in which 100 μl of cell suspension was removed to calculate maximum potential ^{51}Cr release. Samples were counted in a Picker Pace 1 gamma counter. Percent specific lysis was calculated as follows (see Fig. 11):

$$\% \text{ specific lysis} = \frac{\text{sample cpm} - \text{spontaneous cpm}}{\text{maximum cpm} - \text{spontaneous cpm}} \times 100$$

REFERENCES

1. Ritz, J., and Schlossman, S. F. (1982) Utilization of monoclonal antibodies in the treatment of leukemia and lymphoma. *Blood 59*: 1–11.
2. Miller, R. A., and Levy, R. (1981) Response of cutaneous T cell lymphomas to therapy with hybridoma monoclonal antibody. *Lancet 2*:226-230.
3. Miller, R. A., Maloney, D. G., Warnicki, E. R., and Levy, R. (1982) Treatment of B cell lymphoma with monoclonal anti-idiotype antibody. *N. Engl. J. Med. 306*:517-522.
4. Sehon, A. H. (1982) Suppression of IgE antibodies with conjugates of haptens or allergens and synthetic hydrophilic polymers. *Ann. N.Y. Acad. Sci. 392*:45-70.
5. Wilkinson, I., Jackson, C-J. C., Lang, G. M., Holford-Strevens, V., and Sehon, A. H. (1986) Tolerance induction by conjugates of xenogeneic monoclonal IgG (xIgG) and monomethoxypolyethylene glycol. (mPEG). In *Proceedings of the 6th International Congress of Immunology*. Abstract no. 3.74.5, p. 493.
6. Herlyn, D., Ross, A. H., and Koprowski, H. (1986) Anti-idiotypic antibodies bear the internal image of a human tumor antigen. *Science 232*:100-102.
7. Schreiher, H. (1984) Idiotype network interactions in tumor immunity. *Adv. in Cancer Res. 41*:291-321.
8. Jerne, N. K., Roland, J., and Cazenave, P. A. (1982) Recurrent idiotypes and internal images. *Eur. Molec. Biol. J. 1*:243-247.
9. Koprowski, H., Herlyn, D., Lubeck, M., DeFreitas, E., and Sears, H. F. (1984). Human anti-idiotypic antibodies in cancer patients. Is the modulation of the immune response beneficial for the patient? *Proc. Natl. Acad. Sci. 81*:216-219.
10. Springer, J. F., Desai, P. R., Murthy, M. S., Tegtmeyer, H., and Scanlon, E. F. (1979) Human carcinoma-associated precursor antigens on blood group MN system and the hosts' immune response to them. *Prog. Allergy 26*:42-48.
11. Meeker, T., Lowder, J., Cleary, M. L., Stewart, S., Warnke, R., Sklar, J., and Levy, R. (1985) Emergence of idiotype variants during treatment of B cell lymphoma with anti idiotype antibodies. *New Engl. J. Med. 312*: 1658-1665.
12. Longenecker, M. B., Rahman, A. F. R., Leight, J. B., Purser, R. A., Greenberg, A. H., Willians, D. J., Keller, O., Petrik, P. K., Thay, T. Y., Suresh, M. R., and Noujaim, A. A. (1984) Monoclonal antibody against a cryptic carbohydrate antigen of murine and human lymphocytes. *Int. J. Cancer 33*: 123-129.
13. Shysh, A., Eu, S. M., Noujaim, A. A. Suresh, M. R., and Longenecker, B. M. (1985) Radioimmunodetection of murine manamaryadenocarcinoma (TA3/

Ha) lung and liver metastases with radioiodinated PNA. *Int. J. Cancer 35*: 113-119.

14. Spikes, J. D. (1984) In *Porphyrin Localization and Treatment of Tumors* (Doiron, D. R., and Gomer, Ch., Eds.). Alan R. Liss, Inc., New York, pp. 19-39.
15. Kessel, D., Chang, C. K., and Musselman, B. (1985) Chemical, biologic and biophysical studies on hematoporphyrin derivative. In: *Methods in Porphyrin Photosensitization* (Kessel, D., Ed.). Plenum Press, New York, pp. 213-227.
16. Dougherty, T. J. (1981) Photoradiation therapy for cutaneous and subcutaneous maliganancies. *J. Invest. Dermatol. 77*:122-124.
17. Dougherty, T. J., Kaufman, J. H., Godlfarb, A., Weishaupt, K. R., Boyle, D., and Mittleman, A. (1978) Photoradiation therapy for the treatment of maligmant tumors. *Cancer Res. 38*:2628-2635.
18. Ha, X.-W., Sun, S.-M., Xie, J.-G., Fan, X.-J., Zhang, Y.-H., Mei, Q.-C., Shen, H., and Xu, S.-L. (1983) Clinical use of hematoporphyrin derivative in malignant tumors. *Chin. Med. J. 96*;743-739.
19. Mew, D., Wat, C.-K., Towers, G. H. N., and Levy, J. G. (1983) Photoimmunotherapy: treatment of animal tumors with tumor-specific monoclonal antibody-hematoporphyrin conjugates. *J. Immunol. 130*:1473-1477.
20. Mew, D., Lumn, V., Wat, C.-K., Towers, G. H. N., Sun, C. Oh. C., Walter, R. J., Wright, W., Berns, M. W., and Levy, J. G. (1985) Ability of specific monoclonal antibodies and conventional antisera conjugated to hematoporphyrin to label and kill selected cell lines subsequent to light activation. *Cancer Res. 45*:4380-4386.
21. Takei, F., Levy, J. G., and Kilburn, D. G. (1976) In vitro induction of cytotoxicity against syngeneic mastocytoma and its suppression by spleen and thymus cells from tumor bearing mice. *J. Immunol. 116*:288-293.
22. Takei, F., Levy, J. G., and Kilburn, D. G. (1977) Characterization of suppressor cells in mice bearing syngeneic mastocytoma. *J. Immunol. 118*: 412-417.
23. Takei, F., Levy, J. G., and Kilburn, D. G. (1978) Characterization of a soluble factor which specifically suppresses the in vitro generation of cells cytotoxic for syngeneic tumor cells in mice. *J. Immunol. 120*:1218-1224.
24. Maier, T., Stammers, A., Tench, and Levy, J. G. (1983) Characterization of a monoclonal antibody directed to a T cell suppressor factor. *J Immunol. 131*:1843-1848.
25. Mills, C. D., and North, R. J. (1985) $Ly1^+$ suppressor T cells inhibit the expression of passively transferred anti-tumor immunity by suppressing the generation of cytolytic T cells. *Transplantation 39*:202-208.
26. Fujiwara, H., Hamaoka, T., Shearer, G. M., Yamamoto, H., and Terry, W.D. (198) The augmentation of in vitro and in vivo tumor-specific T cell mediated immunity by amplifier T lymphocytes. *J. Immunol. 124*:863-869.
27. Fernandez-Cruz, E., Gilman, S. E., and Feldman, J. D. (1982) Immunotherapy of a chemically induced sarcoma in rats: characterization of the

effector T cell subset and nature of suppression. *J. Immunol. 128*:1112-1121.

28. Mule, J. J., Rosenstein, M., Shu, S., and Rosenberg, S. A. (1985) Eradication of a disseminated syngeneic mouse lymphoma by systemic adoptive transfer of immune lymphocytes and its dependence on host components. *Cancer Res. 45*:526-531.
29. Evans, R., and Duffy, T. M. (1985) Amplification of immune T lymphocyte function in situ: the identification of active components of the immunologic network during tumor rejection. *J. Immunol. 135*:1498-1504.
30. Greene, M. I., Fujimoto, S., and Sehon, A. H. (1977) Regulation of the immune response to tumor antigens. *J. Immunol. 119*:747-764.
31. Fujimoto, S., Matsugawa, T., Nakagawa, K., and Tada, T. (1978) Cellular interaction between cytotoxic and suppressor T cells against syngeneic tumors in the mouse. *Cell. Immunol. 38*:378-387.
32. Nagarkatti, M., and Kaplan, A. M. (1985) The role of suppressor T cells in BCNU-mediated rejection of syngeneic tumor. *J. Immunol. 135*:1510-1517.
33. Kern, D. E., Klarnet, J. P., Jensen, M. C., and Greenberg, P. D. (1986) Requirement for recognition of class II molecules and processed tumor antigen for optimal generation of syngeneic tumor-specific class I restricted CTL. *J. Immunol. 136*:4303-4310.
34. Ninnemin, J. L. (1978) Melanoma-associated immunosuppression through B cell activation of suppressor T cells. *J. Immunol. 120*:1573-1579.
35. Chiorazzi, N., Fu, S. M., Montazeri, H. G., Kunkel, H. G., Lai, K., and Gee, T. (1979) T cell helper defect in patients with chronic lymphocytic leukemia. *J. Immunol. 122*:1087-1090.
36. Ramey, W. G., Kaskin, G. A., Munther, A. S., Swistel, A. J., Burrows, W. B., and Fitzpatrick, H. F. (1980) Detection of circulating lung tumor antigen sensitive T lymphocytes in the early stages of lung cancer. *Surgery 88*:202-206.
37. Kelly, B. S., Stredulinsky, U., Van den Hoek, J., and Levy, J. G. (1981) Antibodies in the sera of patients with bronchogenic carcinoma that react with antigen from a tumor cell line. *Cancer Immunol. Immunother. 12*:5-10.
38. Kutteh, W. H., and Doellgast, G. J. (1986) Autologous antibodies eluted from membrane fragments in human ovarian epithelial neoplastic effusions. *J. Natl. Cancer Inst. 76*:797-804.
39. Lewis, M. j., Phillips, T. M., and Rowden, G. (1978) Beneficial and detrimental effects of humoral immunity in malignancy. *Pathobiol. Annu. 8*:217-239.
40. Vlock, D. R., Der Simonian, R., and Kirkwood, J. R. (1986) Prognostic role of antibody reactivity to melanoma. *J. Clin. Invest. 77*:1116-1121.
41. Steele, J. K., Stammers, A. Tench, and Levy, J. G. (1985) Isolation and characterization of a tumor specific T suppressor factor from a T cell hybridoma. *J. Immunol. 134*:2767-2778.

42. Steele, J. K., Chu, N. R., Chan, A., North, J., and Levy, J. G. (1987) Isolation of an antigen specific T suppressor factor which suppresses the in vivo response of DBA/2 mice to ferredoxin. *J. Immunol., 139*:469-474.
43. Steele, J. K., Singhai, R., Stammers, A. Tench, and Levy, J. G. (1986) Immunization of DBA/2 mice with a T cell hybridoma-derived TsF increases immune resistant to the syngeneic tumors P815 and L1210. *J. Immunol. 137*:3025-3030.
44. Steele, J. K., Stammers, A. Tench, and Levy, J. G. (1985) Preliminary characterization of human T cell suppressor factor (HTsF) isolated from tonsil cells by monoclonal antibody immunoadsorbence. *J. Immunol. 135*: 1201-1207.
45. Kurzer, F., and Doraghi-Zadeh (1967) Advances in the chemistry of carbodiimide. *Chem. Rev. 67*:107-152.
46. Doleschall, G., and Lempert, K. (1963) On the mechanisms of the carboxyl condensation by carbodiimides. *Tetrahedron Letters*: 1195-1199.
47. Scatchard, G. (1949) The attractions of proteins for small molecules and ions. *Ann. N.Y. Acad. Sci. 51*:660-672.

7

Synthesis of Antibody Conjugates with Cobra Venom Factor Using Heterobifunctional Cross-Linking Reagents

CARL-WILHELM VOGEL
Vincent T. Lombardi Cancer Center and International Center for Interdisciplinary Studies of Immunology, Georgetown University School of Medicine, Washington, D.C.

Most of the current approaches of immunotargeting utilize antibody conjugates with toxic substances, such as protein toxins of bacterial or plant origin or chemotherapeutic drugs (for review, see Ref. 1). An alternative to the antibody-targeted delivery of toxic substances is antibody-targeted delivery of biological response modifiers, such as cobra venom factor (CVF), interferon, formyl-methionyl-leucyl-phenylalanine (f-met-leu-phe), and others (2,3). These substances typically lack direct cytotoxic effects while exerting antitumor effects through activation or stimulation of one or more of the host's defense mechanisms. In this chapter, antibody conjugates with CVF will be reviewed. Emphasis is placed on the methods of synthesis of antibody-CVF conjugates using heterobifunctional cross-linking reagents and the effect that these cross-linking reagents have on the activity and properties of the resulting conjugates.

CVF is the complement-activating protein in cobra venom. It is a glycoprotein of M_r = 136,000 (4,5) that structurally resembles C3 and its physiological activation products C3b and C3c (6). In mammalian serum, CVF functions like C3b, which is physiologically formed during the activation of the alternative complement pathway (for review, see Ref. 7). Like C3b, CVF binds in serum to Factor B (8,9). When in complex with CVF, Factor B is cleaved by Factor D into Bb, which remains bound to CVF, and Ba, which is released (10,11). The bimolecular complex CVF,Bb, like C3b,Bb is an alternative complement pathway C3/C5 convertase (EC 3.4.21.47). The catalytic site resides in the Bb subunit of both enzymes which cleaves the alpha chains of C3 and C5.

Despite the identical substrate specificity and a similar molecular architecture of the two enzymes (12,13), the enzymes differ in several important properties. While both enzymes exhibit spontaneous decay-dissociation into the two respective subunits, the half-life of this decay-dissociation at 37°C is 1.5 min for C3b,Bb (14) and 7 hr for CVF,Bb (15). C3b,Bb is disassembled by Factor H (16), and C3b is inactivated by the combined action of Factor H and Factor I (17). In contrast, CVF,Bb is resistant to these regulatory complement proteins (18,19). C3b,Bb requires additional C3b to act on C5 (20,21), whereas CVF,Bb can cleave C5 directly (22,23). Due to these properties, the CVF,Bb enzyme continuously activates C3 and C5. For this reason, CVF is commonly used in immunological research to decomplement laboratory animals (24,25).

The physicochemical stability of the CVF,Bb enzyme and its resistance to inactivation by the regulatory proteins Factor H and Factor I were the rationale for coupling CVF to monoclonal antibodies with specificity for cell surface antigens. By targeting CVF to a cell surface, the stable CVF-dependent C3/C5 convertase will form on the cell in the presence of serum, causing continuous activation of C3 and C5. This exhaustive complement activation will cause cell death. Therefore, the targeting of CVF functionally represents the targeting of exhaustive complement activation. This concept has been shown to be successful with melanoma cells, leukemia cells, lymphocytes, and erythrocytes as target cells (see Sec. V).

I. SYNTHESIS AND ACTIVITY OF ANTIBODY CONJUGATES WITH COBRA VENOM FACTOR

The synthesis of antibody conjugates with cobra venom factor requires derivatization of both proteins with a heterobifunctional cross-linking reagent, since neither protein contains a free sulfhydryl group. The antibody was always used for the introduction of free sulfhydryl groups using N-succinimidyl-3-(2-pyridyldithio)propionate (SPDP) (26), while CVF was always used to introduce sulfhydryl-reactive groups. This was performed with several heterobifunctional cross-linking reagents differing in their sulfhydryl-reactive groups. The sulfhydryl-reactive groups introducted into CVF included the pyridyldithio group (using SPDP), the maleimide group (using succinimidyl-4-(N-maleimidomethyl)-cyclohexane-1-carboxylate (SMCC), γ-N-maleimidobutyryl-N-hydroxysuccinimide ester (GMBS), m-maleimidobenzoyl-N-hydroxysuccinimide ester (MBS), or succinimidyl-4-(p-maleimidophenyl)butyrate (SMPB)), and the iodide group (using iodoacetyl-N-hydroxysuccinimide ester (IAHS) or N-succinimidyl-(4-io-

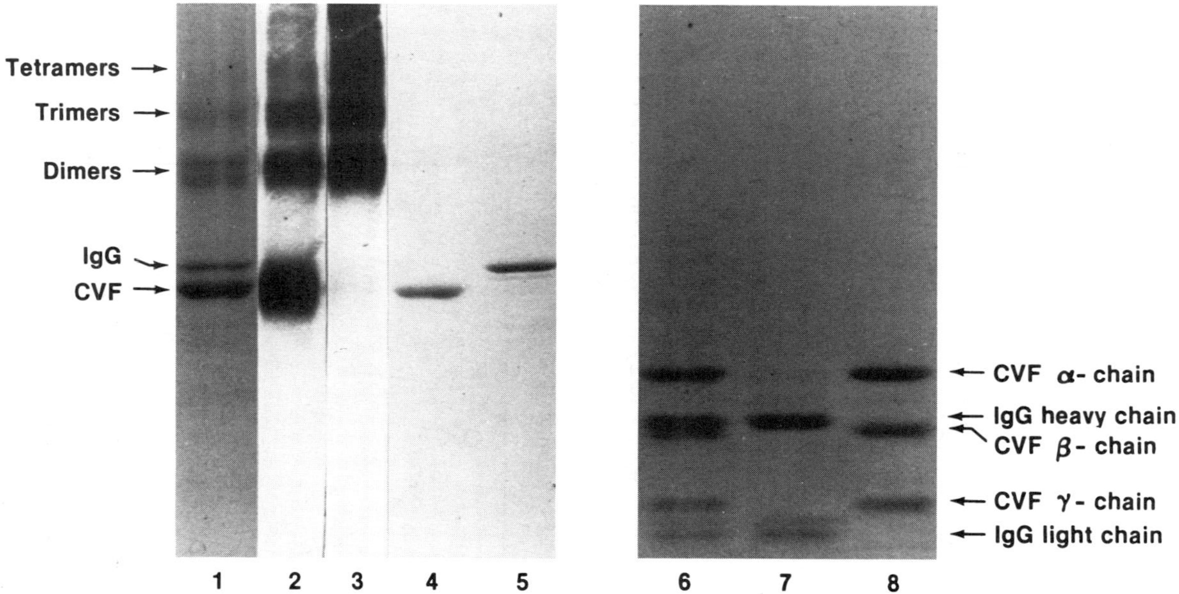

Figure 1 Characterization of hybrid proteins consisting of a monoclonal IgG antibody and CVF by SDS gradient polyacrylamide gel electrophoresis under nonreducing (left panel) and reducing conditions (right panel). Lane 1 shows a typical reaction mixture stained with Coomassie blue. The presence of free IgG and CVF (noncoupled monomers) and of different oligomeric hybrids is evident. Lane 2 shows an autoradiograph of a similar reaction mixture containing ^{125}I-labeled CVF and unlabeled IgG. Lane 3 shows an autoradiograph of the same reaction mixture after removal of free ^{125}I-CVF and IgG by gel filtration. Lane 4 (CVF) and lane 5 (IgG) show the individual proteins prior to coupling. Lane 6 shows the reaction mixture of lane 1 under reducing conditions. Note the complete reduction of the hybrids resulting in a mixture of the heavy and light chains of IgG (lane 7) and the alpha, beta, and gamma chains of CVF (lane 8), indicating the disulfide nature of all intermolecular cross-links. (From Ref. 27.)

doacetyl)aminobenzoate (SIAB)). For the chemical structures of all seven heterobifunctional cross-linking reagents, see Ref. 3.

Figure 1 shows a typical reaction mixture after coupling of cross-linker-derivatized CVF with SH-derivatized IgG antibody (Ab). The reaction mixture contains free CVF and IgG (noncoupled monomers) and several bands of conjugates. Based on the molecular weight of the bands, they represent dimeric (Ab-CVF; $M_r \sim 300{,}000$), trimeric (Ab_2-CVF, Ab-CVF_2; $M_r \sim 450{,}000$), tetrameric (Ab_3-CVF, Ab_2-CVF_2, Ab-CVF_3; $M_r \sim 600{,}000$), and some higher oligomeric hybrids (Fig. 1). An increased degree of substitution of the two reactants with the cross-linker and an increased concentration of the two derivatized proteins in the reaction mixture decrease the amount of remaining free reactants and cause a shift of the ratio of the different conjugates toward higher oligomers. Conversely, a decrease in the degree of substitution and a decrease of the protein concentration in the reaction mixture will result in an increased amount of noncoupled CVF and IgG and in a relatively increased proportion of dimeric conjugates.

Free CVF and IgG can be removed from conjugates by gel filtration on Ultrogel AcA 22 or TSK-4000 columns (Figs. 1 and 2). However, the separation of

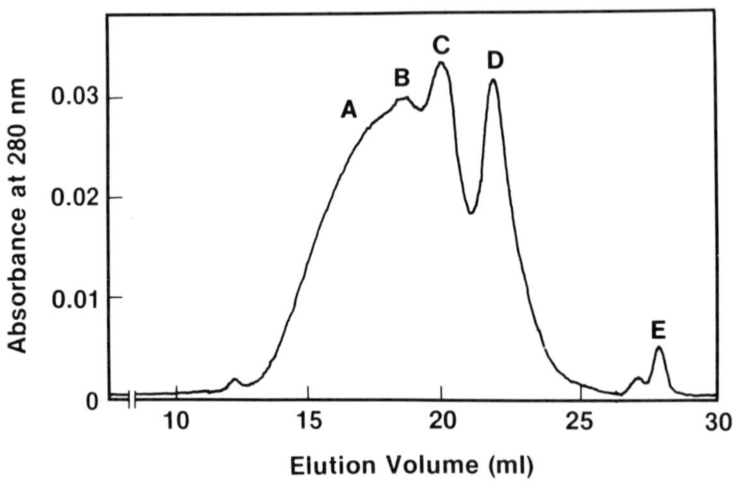

Figure 2 Size exclusion chromatography of a reaction mixture on a TSK-4000 column. Peak D contains free CVF and IgG. Peak C contains the dimeric hybrids, which are only poorly resolved from trimeric hybrids (Peak B). Tetrameric and higher oligomeric hybrids represent a shoulder (A) to the trimer peak. Peak E occurs at the total volume of the column and contains no protein. (From Refs. 27 and 28.)

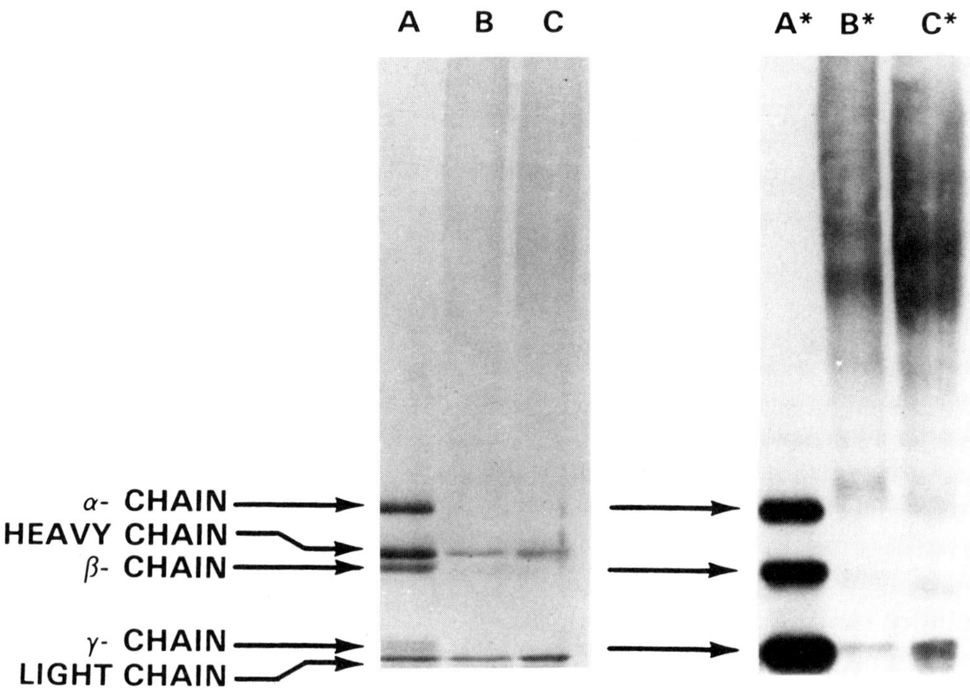

Figure 3 Partial resistance to reduction of conjugates prepared with cross-linking reagents resulting in thioether linkages. Shown is an SDS gradient polyacrylamide gel under reducing conditions (left panel) and the corresponding autoradiograph (right panel) of antibody-CVF conjugates prepared with SPDP (lane A), MBS (lane B), and IAHS (lane C). The SPDP-linked conjugates are subject to complete reduction resulting in the three polypeptide chains of CVF and the heavy and light chains of the IgG antibody (lanes A and A*; compare Fig. 1) (the autoradiograph shows only the three chains of CVF, since the ^{125}I-label was only in the CVF). MBS or IAHS-linked conjugates are partially resistant to reduction showing only low amounts of free polypeptide chains. Note that far more heavy and light chains are visible than polypeptide chains derived from CVF suggesting the presence of intramolecular cross-links in the MBS- and IAHS-derivatized CVF (compare Sec. II). (From Ref. 29 and modified from Ref. 30.)

individual oligomeric conjugates (dimers, trimers, tetramers) is not possible by this technique due to the given molecular weights of the conjugates (Fig. 2). In the case of SPDP-linked conjugates resulting in a disulfide bond in the intermolecular cross-links, the conjugates could be reduced to the individual chains of the coupled proteins (alpha, beta, and gamma chains of CVF; heavy and light chains of IgG) (Figs. 1 and 3). In the case of conjugates prepared with cross-linkers introducing a maleimide or iodide group into CVF, the resulting intermolecular cross-links contain a nonreducible thioether bond. Such conjugates are only partially susceptible to reduction; only those chains of the two proteins not involved in any cross-links are present as free chains after reduction (Fig. 3).

The degree of substitution of CVF or IgG with a cross-linker can partially be controlled by the molar ratio of cross-linker to protein (Table 1). For SPDP, it was observed that, within limits, an increase in the molar ratio resulted in a higher degree of substitution. For cross-linkers containing maleimide or iodide groups as their sulfhydryl-reactive moiety, such as MBS or IAHS, it was generally found that somewhat higher molar ratios than for SPDP were required to introduce a similar number of detectable cross-linkers. In addition, increasing the molar ratio of these cross-linking reagents did not cause a corresponding increase in the number of detectable cross-linker molecules in the derivatized proteins (Table 1). These results were found to be due to the occurrence of intramolecular cross-linking (see Sec. II).

The introduced free sulfhydryl groups oxidize within hours when exposed to air, causing the formation of disulfide-linked homooligomers of the derivatized protein (Fig. 4). To minimize this homooligomer formation, the coupling reac-

Table 1 Effect of Molar Excess of Cross-linking Reagents on Detectable Sulfhydryl-reactive Groups and Hemolytic Activity of CVF

Cross-linker	Molar excess	Sulfhydryl-reactive groups/molecule	Hemolytic activity
none	–	0	100%
SPDP	10X	3.9	53%
	20X	8.6	42%
	40X	12.8	23%
MBS	20X	6.6	9%
	40X	6.1	7%
	80X	7.7	3%
IAHS	40X	11.4	67%
	80X	9.3	29%
	160X	9.5	7%

Protein concentration 2.3 mg/ml.

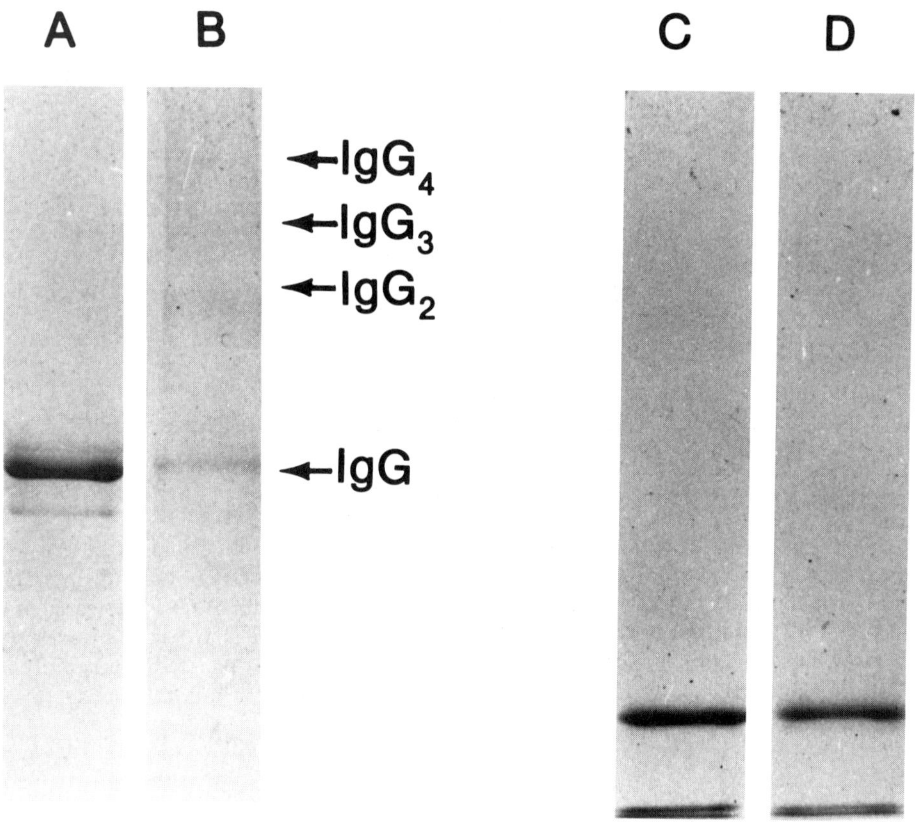

Figure 4 Homooligomer formation of sulfhydryl-derivatized IgG. Shown are SDS gradient polyacrylamide gels under nonreducing (left panel) and reducing conditions (right panel) of purified IgG (lanes A and C) and of sulfhydryl-derivatized IgG (lanes B and D) after storage for several days. (From Ref. 27.)

tions were performed under nitrogen. Furthermore, the sulfhydryl-modified IgG was immediately used for coupling. Under these conditions, homooligomer formation is insignificant as evidenced by the presence of approximately equal amounts of noncoupled CVF and IgG after the coupling reaction and by the incorporation of ^{125}I-CVF into conjugates (Fig. 1).

To study the effect of derivatization and conjugation on the functional activities of the two proteins, the hemolytic activity of CVF and the antigen-binding activity of an antimelanoma monoclonal antibody were measured. Figure 5 depicts the effect of increasing concentrations of two cross-linkers (SPDP, MBS) on the hemolytic activity of CVF. While CVF shows a dose-de-

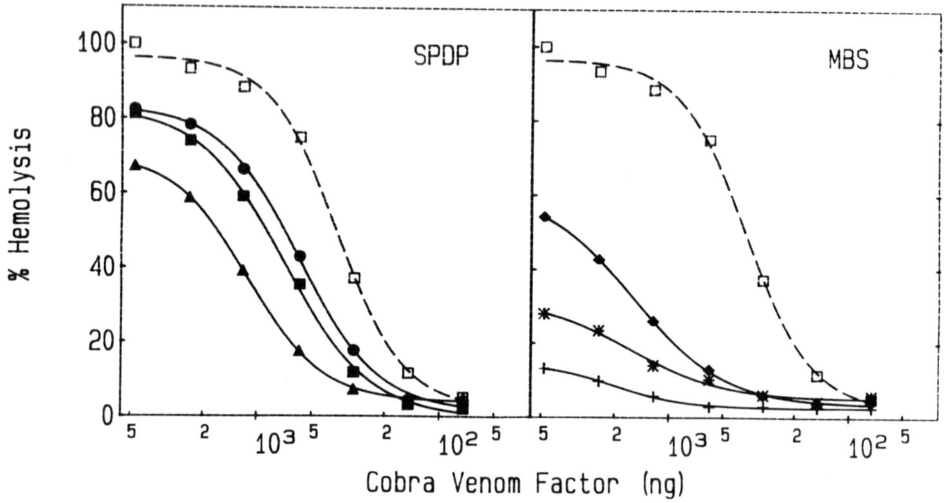

Figure 5 Effect of increasing derivatization with heterobifunctional cross-linkers on the ability of CVF to activate the alternative pathway of complement. Shown is the extent of hemolysis achieved by equal amounts of CVF derivatized with a 10X (●), 20X (■), and 40X (▲) molar excess of SPDP (left panel) or with a 20X (♦), 40X (∗), and 80X (+) molar excess of MBS (right panel). The hemolysis by equimolar amounts of underivatized CVF (□) is shown in both panels. (Portions taken from Ref. 29.)

pendent loss of activity with increasing concentration of of either cross-linker, the functional inactivation by MBS is substantially greater (compare also Table 1). Figure 6 demonstrates that the hemolytic activity of CVF upon derivatization with 7.6 SPDP molecules or 6.4 IAHS molecules was reduced by not more than 30%. The subsequent coupling to the IgG antibody further reduced the hemolytic activity by an additional 40%, indicating that the steric inactivation by conjugation is the more important factor in decreasing the functional activity than the chemical modification with the cross-linking reagent.

Figure 7 similarly demonstrates the effect of increasing degrees of derivatization of the antimelanoma monoclonal antibody with IAHS or SPDP on its binding activity. It is apparent that, while a low degree of derivatization does not cause any detectable decrease in the binding activity, higher degrees of derivatization will affect the antibody binding. Figure 7 also demonstrates that a substantially higher degree of derivatization with SPDP is required to achieve the same reduction of binding activity than observed with IAHS. The subsequent conjugation of the derivatized antibody to CVF, in contrast to the effect on the

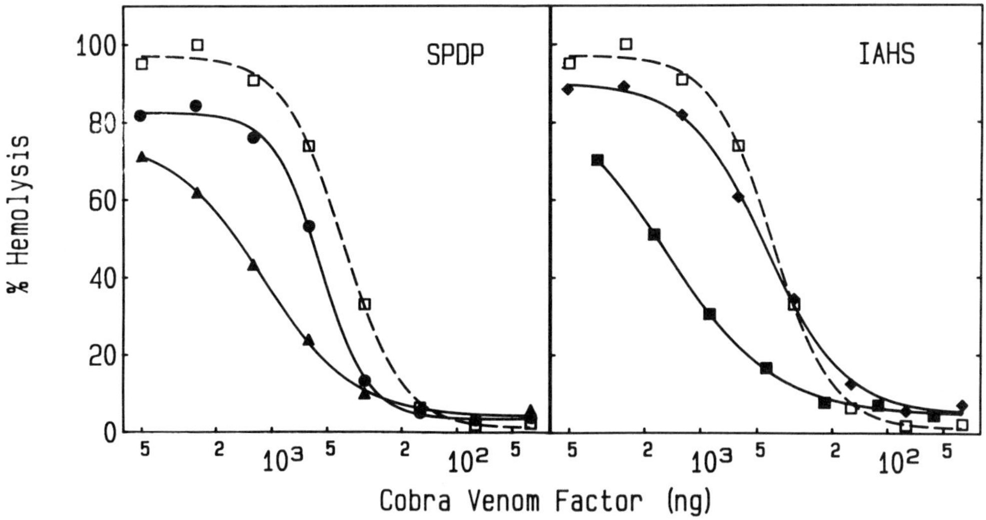

Figure 6 Effect of derivatization and conjugation on the ability of CVF to activate the alternative pathway of complement. Shown is the extent of hemolysis achieved by equimolar amounts of CVF (□), SPDP-derivatized CVF (●), and antibody-CVF conjugates (based on CVF content) (▲) (left panel) and of CVF (□) IAHS-derivatized CVF (♦), and antibody-CVF conjugates (■) (right panel). (Portions taken from Ref. 27 and 28.)

hemolytic of CVF, does not cause any detectable further decrease in the binding activity of the antibody (Fig. 8). This lower susceptibility of the IgG antibody to steric inactivation by conjugation is most likely due to the fact that there are two antigen binding sites at the distal ends of the Fab regions of the flexible IgG molecule. CVF lacks this flexibility; in addition, it needs to bind two rather bulky proteins (Factor B: $M_r \sim 93{,}000$; C5: $M_r \sim 200{,}000$). Therefore, inactivation of CVF by steric hindrance due to the coupled IgG molecule is far more likely.

The functional inactivation of both proteins by derivatization with the cross-linking reagents is a consequence of the chemical modification of primary amino groups of the proteins with the cross-linker. Assuming random and independent reaction of cross-linker molecules with amino groups and a low degree of substitution compared to the total number of amino groups (CVF or IgG contain approximately 75 primary amino groups per molecule), the process can be described by Poisson distribution. At a given average derivatization with cross-linker molecules the actual distribution is shown in Figure 9. Increasing the average degree of substitution will result in the inactivation of a higher per-

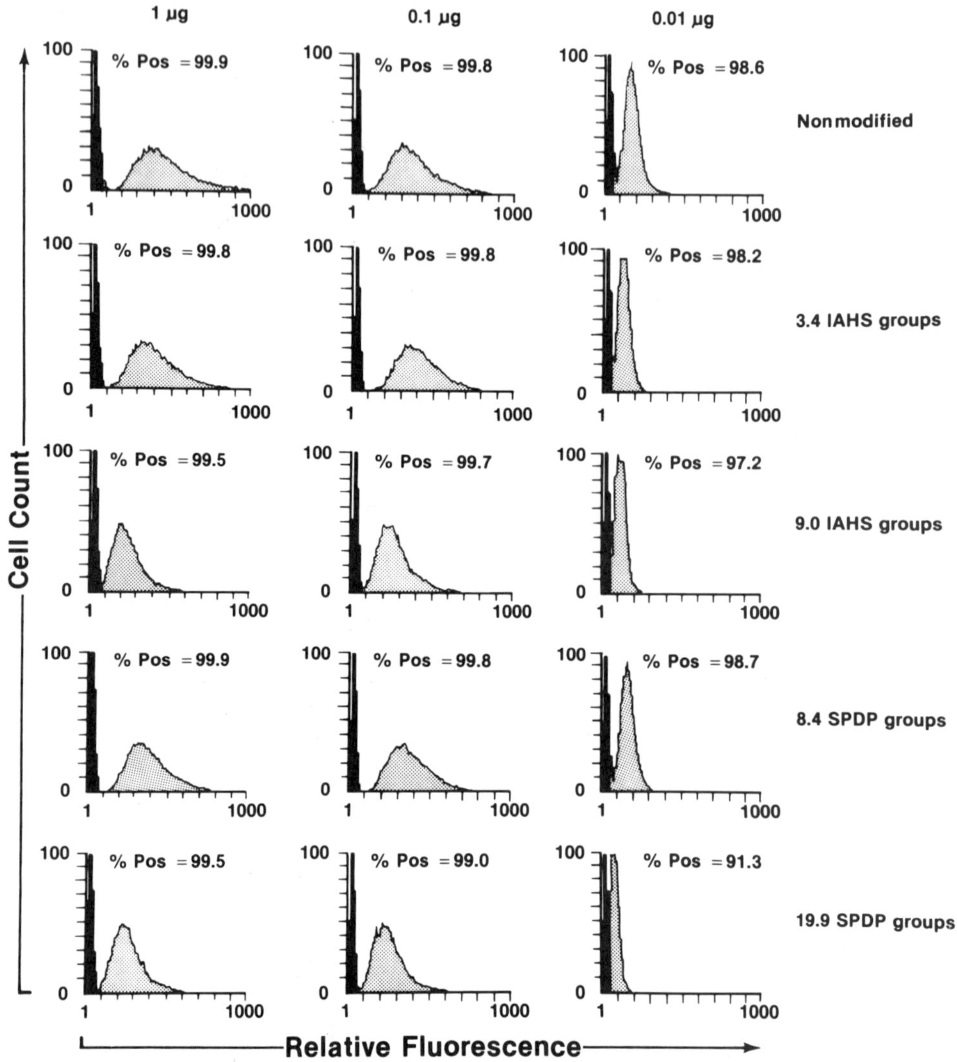

Figure 7 Effect of derivatization with heterobifunctional cross-linkers on the binding activity of the 9.2.27 monoclonal antimelanoma antibody. Shown is the relative fluorescence distribution by flow cytofluorometry of antigen-positive FEMX-Met II human melanoma cells after incubation with three different amounts of either the nonmodified monoclonal antibody or of the antibody modified with different numbers of IAHS or SPDP groups (shaded areas). Note that an average derivatization of 8.4 SPDP groups per antibody molecule has virtually no detectable effect on the binding activity. Derivatization with 3.4 IAHS groups shows only a marginal reduction of the binding activity. In contrast, derivatization with either 9.0 IAHS groups or 19.9 SPDP groups per antibody molecule reduces the binding activity as indicated by a left-shift of the

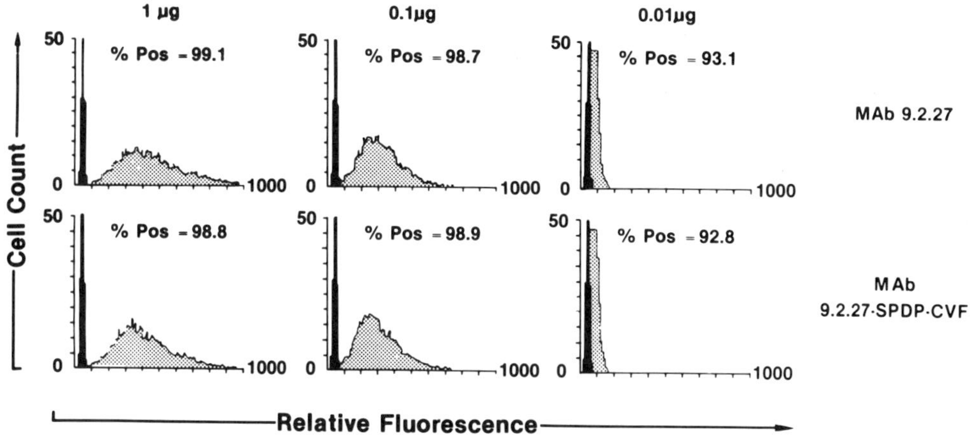

Figure 8 Effect of conjugation on the binding activity of the 9.2.27 monoclonal antimelanoma antibody. Shown is the relative fluorescence distribution by flow cytofluorometry of antigen-positive FMEX-Met II melanoma cells after incubation with three different amounts of the nonmodified monoclonal antibody (upper panels) or of antibody-CVF conjugates prepared from SH-derivatized IgG and SPDP-derivatized CVF (lower panels) (shaded areas). Note that the mean relative fluorescence is very similar for all three amounts of antibody or antibody conjugates, indicating virtually no reduction of the amount of bound IgG. The percentage of fluorescence-positive cells is also indicated in each panel. The relative fluorescence distribution obtained with a control antibody without affinity for the FMEX-Met II melanoma cells is also shown (black areas). As expected, identical results were obtained when the SH-derivatized IgG was coupled to MBS- or IAHS-derivatized CVF (30). (From Refs. 27 and 30.)

---

peak fluorescence channels. The percentage of fluorescence-positive cells is also indicated in each panel. The relative fluorescence distribution obtained with a control antibody without affinity for the FMEX-Met II melanoma cells is also shown (black areas). (From Ref. 29.)

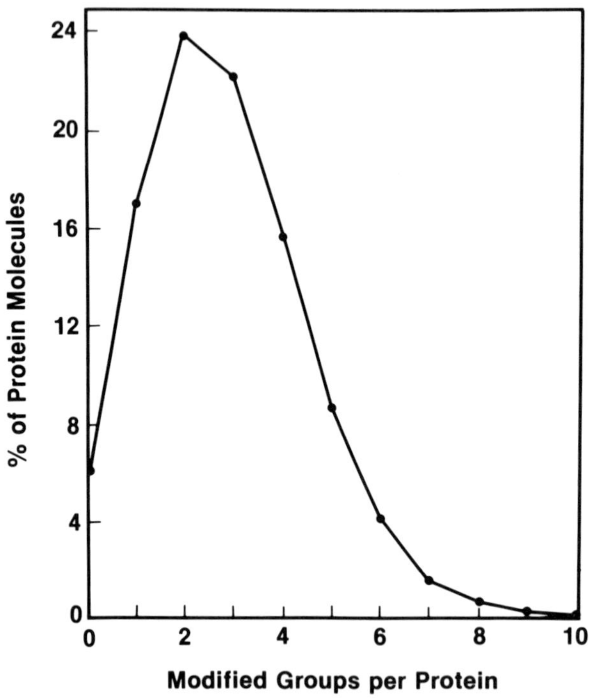

Figure 9 Shown is the actual distribution of the number of cross-linker groups per protein molecule at a mean derivatization of 2.8 groups per molecule as determined by Poisson distribution. (From Ref. 27.)

centage of the molecules. On the other hand, a comparatively low degree of average substitution will result in a greater percentage of molecules remaining unmodified (Fig. 10). For these reasons, an average degree of derivatization of approximately three to four cross-linker molecules per IgG or CVF molecule is recommended, which results in less than 5% unmodified molecules (Fig. 10). At this degree of derivatization the activity of CVF was only somewhat reduced while no loss of antigen binding of the antibody was apparent (compare Figs. 5 and 7). The subsequent coupling of the two derivatized proteins caused further and rather substantial inactivation of CVF (usually greater than 50% of the precoupling activity of the derivatized CVF), while the binding activity of the antibody portion remained unchanged (compare Figs. 6 and 8).

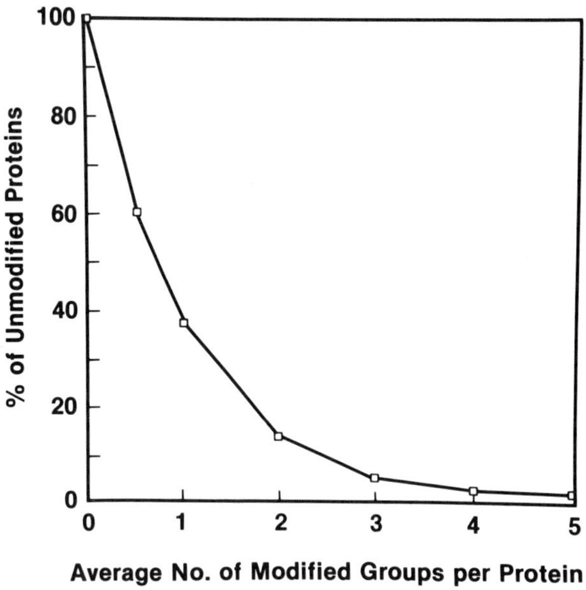

Figure 10 Shown is the percent of unmodified protein molecules as a function of the mean number of cross-linker groups per protein as determined by Poisson distribution. (From Ref. 27.)

II. OCCURRENCE OF INTRAMOLECULAR CROSS-LINKS

The substantially greater ability of maleimide- or iodide-containing cross-linking reagents to inactivate proteins upon derivatization (see Figs. 5 and 7) and the observation of increasing cross-linker concentrations not causing increasing numbers of detectable cross-linker molecules per protein molecule (see Table 1) led to investigation of the molecular basis for these findings. As is shown in Figure 11, heterobifunctional cross-linking reagents containing a maleimide group (MBS, SMCC) or an iodide groups (IAHS) as their sulfhydryl-reactive group cause intramolecular cross-linking of the three chains of CVF. All possible combinations of two covalently linked chains as well as covalent linking of all three chains is evident under reducing conditions. Nonreducing conditions reveal even the presence of covalently linked CVF dimers. This intramolecular cross-linking does not occur with SPDP, which has a pyridyldithio group as its sulfhydryl-reactive group. The intramolecular cross-linking is due to a relative lack of specificity of the maleimide group and iodide group for sulfhydryl groups. Both groups can react with amino groups (31,32), which are present in a high local concentration on the protein leading to intramolecular cross-linking and

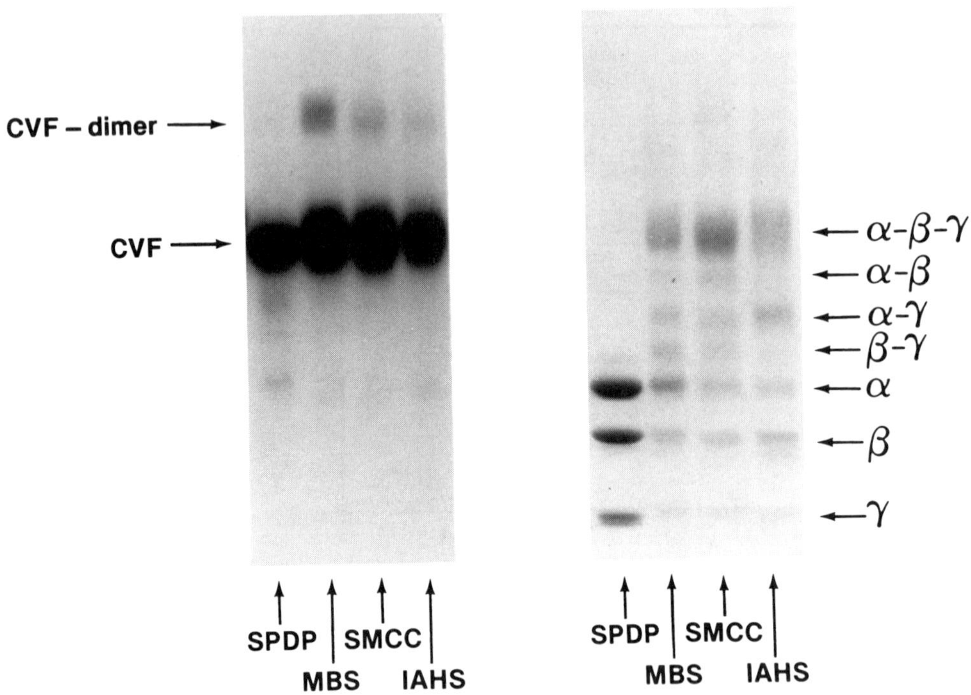

Figure 11 Intramolecular cross-links in CVF after derivatization with different heterobifunctional reagents. Shown are autoradiograms of SDS gradient polyacrylamide gels under nonreducing (left panel) and reducing conditions (right panel) of CVF derivatized with SPDP, MBS, SMCC, and IAHS. Derivatization with MBS, SMCC, and IAHS caused intramolecular cross-links leading to all possible combinations of covalent associations of the three chains of CVF (right panel) and even to formation of covalent CVF dimers (left panel). (From Refs. 3 and 29.)

even dimer formation. In contrast, the pyridyldithio group is highly specific for sulfhydryl groups. No intramolecular cross-linking or dimer formation occurs using SPDP; and under reducing conditions, the alpha, beta, and gamma chains of CVF are visible (Fig. 11).

To demonstrate that the occurrence of intramolecular cross-links is not specific for CVF, similar analyses were performed with IgG and the plant toxin ricin, a two-chain toxin frequently employed in immunoconjugates (33-35). As is shown in Figure 12, IgG derivatized with IAHS shows under reducing conditions all possible covalent combinations of light and heavy chains, while IgG deriva-

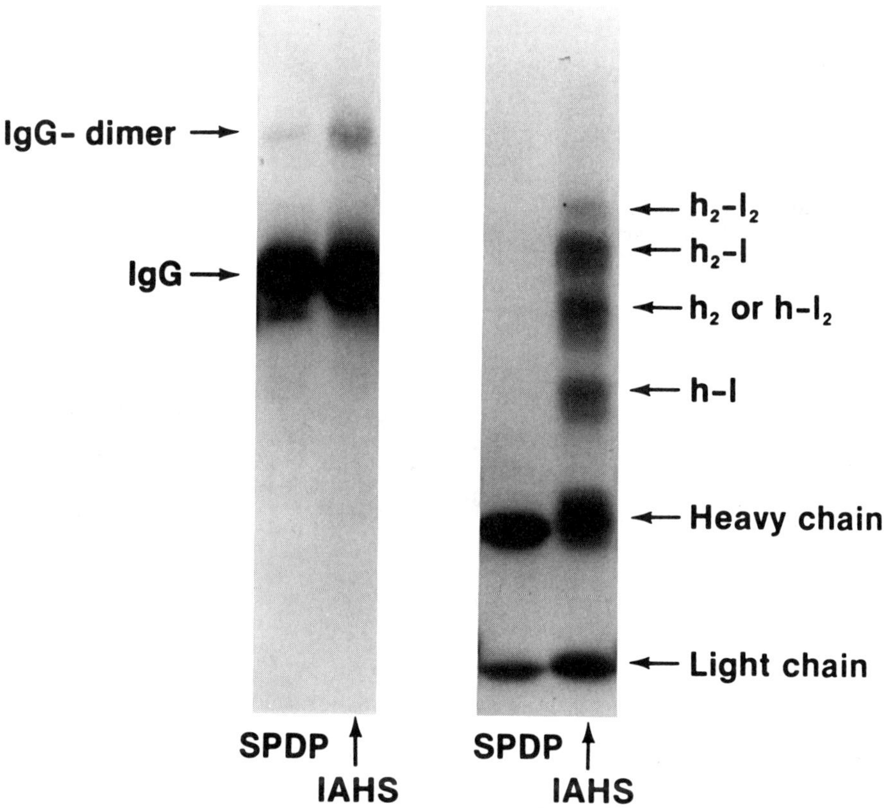

Figure 12 Intramolecular cross-links in IgG after derivatization with two heterobifunctional reagents (SPDP or IAHS). Shown are autoradiograms of SDS gradient polyacrylamide gels under nonreducing (left panel) and reducing conditions (right panel). Derivatization with IAHS caused intramolecular cross-links leading to all possible combinations of covalent associations of the IgG heavy and light chains (right panel) and even to the formation of covalent IgG dimers (left panel). (From Ref. 29.)

tized with SPDP shows only the free heavy and light chains. Similarly, nonreducible ricin (covalently linked A chain/B chain dimer) is detectable under reducing conditions after derivatization of ricin with MBS (Fig. 13). However, the extent of intramolecular cross-linking of ricin is substantially lower than observed with CVF and IgG. This decreased intramolecular cross-linking is most likely a consequence of the lower molecular weight of ricin ($M_r \sim 62{,}000$) and the correspondingly lower local concentration of amino groups.

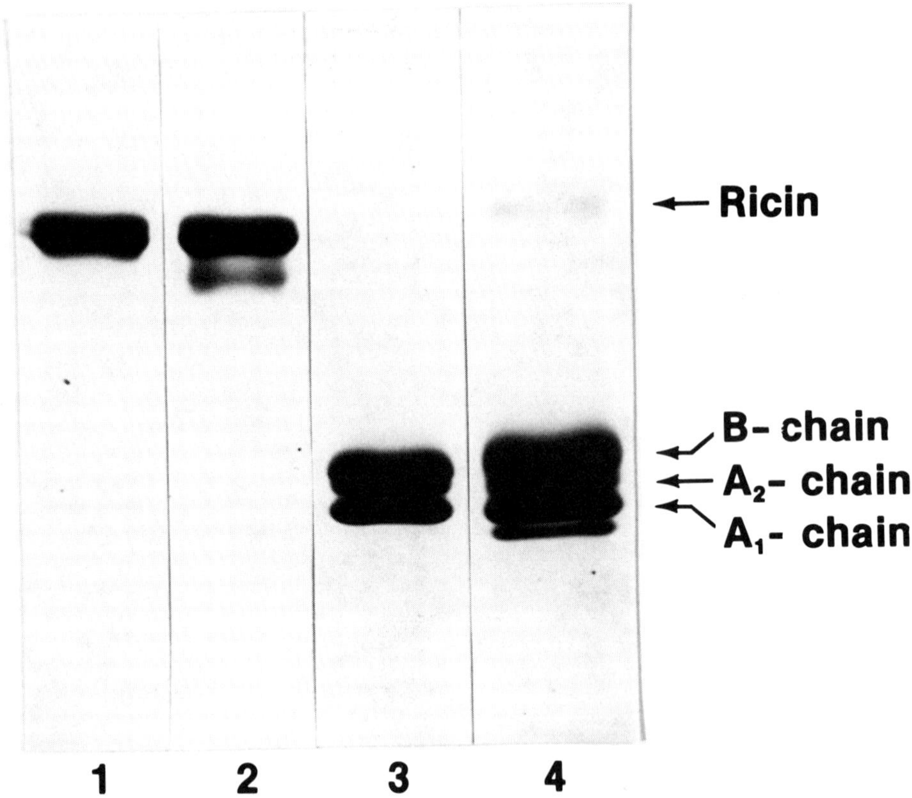

Figure 13 Intramolecular cross-links in ricin after derivatization with MBS. Shown is a polyacrylamide gel after Coomassie staining under nonreducing (left panel) and reducing conditions (right panel). The derivatization with MBS caused the formation of nonreducible ricin (covalent A chain/B chain dimer) (lane 4). (From Ref. 29.)

III. INTERACTION WITH PLASMA PROTEINS

Investigations on the effect of different heterobifunctional cross-linking reagents on the properties of the resulting antibody-CVF conjugates showed that conjugates prepared with IAHS bound covalently to plasma proteins, causing an increase in the apparent molecular weight when incubated with serum in vitro or when injected into mice (3,36-40). This observation led to a study characterizing the interaction of cross-linker-derivatized CVF and IgG with plasma proteins. Figure 14 shows that CVF and IgG after derivatization with SPDP, MBS, SMCC,

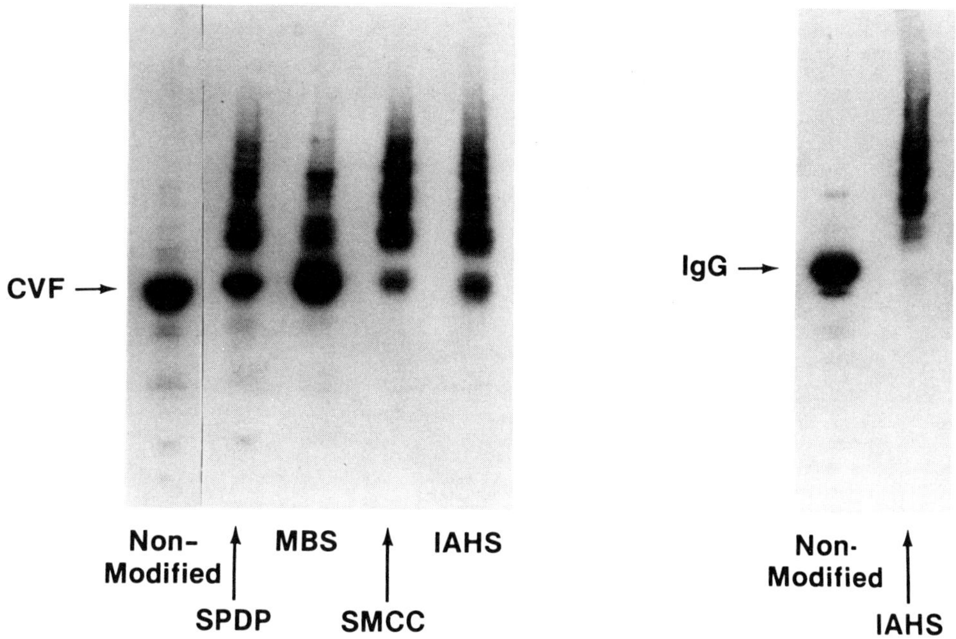

Figure 14 Covalent binding to plasma proteins of cross-linker-derivatized CVF (left panel) and IgG (right panel) after incubation for 30 hours at 37°C in human serum. Shown are autoradiographs of samples after SDS gradient polyacrylamide gel electrophoresis under nonreducing conditions. (From Ref. 40.)

or IAHS covalently bind to plasma proteins when incubated with human serum in vitro. Similar results were obtained when the derivatized proteins were injected into mice (Fig. 15). This in vivo experiment demonstrates the typical finding of complete binding of proteins derivatized with iodide-containing cross-linkers (IAHS and SIAB) to plasma proteins with the greatest increase in the apparent molecular weight. Under reducing conditions, SPDP-derivatized CVF shows the three free chains of CVF, indicating that the binding to plasma proteins is due to reducible disulfide bonds (Fig. 16). Apparently, free sulfhydryl groups present in plasma proteins react with the pyridyldithio groups of SPDP-derivatized CVF. The cross-links to plasma proteins of CVF and IgG derivatized with maleimide- or iodide-containing cross-linkers (similar to the intramolecular cross-links) are not susceptible to reduction (Fig. 16). Consequently, the chemical nature of the reactive groups of plasma proteins reacting with the maleimide and iodide groups cannot be easily identified. The results obtained with SPDP-derivatized CVF suggests that free sulfhydryl groups of plasma pro-

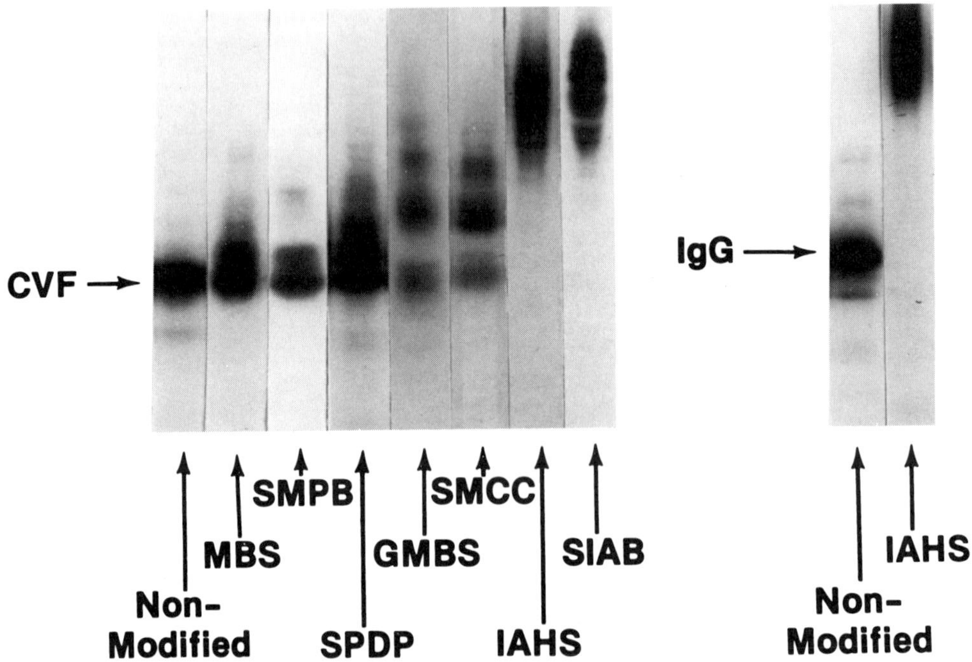

Figure 15 Covalent binding to plasma proteins of cross-linker-derivatized CVF (left panel) and IgG (right panel) after i.v. injection into BALB/c mice. Shown are autoradiographs of serum samples obtained 10 hours after injection and subjected to SDS gradient polyacrylamide gel electrophoresis. Note the complete binding of CVF or IgG derivatized with iodide-containing cross-linkers (IAHS, SIAB), exhibiting the greatest increase in the apparent molecular weight. (From Ref. 40.)

teins are involved. However, the particularly strong reaction of iodide-derivatized proteins suggest that other than free sulfhydryl groups are responsible for the covalent binding. Iodide is the least specific of the sulfhydryl-reactive groups of the heterobifunctional cross-linkers used. Imidazole, thioether, and primary amino groups are known to react with iodide (31,32). The slightly alkaline pH of the buffer used for derivatization and the fact that primary amino groups are present at a very high concentration in serum (the protein concentration of serum is approximately 60 mg/ml) strongly suggests that cross-linking to IAHS- or SIAB-derivatized proteins also involves primary amino groups of plasma proteins. To verify that both sulfhydryl and amino groups of plasma proteins are involved in the cross-linking, the iodide groups of CVF derivatized

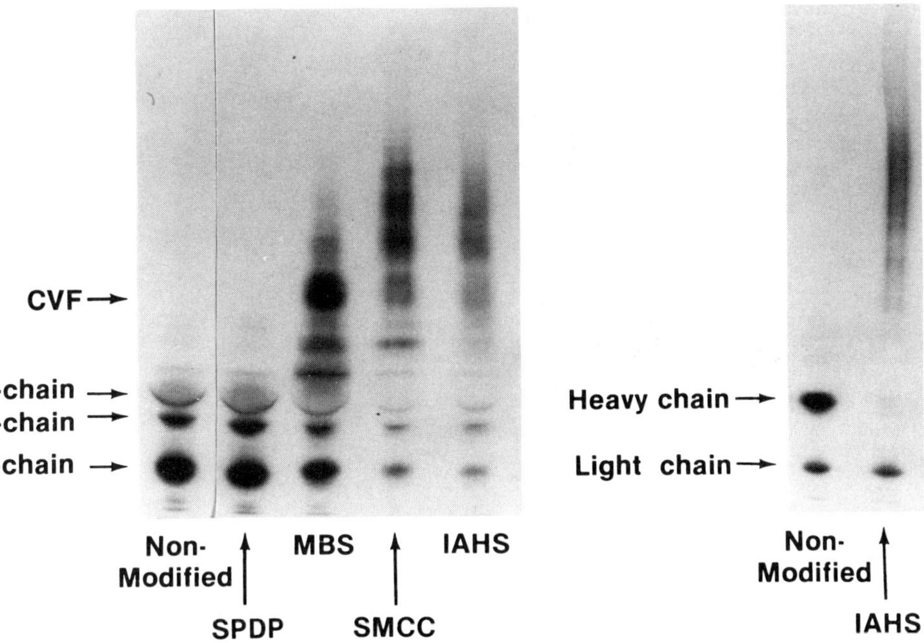

Figure 16 Covalent binding to plasma proteins of cross-linker-derivatized CVF (left panel) and IgG (right panel) after incubation in human serum. Shown is an autoradiograph of the same serum samples as in Figure 14 after SDS gradient polyacrylamide gel electrophoresis under reducing conditions. (From Ref. 40.)

with IAHS were blocked with either cysteine or ethanolamine prior to incubation with serum. Figure 17 shows that this pretreatment with cysteine or ethanolamine completely inhibited the covalent binding to plasma proteins.

We had previously noted that CVF derivatized with IAHS or SIAB exhibited a substantially prolonged plasma half-life (∿33 hours) compared to unmodified CVF or CVF derivatized with SPDP or SMCC (∿14 hours) (3,38-40). Figure 18 shows that the plasma half-life of IAHS-derivatized CVF pretreated with ethanolamine is identical to that of underivatized CVF. This observation demonstrates that the covalent binding to plasma proteins through excess iodide groups causes the prolonged plasma half-life. While this may be an unwanted effect, derivatization with iodide groups may also present a potential for modulating the pharmacokinetic properties of immunoconjugates. In contrast to IAHS derivatization of CVF, derivatization of an IgG monoclonal antibody with IAHS decreased the plasma half-life from ∿71 hours to ∿36 hours (Fig. 19). This observation sug-

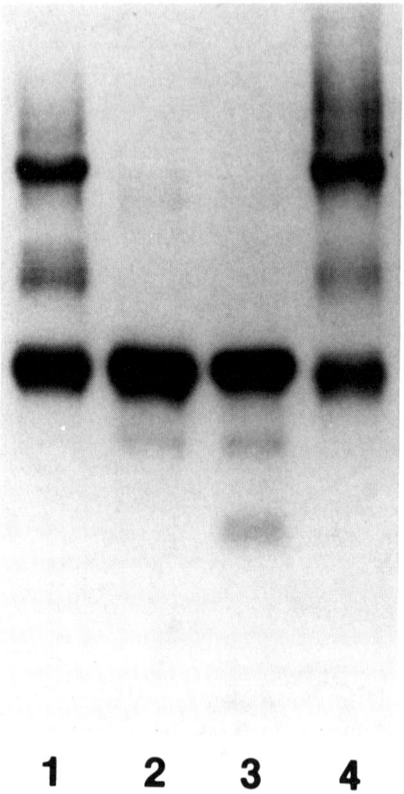

Figure 17 Prevention of covalent binding to plasma proteins of IAHS-derivatized CVF by blocking of iodide groups. Shown is an autoradiograph of IAHS-modified CVF (lane 1), IAHS-derivatized CVF treated with 500 mM ethanolamine at pH 9.0 for 24 hours (lane 2), IAHS-modified CVF treated with 100 mM cysteine for 24 hours at pH 7.2 (lane 3), and IAHS-derivatized CVF incubated for 24 hours in sodium bicarbonate buffer, pH 9.0 (pH control) (lane 4) after incubation for 18 hours in human serum with subsequent SDS gradient polyacrylamide gel electrophoresis under nonreducing conditions. (From Ref. 40.)

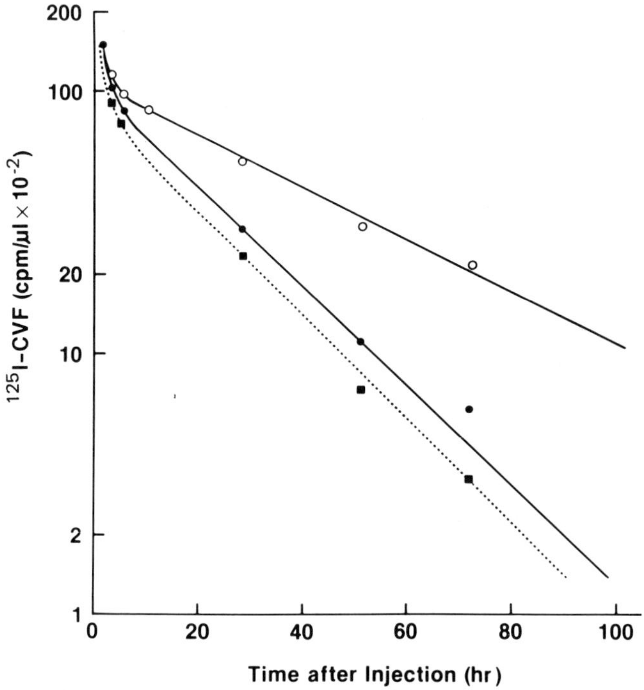

Figure 18 The effect of derivatization of CVF with IAHS on the plasma half-time with and without prior blocking of iodide groups with ethanolamine at pH 9. Radiolabeled proteins were injected i.v. into BALB/c mice. At time intervals as indicated, blood samples were taken and the plasma was counted for radioactivity. Derivatization of CVF with IAHS (○) increased the plasma half-time to approximately 33 hours. Prior blocking of the iodide groups (●) prevented the increase of the plasma half-time. The plasma half-time of IAHS-derivatized and ethanolamine-blocked CVF was indistinguishable from the plasma half-time of native CVF (■, dashed line) (approximately 14 hours). (From Ref. 40.)

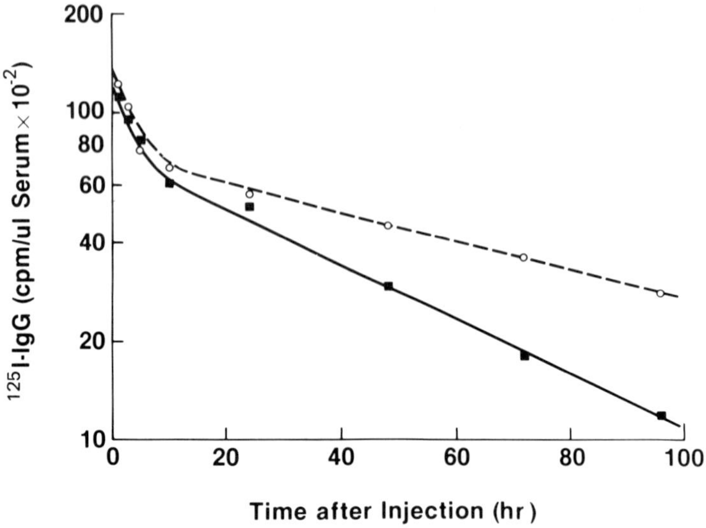

Figure 19 Effect of derivatization with IAHS on the plasma half-time of monoclonal IgG. The experiment was performed as described in thelegend to Figure 18 with nonderivatized IgG (○, dashed line) (half-time: 71 hours) and IAHS-derivatized IgG (■, solid line) (half-time: 36 hours). (From Ref. 40.)

Table 2 Effect of Heterobifunctional Cross-linking Reagents on the Biodistribution (% cpm/wet organ) of Derivatized CVF and IgG in BALB/c Mice 96 hr After i.v. Injection

	% cpm/organ				
Injected protein	Liver	Spleen	Kidneys	Heart	Lungs
CVF	57.8 ± 4.9	5.2 ± 0.7	19.0 ± 1.5	6.3 ± 1.7	11.6 ± 4.4
CVF-SPDP	55.9 ± 5.8	4.6 ± 0.4	17.8 ± 3.3	4.3 ± 0.8	17.3 ± 7.6
CVF-GMBS	69.1 ± 3.5	4.5 ± 0.2	11.2 ± 0.4	5.6 ± 1.8	9.6 ± 1.8
CVF-SMCC	63.4 ± 2.7	6.6 ± 0.4	14.7 ± 1.4	5.9 ± 0.3	10.0 ± 1.2
mean	61.6	5.2	15.7	5.5	12.1
CVF-SIAB	49.6 ± 5.3	7.8 ± 0.5	12.7 ± 1.0	11.9 ± 4.9	18.0 ± 0.9
CVF-IAHS	48.7 ± 2.7	8.1 ± 0.1	14.4 ± 0.5	11.1 ± 2.4	17.8 ± 0.8
mean	49.2	8.0	13.6	11.5	17.9
IgG	50.8 ± 2.9	12.8 ± 1.8	12.7 ± 1.0	8.3 ± 2.8	15.3 ± 4.3
IgG-IAHS	55.0 ± 0.7	9.0 ± 0.8	13.8 ± 0.8	8.4 ± 1.1	13.9 ± 0.1

The data are derived from the same experiment described in Table 3.
Source: Ref. 40.

Table 3 Effect of Heterobifunctional Cross-linking Reagents on the Biodistribution (% cpm/g) of Derivatized CVF and IgG in BALB/c Mice 96 hr After i.v. Injection

	% cpm/g				
Injected protein	Liver	Spleen	Kidneys	Heart	Lungs
CVF	20.5 ± 4.5	8.0 ± 0.0	28.5 ± 1.5	16.5 ± 0.5	26.0 ± 6.0
CVF-SPDP	17.7 ± 4.2	6.3 ± 2.0	25.0 ± 6.5	12.7 ± 2.5	38.7 ± 13.0
CVF-GMBS	27.9 ± 2.4	7.1 ± 1.4	16.2 ± 1.5	17.8 ± 2.5	30.9 ± 3.1
CVF-SMCC	21.5 ± 0.5	9.0 ± 1.0	20.0 ± 2.0	19.8 ± 1.5	28.8 ± 4.7
mean	21.9	7.6	22.4	16.7	31.1
CVF-SIAB	13.0 ± 0.9	7.0 ± 0.4	12.3 ± 0.4	25.5 ± 7.3	42.1 ± 5.9
CVF-IAHS	14.5 ± 3.6	10.0 ± 2.0	18.0 ± 2.0	27.0 ± 1.0	33.0 ± 3.0
mean	13.8	8.5	15.2	26.3	37.6
IgG	16.0 ± 0.8	15.0 ± 1.4	17.0 ± 0.8	21.7 ± 4.4	30.0 ± 2.5
IgG-IAHS	16.5 ± 0.5	11.5 ± 0.5	16.5 ± 0.5	23.0 ± 4.0	31.5 ± 4.5

The data are derived from the same experiment described in Table 2.
Source: Ref. 40.

gests that the plasma protein(s) to which the iodide-derivatized proteins became bound determines the plasma half-life. Tables 2 and 3 indicate that derivatization with iodide-containing cross-linkers not only affects the plasma half-life but also the biodistribution. CVF derivatized with SIAB or IAHS shows decreased uptake by liver and kidneys and increased uptake by spleen, heart, and lungs. In contrast, the biodistribution of IgG is not affected by derivatization with IAHS. Apparently, the preferential route of elimination from the bloodstream is the same for IgG and the plasma protein(s) to which it binds after derivatization with IAHS; only the rate of elimination is affected.

IV. ADDITIONAL OBSERVATIONS OF PRACTICAL INTEREST

A. Stability of Sulfhydryl-reactive Groups

Table 4 shows the stability of sulfhydryl-reactive groups at pH 7.5 and 4°C after introduction into CVF. As is evident from the table, the pyridyldithio group of SPDP as well as the maleimide group of SMCC and the iodide groups of IAHS were still detectable after 5 days of storage at 4°C. In contrast, the number of maleimide groups detectable on MBS-derivatized CVF shows a marked decrease during the first 24 hours and continued to decrease thereafter, although at a much

Table 4 Stability of Sulfhydryl-reactive Groups

Cross-linker	Day 0	Day 1	Day 3	Day 5
SPDP	100%	102%	102%	102%
IAHS	100%	100%	81%	102%
SMCC	⩾100%	⩾100%	113%	106%
MBS	100%	40%	32%	29%

CVF was derivatized with 3-6 cross-linker molecules (day 0) and kept at 4°C. After 1, 3, and 5 days the number of detectable sulfhydryl-reactive groups was determined (average derivatization at day 0 = 100%).
Source: Ref. 29.

slower rate. These observations indicate that proteins derivatized with most heterobifunctional cross-linking reagents can be stored for several days before conjugation. The instability of the maleimide group of MBS-derivatized CVF might be due to the aromatic ring, which is directly attached to the maleimide moiety (41).

B. Protein Determination of Cross-linker-derivatized Proteins

It is frequently necessary to determine the protein concentration of the protein solution after the derivatization with the cross-linker. Since the presence of the cross-linker moieties might affect the protein determination, the effects of different heterobifunctional cross-linking reagents on three standard methods of protein determination were investigated. The results were compared to the protein concentration determined by amino acid analysis, which served as absolute standard. Table 5 shows that protein determination with the Lowry assay was not affected by the cross-linker moieties. Simiarly, absorbance at 280 nm was found to be a reliable method unless the cross-linker contained an aromatic structure such as MBS. The absorbance of the aromatic ring contributes to the absorbance at 280 nm, causing a false high determination of the protein concentration. Using the Bradford assay no specific effect of any cross-linker was observed. However, this assay showed the least agreement with the other methods of protein determination.

C. Stability of Antibody-CVF Conjugates to In Vitro Storage

Storage for 1.5 years at 4-6°C did not alter the band pattern on SDS polyacrylamide electrophoresis of a conjugate preparation synthesized with SPDP. Similarly, no measurable reduction of the functional activity was observed (27).

Table 5 Effect of Derivatization with Heterobifunctional Cross-linkers on Protein Determination Assays

Protein	Method of protein determination			
	Amino acid analysis	Absorbance at 280 nm	Folin assay	Bradford assay
CVF	100%	97%	110%	224%
CVF-SPDP	100%	90%	94%	160%
CVF-IAHS	100%	95%	87%	155%
CVF-SMCC	100%	106%	103%	193%
CVF-MBS	100%	149%	92%	157%

CVF was derivatized with 3-6 cross-linker molecules (same samples as Table 4). All solutions had an approximate protein concentration of 3 mg/ml. The protein concentration of each sample was determined by amino acid analysis (taken as reference = 100%), by absorbance at 280 nm using an $E_{1\,cm}^{0.1\%} = 0.99$ for CVF (6), by the Folin method (56), and by the Bradford method (57).
Source: Ref. 29.

V. SELECTIVE CYTOTOXIC ACTIVITY

The purpose of this review is to concentrate on the synthesis of antibody conjugates with CVF and implications for their activity. Several aspects of the work reviewed here may not only apply to antibody-CVF conjugates but to antibody conjugates with other proteins. In the following, the experimental systems where antibody-CVF conjugates have been successfully employed as selective cytotoxic agents will briefly be mentioned but not reviewed in great detail. The reader is referred to the original literature.

Antibody-CVF conjugates had first been made with the 9.2.27 murine monoclonal antibody to a high molecular weight human molecular weight antigen (3,28,42). They were shown to induce specific cytotoxicity of antigen-positive melanoma cells in the presence of serum. In the absence of serum as a source of complement, no cytotoxic effects of the antibody-CVF conjugates were observed. The complement activation occurred through activation of the alternative pathway by cobra venom factor since the conjugates were fully active in the presence of C4-deficient serum. Subsequently, these conjugates were also tested in an initial in vivo system using nude mice with intraperitoneally growing human melanoma cells. It was shown that a single injection of antibody-CVF conjugates caused a prolongation of the period until tumor outgrowth was macroscopically detectable (37).

Two groups have subsequently shown that antibody-CVF conjugates can induce lysis of erythrocytes. One group used CVF conjugates with a monoclonal antibody to human C3b and showed lysis of C3b-coated erythrocytes (43). The other group employed a polyclonal antibody to human erythrocytes coupled to CVF. This conjugate induced C3b deposition and hemolysis in the presence of Mg^{2+} and EGTA (44).

In a second model system using nucleated cells as target, it was shown that antibody-CVF conjugates induce complement-mediated killing of antigen-positive human lymphocytes and leukemia cells (45-49). The authors showed that they could use human complement to induce killing of human target cells with the antibody-CVF conjugates. They compared the selectivity and potency of the antibody-CVF conjugates with antibody-ricin conjugates as potential agents for bone marrow purging. They conclude that, on a molar basis, antibody-CVF conjugates are somewhat less potent than antibody-ricin conjugates but appear to be superior agents due to their virtual lack of toxicity for antigen-negative cells (47-49). The authors also report that differences of complement susceptibility exist among different cell lines, which are unrelated to the antigen density. In the light of these results, lymphoid cells seem to be a particularly suitable target for antibody-CVF and complement-mediated killing. Compared to the above-mentioned melanoma cells (42), the lymphoid cells required approximately 100 times less antibody-CVF conjugates to achieve optimal killing (48,49).

VI. APPENDIX

Purification of Cobra Venom Factor

CVF was purified from lyophilized *Naja naja siamiensis* venom (Miami Serpentarium Laboratories, Salt Lake City, UT) as described (4). 1.5 g of venom was dissolved in 11 ml buffer A (50 mM Tris-HCl, 100 mM NaCl, pH 7.5), stirred for 30 min at 25°C, and kept at 25°C for several hours. The solution was centrifuged at 4°C for 20 min to remove insoluble material and applied to a Bio-Gel A-0.5 m (mesh 200-400) (Bio-Rad, Richmond, California) gel filtration column (2.8 × 116 cm) equilibrated with buffer A at 4°C at a linear flow rate of 1.3 ml/hr per cm^2. Fractions containing CVF activity were pooled, concentrated by ultrafiltration (Amicon XM-50 membrane, Danvers, Massachusetts), and dialyzed against buffer B (4.3 mM Na-phosphate, pH 7.2). The pools from two identical runs of the gel filtration column were combined and applied to a DEAE-Sephacel (Pharmacia, Piscataway, NJ) column (1.6 × 21 cm) equilibrated with buffer B at 4°C. The column was washed with several column volumes of buffer B and protein was eluted with a linear NaCl gradient (350 ml buffer B/350 ml buffer B at a conductivity of 28.5 mS) at a linear flow rate of 17 ml/hr per cm^2. Fractions containing CVF activity were pooled and concentrated as described above and dialyzed against buffer C (10 mM Na-phosphate, pH 5.0). Usually, a precipitate formed during dialysis, which was removed by centrifugation. The supernatant was applied to a CM-cellulose (Whatman, Clifton, NJ) column (1.6 × 17 cm) equilibrated at 4°C with buffer C. After the column was thoroughly washed, protein was eluted with a linear NaCl gradient (350 ml buffer C/350 ml buffer C at a conductivity of 40 mS) at a linear flow rate of 17 ml/hr per cm^2. Fractions containing CVF activity were pooled and directly applied to a Cibacron blue-agarose (mesh 100-200) column (Bio-rad) (3.2 × 12.5 cm) equilibrated with buffer C at 4°C. After the sample was applied, protein was eluted with 700 ml of buffer D (10 mM Na-phosphate adjusted with NaCl to a conductivity of 29 mS, pH 6.5) at a linear flow rate of 3.7 ml/hr per cm^2. This buffer elutes CVF which was pooled, concentrated and stored at −70°C in 100 mM Na-phosphate, 100 mM NaCl, pH 7.5. All conductivity measurements were performed at room temperature.

Heterobifunctional Cross-linking Reagents

Iodoacetyl-N-hydroxysuccinimide ester (IAHS) was synthesized from iodoacetic acid (3.25 g, 17.5 mmoles) and N-hydroxysuccinimide (2.0 g, 17.5 mmoles) in 180 ml of anhydrous dioxane in the presence of dicyclohexylcarbodiimide (3.6 g, 17.5 mmoles). The reaction mixture was stirred at room temperature for 1 hour. Subsequently the solution was filtered to remove the precipitated dicyclohexylurea. The filtrate containing the IAHS was evaporated to dryness. The IAHS was purified by repeated recrystallization from chloroform until the supernatant did no longer show a pinkish color (usually 3 times). The method of synthesis has been published (30) and represents a slight modification of an earlier procedure (50). The structure of IAHS was confirmed by IR and NMR spectroscopy and by elemental analysis (30): C 25.53% (25.46%), N 4.97% (4.95%), O 22.69% (22.61%), H 2.08% (2.14%), I 44.46% (44.84%); calculated values are in parentheses. SPDP was purchased from Pharmacia. All other cross-linking reagents were purchased from Pierce, Rockford, ME.

Other Materials

The 9.2.27 anitmelanoma antibody of the murine IgG2a subclass (51) was purified from ascites by protein A affinity chromatography. Human FMEX-Met II melanoma cells were kept in continuous culture using DMEM medium supplemented with 10% (v/v) heat inactivated fetal calf serum, 1% (v/v) non-essential amino acids, 1% (v/v) sodium pyruvate, and 2% (v/v) L-glutamine (GIBCO, Grand Island, NY). Guinea pig erythrocytes and guinea pig serum were obtained by cardiac puncture of adult Hartley guinea pigs. Ricin was purchased from Sigma, St. Louis, MO.

Synthesis and Purification of Antibody Conjugates with CVF

The method described here follows previously described protocols (27,42). Sulfhydryl-reactive groups were introduced into CVF and IgG by incubating either protein for 30 min at room temperature at a protein concentration of 2-3 mg/ml in 100 mM Na-phosphate, 100 mM NaCl, pH 7.5, in the presence of 6-10 molar excess of SPDP. The other cross-linking reagents were usually reacted at a higher molar excess (20X or 40X). Unreacted cross-linker and reaction products were removed by gel filtration on Sephadex G-25 (Pharmacia). Prior to the subsequent reduction and coupling reactions, the derivatized proteins were usually concentrated in order to maintain a sufficiently high protein concentration. Free sulfhydryl groups were introduced by reduction of the SPDP-derivatized IgG with 45 mM DTT in 100 mM Na-acetate, 100 mM NaCl, pH 4.5. After 20 min at room temperature, the sulfhydryl-derivatized IgG was purified and transferred into the above pH 7.5 buffer by gel filtration on Sephadex G-25. The subsequent coupling of the cross-linker-derivatized CVF with the sulfhydryl-derivatized IgG at an approximate 1:1 molar ratio was performed overnight at room temperature in pH 7.5 buffer under nitrogen with occasional careful agitation. To prevent oxidation of the introduced free sulfhydryl groups the derivatized IgG was collected from the Sephadex column directly into the coupling solution with the cross-linker-modified CVF. The removal of noncoupled CVF and IgG from the conjugates was performed by gel filtration either on Ultrogel AcA 22 (LKB, Gaithersburg, MD) at 4°C or on a TSK-4000 column at room temperature using an HPLC instrument. Analysis of conjugates was performed by SDS gradient polyacrylamide 3-9% (w/v) gel electrophoresis with subsequent Coomassie staining. In the case of radiolabeled conjugates, autoradiography of dried gels was performed using XAR-5 X-ray film (Kodak, Rochester, NY).

Determination of Sulfhydryl-reactive Groups

The degree of derivatization with pyridyldithio groups was determined by spectrophotometric measurement of released pyridine-2-thione at 343 nm after reduction of an aliquot of the protein solution with 5 mM DTT (final concentration) (26). The extinction coefficient of pyridine-2-thione at 343 nm is 8.08×10^3 M/cm. The protein content was determined by its absorbance at 280 nm corrected for the contribution of the introduced pyridyldithio groups using the empirical formula:

$$A_{280}(\text{protein}) = A_{280}(\text{observed}) - (B \times 5.1 \times 10^3)$$

where B is the molar concentration of the pyridine-2-thione in the solution.

The determination of maleimide groups was performed by reacting the derivatized protein with a known amount of beta-mercaptoethanol. Subsequently, the remaining beta-mercaptoethanol was determined with Ellman's reagent (5,5′-dithiobis-(2-nitrobenzoic acid); DTNB) (30,52,53). The molar quantity of maleimide groups present equals the molar quantity of beta-mercaptoethanol consumed. An aliquot of maleimide-modified protein (100 μl containing approximately 2.8 nmol of protein) was flushed with nitrogen and reacted with 18 μl of 1.4 mM (25.2 nmol) deoxygenated beta-mercaptoethanol for 20 min at room temperature. Subsequently, 1.0 ml of deoxygenated 0.2 M Tris, pH 8.2, and 100 μl of freshly prepared 0.01 M DTNB in deoxygenated methanol were added to the sample and allowed to react for 30 min at room temperature. The absorbance was read at 412 nm. A maximum absorbance value was obtained by substituting the modified protein with 100 μl of buffer. A blank value was obtained by substituting DTNB with 100 μl methanol. In the case of proteins not containing free sulfhydryl groups (such as CVF or IgG), the substitution of the beta-mercaptoethanol by water resulted in another blank value. This control is not always necessary once it has been established that a protein does not contain free sulfhydryl groups.

The determination of iodide groups was performed by the same protocol as described for maleimide groups, with the exception that the incubation period of the sample with beta-mercaptoethanol was increased to 2 hr since the reaction of the iodide groups with the beta-mercaptoethanol is much slower than with maleimide groups (30,50). The percentage (f) of protein molecules derivatized with (r) numbers of cross-linker groups at a mean derivatization (m) was calculated according to Poisson distribution (54):

$$f = \frac{e^{-m} \cdot m^{r}}{r!}$$

Hemolytic Assay for CVF

The ability of CVF to activate the alternative pathway of complement was determined by measuring the extent of bystander lysis of guinea pig erythrocytes in guinea pig serum. The assay was performed as described (4,27). Briefly, various amounts of CVF, cross-linker-derivatized CVF, and antibody-CVF conjugate in 10 μl of phosphate-buffered saline were incubated with 10^7 guinea pig erythrocytes and 20 μl normal guinea pig serum in a total volume of 50 μl. After 30 min at 37°C, 1 ml of cold phosphate-buffered saline was added. After centrifugation in a table-top centrifuge the absorbance of the released hemoglobin was determined at 412 nm in the supernatant, and the percent of hemolysis was calculated.

Flow Cytofluorometry

Single-cell suspensions of human FMEX-Met II melanoma cells at 10^6 cells/ml in phosphate-buffered saline containing 1% (w/v) bovine serum albumin were incubated with the 9.2.27 monoclonal antibody or the 9.2.27 monoclonal antibody-CVF conjugate at 1.0, 0.1, or 0.01 μg IgG protein per 10^6 cells for 30 min at 4°C. After two washes, 10^6 cells were resuspended in 100 μl of the above albumin buffer containing 3 μg of fluorescein-conjugated goat anti-mouse IgG (Tago, Inc., Burlingame, CA). Following a 30-min incubation at 4°C the cells were washed and kept at 4°C until analysis on the cytofluorograph (model 50H, Ortho Diagnostic Systems, Westwood, MA) (27,55). A minimum of 1000 cells from each sample was examined. The percentage of positive cells and the distribution of the surface immunofluorescence were recorded. A mouse IgG2a myeloma protein served as negative control (RPC-5; Bionetics, Kensington, MD).

Other Methods

Protein determinations were performed by UV absorbance at 280 nm, by amino acid analysis (6), and by the Lowry (56) and Bradford methods (57). Radioiodination of proteins was performed with $Na^{125}I$ (Amersham, Arlington Heights, IL) using immobilized chloramine-T (Iodo-Beads; Pierce) (58).

ACKNOWLEDGMENTS

I would like to acknowledge the many contributions of my co-workers, in particular of my graduate students Scott D. Wilkie, Eugene C. Petrella, and Alice H. Grier, as evident from the authorship of cited publications. Work performed in my laboratory was supported by NIH Grants CA35525 and HL29523, by ONR Grant N00014-83-K-2001, by the NIH Support Grant for the Lombardi Cancer Research Center CA14626, and by Research Career Development Award CA01039 from the National Cancer Institute, United States Department of Health and Human Services.

REFERENCES

1. Vogel, C.-W. (ed.) (1987) *Immunoconjugates. Antibody Conjugates in Radioimaging and Therapy of Cancer*. Oxford, New York.
2. Vogel, C.-W. (1987) Current approaches of immunotargeting. In *Immunoconjugates. Antibody Conjugates in Radioimaging and Therapy of Cancer* (Vogel, C.-W., Ed.). Oxford, New York, pp. 3-7.
3. Vogel, C.-W. (1987) Antibody conjugates without inherent toxicity: the targeting of cobra venom factor and other biological response modifiers. In *Immunoconjugates. Antibody Conjugates in Radioimaging and Therapy of Cancer* (Vogel, C.-W., Ed.). Oxford, New York, pp. 170-188.
4. Vogel, C.-W., and Müller-Eberhard, H. J. (1984) Cobra venom factor: improved method for purification and biochemical characterization. *J. Immunol. Meth. 73*:203-220.

5. Eggertsen, G., Lind, P., and Sjöquist, J. (1981) Molecular characterization of the complement activating protein in the venom of the Indian cobra (*Naja n. siamensis*). *Mol. Immunol. 18*:125-133.
6. Vogel, C.-W., Smith, C. A., and Müller-Eberhard, H. J. (1984). Cobra venom factor: structural homology with the third component of human complement. *J. Immunol. 133*:3235-3241.
7. Pangburn, M. K., and Müller-Eberhard, H. J. (1984) The alternative pathway of complement. *Springer Semin. Immunopathol. 7*:163-192.
8. Müller-Eberhard, H. J., and Fjellström, K.-E. (1971) Isolation of the anticomplementary protein from cobra venom and its mode of action on C3. *J. Immunol. 107*:1666-1672.
9. Hensley, P., O'Keefe, M. C., Spangler, C. J., Osborne, Jr., J. C., and Vogel, C.-W. (1986) The effects of metal ions and temperature on the interaction of cobra venom factor and human complement factor B. *J. Biol. Chem. 261*:11038-11044.
10. Vogt, W., Dieminger, L., Lynen, R., and Schmidt, G. (1974) Alternative pathway for the activation of complement in human serum. Formation and composition of the complex with cobra venom factor that cleaves the third component of complement. *Hoppe-Seyler's Z. Physiol. Chem. 355*:171-183.
11. Lesavre, P. H., Hugli, T.E., Esser, A. F., and Müller-Eberhard, H. J. (1979) The alternative pathway C3/C5 convertase: chemical basis of factor B activation. *J. Immunol. 123*:529-534.
12. Smith, C. A., Vogel, C.-W., and Müller-Eberhard, H. J. (1982) Ultrastructure of cobra venom factor-depndent C3/C5 convertase and its zymogen, factor B of human complement. *J. Biol. Chem. 257*:9879-9882.
13. Smith, C. A., Vogel, C.-W., and Müller-Eberhard, H. J. (1984) MHC class III products: an electron microscopic study of the C3 convertases of human complement. *J. Exp. Med. 159*:324-329.
14. Medicus, R. G., Götze, O., and Müller-Eberhard, H. J.(1976) Alternative pathway of complement: recruitment of precursor properdin by the labile C3/C5 convertase and the potentiation of the pathway. *J. Exp. Med. 144*:1076-1093.
15. Vogel, C.-W., and Müller-Eberhard, H. J. (1982) The cobra venom factor-dependent C3 convertase of human complement: a kinetic and thermodynamic analysis of a protease acting on its natural high molecular weight substrate. *J. Biol. Chem. 257*:8292-8299.
16. Whaley, K., and Ruddy, S. (1976) Modulation of the alternative complement pathway by β1H globulin. *J. Exp. Med. 144*:1147-1163.
17. Pangburn, M. K., Schreiber, R. D., and Müller-Eberhard, H. J. (1977) Human complement C3b inactivator: isolation, characterization, and demonstration of an absolute requirement for the serum protein β1H for cleavage of C3b and C4b in solution. *J. Exp. Med. 146*:257-269.
18. Lachmann, P. J., and Halbwachs, L. (1975) The influence of C3b inactivator (KAF) concentration on the ability of serum to support complement activation. *Clin. Exp. Immunol. 21*:109-114.

19. Nagaki, K., Iida, K., Okubo, M., and Inai, S. (1978) Reaction mechanisms of beta-1H globulin. *Int. Archs. Allergy Appl. Immunol. 57*:221-232.
20. Daha, M. R., Fearon, D. T., and Austen, K. F. (1976) C3 requirements for formation of alternative pathway C5 convertase. *J. Immunol. 117*: 630-634.
21. Medicus, R. G., Götze, O., and Müller-Eberhard, H. J. (1976) The serine protease nature of the C3 and C5 convertases of the classical and alternative complement pathways. *Scand. J. Immunol. 5*:1049-1055.
22. Von Zabern, I., Hinsch, B., Przyklenk, H., Schmidt, G., and Vogt, W. (1980) Comparison of *Naja n. naja* and Naja h. haje cobra venom factors: correlation between binding affinity for the fifth component of complement and mediation of its cleavage. *Immunobiology 157*:499-514.
23. Miyama, A., Kato, T., Horai, S., Yokoo, J., and Kashiba, S. (1975) Trypsin-activated complex of human factor B with cobra venom factor (CVF), cleaving C3 and C5 and generating a lytic factor for unsensitized guinea pig erythrocytes. I. Generation of the activated complex. *Biken J. 18*: 193-204.
24. Cochrane, C. G., Müller-Eberhard, H. J., and Aikin, B. S. (1970) Depletion of plasma complement in vivo by a protein of cobra venom: its effects on various immunologic reactions. *J. Immunol. 105*:55–69.
25. Ryan, A. F., Catanzaro, A., Wasserman, S. I., Harris, J. A., and Vogel, C.-W. (1986) The effect of complement depletion on immunologically mediated middle ear effusion and inflammation. *Clin. Immunol. Immunopathol. 40*: 410-421.
26. Carlsson, J., Drevin, H., and Axen, R. (1978) Protein thiolation and reversible protein-protein conjugation. *N*-Succinimidyl-3-(2-Pyridyldithio)Propionate, a new heterobifunctional reagent. *Biochem. J. 173*:723-737.
27. Petrella, E. C., Wilkie, S. D., Smith, C. A., Morgan, Jr., A. C., and Vogel, C.-W. (1987) Antibody conjugates with cobra venom factor. Synthesis and biochemical characterization. *Immunol. Meth. 104*: 159-172.
28. Vogel, C.-W. (1988) Antibody conjugates with cobra venom factor as selective agents for tumor cell killing. In *Cytolytic Lymphocytes and Complement: Effectors of the Immune System*, Volume II (Podack, E. R., Ed.). CRC Press, Boca Raton.
29. Wilkie, S. D., Petrella, E. C., and Vogel, C.-W. (1987) Effect of different heterobifunctional cross-linking reagents on the structure and activity of antibody conjugates with cobra venom factor. (Submitted for publication.)
30. Wilkie, S. D. (1984) The effect of different heterobifunctional crosslinking reagents on the stability and pharmacokinetics of monoclonal antibody-cobra venom factor conjugates. M.S. thesis, Georgetown University, Washington, D.C.
31. Gundlach, H. G., Stein, W. H., and Moore, S. (1959) The nature of the amino acid residues involved in the inactivation of ribonuclease by iodoacetate. *J. Biol. Chem. 234*:1754-1760.
32. Gurd, F. R. N. (1967) Carboxymethylation. *Meth. Enzymol. 11*:532-541.

33. Fulton, R. J., Street, N., Uhr, J. W., and Vitetta, E. S. (1987) Immunotoxins containing ricin A and B chains. In *Immunoconjugates. Antibody Conjugates in Radioimaging and Therapy of Cancer* (Vogel, C.-W., Ed.). Oxford, New York, pp. 97-115.
34. Casellas, P., and Jansen, F. K. (1987) Enhancement of A-chain immunotoxins by pharmacological agents. In *Immunoconjugates. Antibody Conjugates in Radioimaging and Therapy of Cancer* (Vogel, C.-W., Ed.). Oxford, New York, pp. 97-115.
35. Spitler, L. E. (1987) Phase I clinical trials with immunotoxins. In *Immunoconjugates. Antibody Conjugates in Radioimaging and Therapy of Cancer* (Vogel, C.-W., Ed.). Oxford, New York, pp. 290-300.
36. Wilkie, S. D., and Vogel, C.-W. (1984) The effect of different heterobifunctional crosslinking reagents on the in vivo stability of antibody-cobra venom factor conjugates. *Fed. Proc. 43*: 1971.
37. Vogel, C.-W., Wilkie, S. D., and Morgan, A. C. (1985) In vivo studies with covalent conjugates of cobra venom factor and monoclonal antibodies to human tumors. In *Modern Trends in Human Leukemia VI* (Neth, R., Gallo, R. C., Greaves, M. F., and Janka, G., Eds.). Springer Verlag, Berlin, pp. 514-517.
38. Petrella, E. C., Wilkie, S. D., Grier, A. H., and Vogel, C.-W. (1985) Covalent conjugates of cobra venom factor (CVF) with monoclonal antibodies: effect of different heterobifunctional reagents on activity and in vivo properties. *Complement 2*:63.
39. Petrella, E. C., Wilkie, S. D., Grier, A. H., and Vogel, C.-W. (1986) Effect of different heterobifunctional crosslinkers on activity and pharmacokinetics of antibody conjugates with cobra venom factor. *J. Cell. Biochem. Suppl. 10B*:97.
40. Wilkie, S. D., Grier, A. H., Petrella, E. C., and Vogel, C.-W. (1987) Effect of different heterobifunctional crosslinking reagents on the pharmacokinetics of antibody conjugates with cobra venom factor. (Submitted for publication.)
41. Hashida, S., Imagawa, M., Inoue, S., Ruan, K.-H., and Ishikawa, E. (1984) More useful maleimide compounds for the conjugation of Fab′ to horseradish peroxidase through thiol groups in the hinge. *J. Applied Biochem. 6*: 56-63.
42. Vogel, C.-W., and Müller-Eberhard, H. J. (1981) Induction of immune cytolysis: tumor-cell killing by complement is initiated by covalent complex of monoclonal antibody and stable C3/C5 convertase. *Proc. Natl. Acad. Sci. USA 78*:7707-7711.
43. Ganu, V., Fernandez-Cruz, E., and Müller-Eberhard, H. J. (1984) Synthesis and properties of a monoclonal antibody-cobra venom factor complex which is stable in vivo. *Fed. Proc. 43*:1772.
44. Parker, C. J., and White, V. F. (1985) Site-specific activation of the alternative pathway of complement (APC): creation of a hybrid molecule consisting of antibody and cobra venom factor (CoF). *Complement 2*:61.

45. Müller, B., and Müller-Ruchholtz, W. (1985) Antibody (Ab)/cobra venom factor (CVF) conjugates supplement the classical human serum complement pathway with alterante pathway cytolysis. *Complement 2*:56.
46. Müller, B., Harpprecht, H., Anderson, M. J. D., and Müller-Ruchholtz, W. (1986) Activation of human complement by covalent conjugates of mouse monoclonal antibodies and cobra venom factors. *Br. J. Cancer 54*:537.
47. Müller, B., and Müller-Ruchholtz, W. (1986) In vitro killing of target cells by antibody/ricin or antibody/cobra venom factor conjugates: comparison of selectivity and potency. *Immunobiology 173*:195-196.
48. Müller, B., and Müller-Ruchholtz, W. (1986) Covalent conjugates of monoclonal antibody and cobra venom factor mediate specific cytotoxicity via alternative pathway of human complement activation. *Leukemia Res., 11*: 461-468.
49. Müller, B. (1987) Kovalente Konjugate aus monoklonalen Antikörpern und den Effektormolekulen Ricin und Cobra Venom Factor: Vergleich ihrer selektiven Cytotoxizität auf Kulturzellinien. Ph.D. thesis, University of Kiel, West Germany.
50. Rector, E. S., Schwenk, R. J., Tse, K. S., and Sehon, A.-H. (1978) A method for the preparation of protein-protein conjugates of predetermined composition. *J. Immunol. Meth. 24*:321-336.
51. Morgan, Jr., A. C., Galloway, D. R., and Reisfeld, R. A. (1981) Production and characterization of monoclonal antibody to a melanoma specific glycoprotein. *Hybridoma 1*:27-36.
52. Habeeb, A. F. S. A. (1972) Reaction of protein sulfhydryl groups with Ellman's Reagent. *Meth. Enzymol. 25*:457-464.
53. Liu, F.-T., Zinnecker, M., Hamaoka, T., and Katz, D. H. (1979) New procedures for preparation and isolation of conjugates of proteins and a synthetic copolymer of D-amino acids and immunochemical characterization of such conjugates. *Biochemistry*: 690-697.
54. Bevington, P. R. (1969) *Data Reduction and Error Analysis for the Physical Sciences*. McGraw-Hill, New York.
55. Morgan, Jr., A. C., Woodhouse, C., Bartholemew, R., and Schroff, R. (1986) Human melanoma-associated antigens: analysis of antigenic heterogeneity by molecular, serologic and flow-cytometric approaches. *Mol. Immunol. 23*: 193-200.
56. Lowry, O. H., Rosebrough, N. J., Farr, A. L., and Randall, R. J. (1953) Protein measurement with the Folin phenol reagent. *J. Biol. Chem. 193*: 265-275.
57. Bradford, M. M. (1976) A rapid and sensitive method for the quantitation of microgram quantities of protein utilizing the principle of protein-dye binding. *Analyt. Biochem. 72*:248-254.
58. Markwell, M. A. K. (1982) A new solid-state reagent to iodinate proteins. *Analyt. Biochem. 125*:427-432.

8

Immunotoxin Preparation and Testing In Vitro

ARTHUR E. FRANKEL, PHILIP C. WELSH, DAVID IAN WITHERS, and DAVID M. SCHLOSSMAN
Duke University Medical Center, Durham, North Carolina

Immunotoxins are monoclonal antibodies covalently linked to peptide toxins. The monoclonal antibody directs the molecule to specific cell targets. Once antibody toxin conjugate has bound the target antigen, the complex must be mobile and enter an endocytic vesicle from which the toxin can escape to the cytosol. The linker must be capable of holding the toxin and antibody together in the extracellular environment and, in the case of some toxin polypeptides, release the toxin from the antibody in the proper intracellular vesicle to permit toxin translocation to the cytotsol. The toxin component has the enzymatic protein synthesis-inactivating activity of the molecule. For plant and fungal toxins, this consists of an irreversible modification of the 60S ribosomal subunit. For bacterial toxins the catalytic function is ADP-ribosylation of EF-2. Peptide chain elongation is interrupted for all these toxins and cellular protein synthesis halts. The optimal toxin for immunotoxins should have a modified or absent normal cellular binding site. Otherwise the immunotoxin will not show significant specificity to antigen-positive cells. The toxin should also have translocation domains to permit the protein to cross the cell membrane and gain access to the cytosolic ribosomes and polysomes.

Prior to the development of monoclonal antibodies, a variety of xenogeneic antisera were used to construct immunotoxins. While selective toxicity was described, there was seldom careful physicochemical or biological characterization performed on the molecules. With the advent of monoclonal antibody technology, it has been possible to perform careful, repeated studies on reagents available in adequate supply for clinical applications.

Monoclonal antibodies used in immunotoxin preparation have included mouse monoclonal antibodies of all classes and several rat monoclonal antibodies (Table 1). All mouse immunoglobulin classes can be used to generate active toxin conjugates. Many workers have avoided IgMs because of the difficulty in accurately assessing stoichiometry of the product and the likelihood of poor tissue penetration of such molecules for treatment of systemic malignancies.

Between 20 and 30% of monoclonal antibodies prepared against several tumor types (breast, ovarian, T leukemia) have yielded cytotoxic conjugates when linked with toxins (5,9,10). Properties of the antibody and target which are critical in determining immunotoxin activity include antibody affinity, antigen density and the rate and route of internalization of the cell surface antigen after antibody toxin conjugate binding (11).

The chemical linkage between the antibody and toxin can have a profound effect on the immunotoxin activity both in vitro and in vivo. At first homobifunctional reagents were used, such as glutaraldehyde (see Table 2). While linkages were slightly improved with the more controllable mixed anhydrides or N-hydroxysuccinimide ester of chlorambucil, optimal cross-linkage has been achieved by generating a free sulfhydryl on the antibody and a reactive chemical moiety on the toxin, which will react selectively with the antibody free thiol group (25). This type of linkage reduces nonspecific cross-linking, which yields inactive conjugates and large protein aggregates. To introduce a free thiol group in the antibody, the heterobifunctional linkers N-hydroxysuccinimidylpyridyldithiopropionate (SPDP) and 2-iminothiolane (2-IT) are commonly used. Fab′

Table 1 Classes of Monoclonal Antibodies Used in Immunotoxin Synthesis

Antibody	Class	Toxin	Reference
9.2.27	Mouse IgG2a	DTA	1
B3/25	Mouse IgG1	RTA	2
H59	Mouse IgM	RTA	3
T11-1C	Mouse IgG2b	Gelonin	4
113F1	Mouse IgG3	RTA	5
11/160	Rat IgG2b	RTA	6
R17217	Rat IgG2a	RTA	7

Table 2 Linkers Used in Immunotoxin Synthesis

Linker	Conjugate	Reference
SPDP	D3-RTA	12
PDPA + EDC	96.5-RTA	15
2IT	OX7-RTA	16
cystamine + EDC	anti-conA-DTA	18
Fab′	Fab′rabbit anti-human Ig-RTA	21
MPI	anti-CEA-RTA	8
SMPT	OX7-SMPT-deglycosylated RTA	24
Fab′ + PDM	Fab′rabbit anti-L1210-PDM-RTA	26
BVI	hpL-DTA	17
Maleimidohexanoic acid + EDC	T101-S-RTA	13
MMB	HB21-PE	19
N-hydroxysuccinimidyl-iodoacetate	OX7-ricin	20
Glutaraldehyde	anti-DNP-DT	28
TDIC	anti-mumps-DT	29
FNPS	anti-LDH-DT	30
diethylmalonimidate	anti-TNP-DT	31
mixed anhydride chlorambucil	anti-human Ig-DT	32
N-hydroxysuccinimidyl-chlorambucil	F154215-ricin	33
insulin B-IT	OX7-insulin B-ricin	23

EDC = ethyldimethylaminocarbodiimide; BVI = methylbromovalerimidate; MMB = methylmercaptobutyrimidate; PDM = phenylenedimaleimide; MPI = methylmercaptopropinimidate; TDIC = toluene diisocyanate; FNPS = difluorodinitrodiphenylsulfone.

fragments and partially reduced whole immunoglobulin have available free thiol groups. The toxin A chains, such as diphtheria toxin A chain (DTA) and ricin A chain (RTA), already possess free thiol groups that can react with the antibody thiol group. The plant hemitoxins, such as pokeweed antiviral protein (PAP), gelonin, and SO-6, require a disulfide bond with the antibody to retain activity and are usually modified with SPDP or 2-IT to produce thiol groups that can react with the antibody thiol group. In contrast, whole toxins, such as Pseudomonas exotoxin A (PE), diphtheria toxin (DT), ricin, or abrin, can be modified with reagents, such as maleimidobenzoyl-N-hydroxysuccinimide ester (MBS), which will yield thioether linkages to antibody thiol groups. Three new linkers have recently been developed which provide special properties to improve immunotoxin potency or pharmacology. The acid-labile linker of Blattler has been constructed to avoid potential disulfide reduction in vivo in the circulation (22). The toxin and antibody would not separate until reaching a pH 4.5 endosome. No tests of this linker in immunotoxins has been described. Marsh and Neville have used an insulin B-chain linker to provide a longer spacer between the antibody and ricin (23). This improved potency severalfold versus an MBS linkage. Finally, Thorpe has developed a protected disulfide linker, N-succinimidyloxycarbonylalphamethylpyridyldithiotoluene (SMPT), which is apparently less sensitive to breakdown in the circulation in vivo but releases the toxin adequately intracellularly to maintain ricin A-chain conjugate potency (24).

The toxins that have been used in immunotoxin synthesis share some general features. Both plant and bacterial toxins consist of two chains, an A chain and a B chain, connected by a linker peptide. The A chain has the enzymatic or catalytic site for protein synthesis inactivation. The B chain has the normal cell-binding domain. Each chain is about 30,000 daltons, and whole toxins are 60,000 daltons. Two notable exceptions to this scheme are Pseudomonas exotoxin A and the plant hemitoxins. Pseudomonas toxin has an A chain-like domain and a B chain-like domain, but these domains are not linked by a single disulfide bond or a trypsin-sensitive peptide (34). The enzymatic and binding domains appear to be separated by a translocation domain. The plant hemitoxins, including saporin, gelonin, phytolaccins, bryodin, and others consist only of the A-chain portion of the toxin and lack a B chain, linking peptide, or interchain disulfide bond.

Immunotoxins have been prepared with whole toxins (Table 3). In most cases effort has been made to block the B-chain binding function by either steric blockade or small molecular weight blockers. These immunotoxins are particularly potent and efficacious, presumably because the B chain contains a translocation enhancement function in addition to a cell-binding function. Unfortunately, they tend to be toxic to normal cells both in vitro and in vivo. Usually whole toxins are linked to monoclonal antibodies by nonreducible link-

Table 3 Whole Toxins Used in Immunotoxin Synthesis

Toxin	Conjugate	Reference
ricin	RF-HBs-1-ricin	34
abrin	horse anti-human lymphocyte-abrin	35
diphtheria	T3-DT	36
Pseudomonas	anti-TAC-PE	37

ers, such as MBS. Recently, recombinant DNA technology has been used to replace the binding region of diphtheria toxin and Pseudomonas exotoxin with alpha-MSH and alpha-TGF, respectively (55,56).

Immunotoxins are most often prepared by isolating the A chain of a plant whole toxin or using the A chain-like plant hemitoxins (Table 4). There is no normal tissue-binding domain in the toxin. The toxin peptide must be linked to the antibody by a reducible linker, such as SPDP or 2-IT. These conjugates are generally less potent than whole toxin conjugates, and their limited potency and efficacy is dependent upon targeting to an antigen that readily internalizes into endocytic vesicles. Importantly, A-chain conjugates appear safe in clinical trials to date. It is unclear whether the balance of safety and efficacy favors A-chain or whole toxin conjugates in the clinical setting at present.

Table 4 A Chain-like Polypeptides Used in Immunotoxin Synthesis

Toxin	Conjugate	Reference
RTA	B3/25-RTA	2
DTA	9.2.27-DTA	1
abrin A	D3-abrin A	38
PAP	J5-PAP	4
gelonin	T11a-gelonin	4
bryodin	OX7-bryodin	39
MCI	OX7-MCI	39
saporin	OX7-saporin	40
restrictocin	MBr1-restrictocin	41
rRTA	454A12-rRTA	42
MSPSA	UCHT1-MSPSA	43

rRTA = recombinant RTA protein; MSPSA = recombinant diphtheria fragment; MCI = momordica charantia inhibitor.

Table 5 Enhancers for Immunotoxin Cytotoxicity

Enhancer	Immunotoxin	Reference
chloroquine	5E9-11-PAP	44
verapamil	HB21-PE	47
adenovirus	EGF-PE	48
monensin	T101-RTA	49
amantadine	T101-RTA	53
ammonium chloride	T101-RTA	49
ricin B	11/160-RTA	45
Fab′anti-RTA-ricin B	Fab′anti-human Ig-RTA	46

By adding small molecular weight molecules, such as ammonium chloride, monensin, verapamil, or amantadine, or adding ricin B chain alone or conjugated to antibody, it is possible to enhance the cytotoxicity of A-chain conjugates so that they approach the potency and efficacy of whole toxin conjugates (Table 5). The exact mechanism by which these enhancers work is unknown, although it is thought that they improve toxin translocation from a prelysosomal compartment to the cytosol. Unfortunately, none of these enhancers appears suitable at present for clinical application. Problems include the poor solubility of the hydrophobic monocarboxyl acid ionophores and the toxicity in vivo of chloroquine amantidine and other amines at concentrations needed for immunotoxin enhancement.

After conjugation free antibody and toxin must be removed, and this purification generally includes size exclusion chromatography or protein A affinity chromatography to exclude free toxin and either ion exchange or toxin affinity chromatography to remove free antibody. For in vitro testing often free antibody is not removed. This can represent 10 to 40% of the protein in the conjugate mixture and can affect potency and efficacy measurements. However, if only relative immunotoxin activities are desired, as in screening monoclonal antibodies, and if the stoichiometry of the conjugation reaction is kept the same, then purification of toxin conjugate from free antibody may not be necessary. For in vivo work one may need further size exclusion chromatography steps to remove aggregates or higher mers (proteins consisting of multiple antibodies or more than three toxin molecules). Further, for in vivo efficacy and pharmacokinetic measurements, one must remove free antibody (50). The optimal method appears to be ion exchange or toxin affinity chromatography. For RTA conjugates Blue Sepharose can be employed because of the affinity of the Cibacron blue dye for RTA (50).

Characterization of immunotoxins includes both physicochemical and biological tests. The physicochemical tests most often employed include size exclusion HPLC to measure the presence of aggregates and nonreducing SDS-PAGE with densitometry to define the mer status (number of toxin molecules bound per antibody molecule) and the presence of free antibody and free toxin. The biological tests in vitro include measurement of cellular protein synthesis after varying time exposures of varying concentrations of immunotoxins. The relative potency of a conjugate can be estimated by comparing the concentration required to inhibit protein synthesis by 50 or 90% with a constant incubation time with immunotoxin. Potency is proportional to the product of the antibody affinity and antigen density. The relative efficacy of a conjugate is measured by determining the rate of protein synthesis inactivation with saturating amounts of immunotoxin. This efficacy can also be measured by the log kill of target cells after prolonged exposure to saturating amounts of immunotoxin. Log kill measurements require a clonogenic assay. Efficacy of a toxin conjugate appears to reflect the ease with which the immunotoxin can enter the cell and translocate to the cytosol. Efficacy appears to reflect a property of the antigen and toxin rather than the antibody. One exception has been presented. Ring has described monoclonal antibodies to several epitopes on a 55 kilodalton breast cancer-associated antigen (9). Antibodies to one of the epitopes make potent immunotoxins, while antibodies to another epitope make inactive immunotoxins. However, he has not measured the affinity of each of these antibodies. Both potency and efficacy may be important in obtaining optimal clinical effect as saturating amounts of immunotoxin may not be deliverable to all tumor sites.

Immunotoxin selection may also be affected by the heterogeneity in sensitivity of antigen-positive target cells to immunotoxin killing. Several investigators have noted varying toxicity of some immunotoxins on antigen-positive tumor cell lines. While this may reflect in many cases simply antigen density (see description of "potency" above), in some cases antigen internalization appears decreased as well. Thus, a cell surface antigen may behave differently on tumor cells of different types or even different patients or different metastases in the same patient. Immunotoxins with antigen present on a majority of a given tumor type and with minimal cellular heterogeneity would be preferred. In addition, minimal evidence for varying tumor cell sensitivity to the immunotoxin is optimal.

The Appendix describes in detail our ongoing efforts to screen different monoclonal antibodies for immunotoxin development. The preparation and testing and interpretation of the results on a single antibody-RTA conjugate will be presented. We elected to use only a single toxin polypeptide, ricin A chain, for our studies. This protein has the advantages of laboratory safety, ease of conjugation, proven activity with a number of antitumor monoclonal antibodies, and a growing body of knowledge regarding its clinical pharmacology.

I. APPENDIX: MATERIALS AND METHODS

A. Ricin A Chain (RTA)

RTA is prepared from whole ricin by reduction with dithiothreitol or 2-mercaptoethanol and separated from ricin B chain on agarose-based matrices (54). Further ion exchange or immunoaffinity steps can be added. We obtained RTA from Dr. Franz Jansen, Centre de Recherches, Clin-Midi, Sanofi, Rue de Prof. Joseph Blayac, 34082 Montpelier, Cedex France. After signing a materials transfer agreement we obtained 50 mg of RTA suitable for 5 to 10 conjugations. Alternative sources, which we have not found suitable due to cost or quality, include Sigma Laboratories and Vector Laboratories. Several biotechnology companies have RTA available. Availability and collaborative arrangements may vary for each company. Contact persons include Dr. Lou Houston, Cetus Corporation, 1400 53rd Street, Emeryville, CA 94608, and Dr. Lynn Spitler, Xoma Corporation, 2910 Seventh Street, Berkeley, CA 94710. We received the RTA in sodium phosphate buffered saline, pH 7.4, PBS, at 10 mg/ml and stored the materal at 4°C until used. We avoided storage for longer than 1 to 2 months, and the RTA solution was microfuged 2 to 4 minutes prior to each use. We measured the optical density of the RTA at 280 nm and assumed that a 1 mg/ml solution yields an otpical denisty of 0.77.

B. Antibodies

Monoclonal antibodies used in this study were the anti-CEA antibody, Ab2, from Abbott Laboratories and the antitransferrin receptor antibody, B3/25, from Hybritech. Both Ab2 and B3/25 are IgG1 mouse monoclonal antibodies. Ab2 was received in PBS at 10 mg/ml and stored at 4°C. B3/25 was received in 50 mM sodium phosphate buffer at 14.7 mg/ml and stored at 4°C. For each antibody a 1 mg/ml solution yielded an optical density of approximately 1.0 at 280 nm.

C. Preparation of RTA Conjugate

1. SPDP Labeling

On the day of conjugation for each antibody, two PD10 columns (Pharmacia) were prewashed with sterile filtered PBS and 1 ml of 1 mg/ml bovine serum albumin (Sigma) in PBS. After the optical density of the eluent had returned to baseline, the columns were labeled "Ab-SPDP" and "RTA" and stored loosely covered at room temperature.

A stock solution of 20 mM SPDP (Pierce) was prepared by dissolving 62.4 mg in 10 ml of 95% ethanol and stored at 4°C. We used a stock solution of SPDP for over 6 weeks without evidence of loss of activity. One molar dithiothreitol

(DTT, Sigma) was prepared in distilled water, and 1-ml aliquots were frozen at −20°C. These aliquots were used for up to 6 months without loss of activity.

Seven mg of monoclonal antibody was mixed with 11.5 μl of 20 mM SPDP in an Eppendorf 1.5-ml microfuge tube and gently rotated on a roller apparatus for 30 minutes at room temperature. This yields a fivefold molar excess of SPDP to antibody. The ratio of SPDP/antibody must be tested empirically on each antibody, so that a final derivatization of 2 to 3 SPDPs per antibody is obtained. After 30 minutes the antibody-SPDP solution was loaded on the "Ab-SPDP" PD10 column and eluted with PBS. One-ml fractions were collected and optical density at 280 nm was measured on each sample. The 2 ml containing 90% of the protein was pooled. A 50-μl sample of the pooled material was mixed with 50 μl of freshly thawed 1 M DTT and 900 μl of distilled water. Optical density was read at 280 and 343 nm in 1-cm quartz cuvettes in a LKB spectrophotometer. The molarity of antibody and attached SPDP was calculated as shown below:

$$\text{molarity SPDP attached} = \frac{\text{OD343}}{8000}$$

$$\text{molarity antibody} = \text{OD280} - 5100 \times \text{molarity SPDP attached}$$

Using a fivefold molar excess of SPDP an average of 2 SPDPs were attached per Ab2 antibody molecule and 1.7 SPDPs per B3/25 antibody molecule. The recovery of Ab2-SPDP from the PD10 column was generally 85%, yielding 6 mg of protein, and the recovery of B3/25-SPDP from the PD10 column was 40%, yielding 2.8 mg of protein.

D. RTA Conjugation

Fifty μl of 1 M DTT was added to 0.7 ml of RTA (10 mg/ml in PBS). The solution was rotated at room temperature in a 1.5-ml Eppendorf tube attached to a roller apparatus. After 30 minutes the solution was loaded on the "RTA" PD10 column and the freshly reduced RTA eluted with PBS. One-ml fractions were collected and the optical density at 280 nm read. Usually one fraction contains the freshly reduced RTA. The usual yield was 58%, yielding four milligrams of protein.

The antibody-SPDP and freshly reduced RTA were then mixed. We had 3.3 M excess of RTA to immunoglobulin or a 1.7 M excess over available SPDP groups on the immunoglobulin for Ab2 and a 3.5 molar excess of RTA to immunoglobulin or 2.0 molar excess of RTA to available SPDP groups on B3/25 immunoglobulin. The mixture was left stationary at room temperature in a 5 ml plastic stoppered test tube for 24 hours. Then sodium azide (Baker) was added to make a final 0.02% sodium azide solution to prevent microbial contamination for each conjugate.

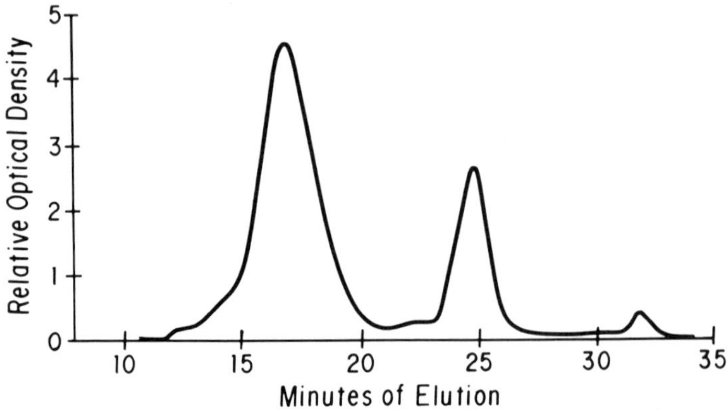

Figure 1 HPLC TSK3000 elution of Ab2-RTA at four ml/min with PBS. First peak is antibody + conjugate. Second peak is free RTA. Third peak is sodium azide.

Within 3 to 4 days the Ab2-RTA solution was loaded on a Waters HPLC outfitted with a TSK G-3000 column and the conjugate eluted with PBS at 4 ml/min. The antibody + conjugate peak was separate from the RTA peak (Fig. 1). The antibody/conjugate fractions were pooled and mixed with sodium azide to a final concentration of 0.02%. The solution was then concentrated to 1 ml on an Amicon stirred ultrafiltration cell model 8010 fitted with a YM10 membrane prewashed with 0.1% bovine serum albumin and then PBS. The yield of Ab2-RTA was 3.3 mg for a recovery of 33% from the conjugation reaction or 25% from the starting material. The B3/25-RTA was loaded on a Pharmacia FPLC with a HR16/50 column packed with Superose 6, and the conjugate was eluted in PBS at 1 ml/min. Again there was good separation of the antibody + conjugate from the RTA. The conjugate fractions were pooled and made 0.02% with sodium azide. The recovery was 3 mg conjugate + antibody or 70% of the expected yield from the conjugation reaction—20% from the starting materials.

A 15-μl aliquot of each conjugate was mixed with 15 μl of 2x nonreducing sample buffer (lacking 2-mercaptoethanol) and boiled 2 minutes and then loaded with standards on a 3% stacking-5% resolving SDS-PAGE using a Biorad minigel apparatus. After running the gel for 35 minutes at 175 volts, the gel was removed and stained with Coumassie blue staining solution and destained as described in the Biorad electrophoresis manual (Fig. 2). Densitometry was performed with a Helena Industries densitometer and area under the peaks compared (Fig. 3). There was a Poisson distribution of mers with an average of 2.1

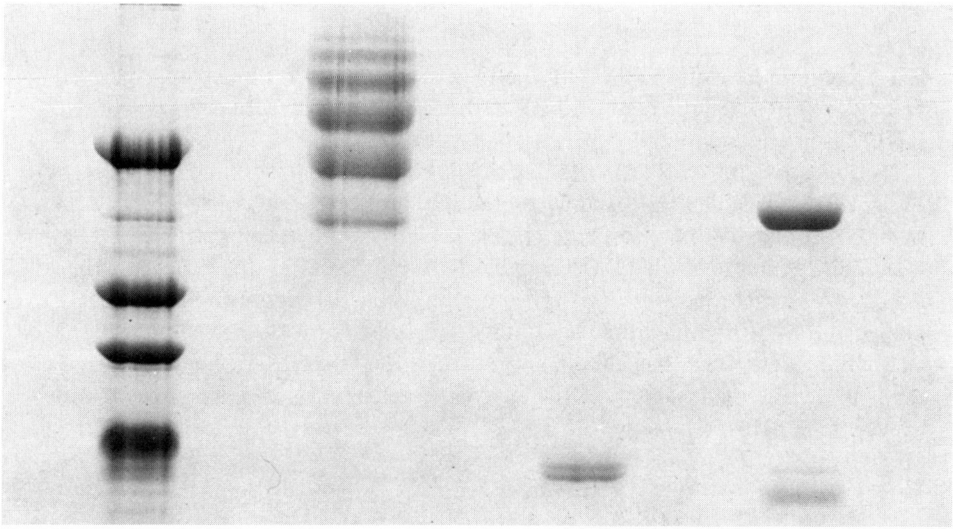

Figure 2 Five-percent nonreducing SDS-PAGE with lanes from left to right: protein molecular weight standards (myosin:205 kilodaltons, phosphorylase B:92.5 kilodaltons, bovine serum albumin:67 kilodaltons, and ovalbumin:44.5 kilodaltons), Ab2-RTA peak from HPLC, RTA, and Ab2.

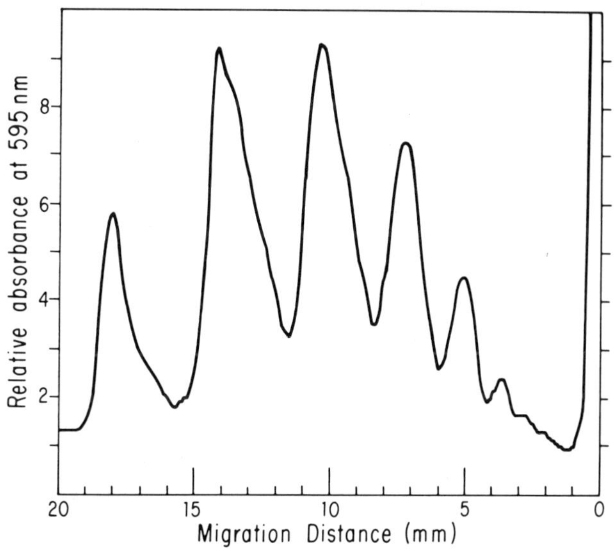

Figure 3 Densitometry scan of Ab2-RTA from Figure 2. Peaks from left to right are antibody, one-mer, two-mer, three-mer, four-mer, five-mer, and higher.

RTAs per immunoglobulin molecule and less than 1% free RTA and approximately 12% free antibody for Ab2-RTA. B3/25-RTA yielded an average of 1.2 RTAs per immunoglobulin with 39% free antibody.

Twelve ml of B3/25-RTA (0.15 mg/ml) in PBS were loaded on a Pharmacia FPLC HR 10/10 column packed with Blue Sepharose. The column was washed with 0.05 molar sodium phosphate buffer, pH 7.5, and the conjugate was eluted with 0.5 M sodium chloride/0.05 M sodium phosphate buffer, pH 7.5 (50). The load, wash, and elution were performed at 1 ml/min. The conjugate peak was pooled and 3-5% nonreducing SDS-PAGE performed (Fig. 4). As can be seen, all the conjugate was in the eluant, and there was less than 1% free antibody in the conjugate pooled fractions. The recovery was 40% from the starting conjugate (post-Superose 6).

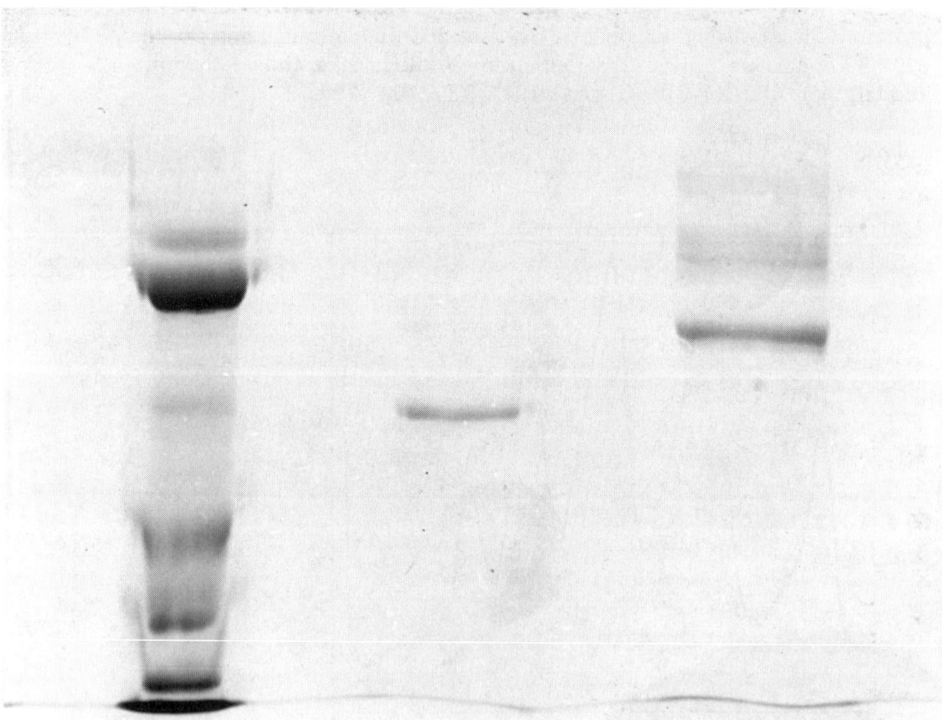

Figure 4 Five-percent nonreducing SDS-PAGE from left to right: protein molecular weight standards as in Figure 2, B3/25 from void peak on Blue Sepharose, B3/25-RTA from eluant on Blue Sepharose.

E. Enzymatic Activity

A test for the enzymatic activity of the toxin before and after conjugation was carried out. Eppendorf 1.5-ml tubes with 20 μl of water or ricin A chain (0.8 mg/ml) in PBS or B3/25-RTA (0.15 mg/ml) in PBS were mixed with 1 μl of 1 M dithiothreitol and left at room temperture for 30 minutes. Sequential 1:2 and 1:10 dilutions of these 3 solutions were made with autoclaved distilled water. 17.5 μl of Promega Biotec nuclease-treated rabbit reticulocyte lysate were mixed with 1 μl of 1 mM amino acids (minus leucine), 1 μl of BMV RNA (0.5 μg/ml), 2.5 μl of [^{3}H]-leucine (200 Ci/mM and 5 mCi/ml, NEN), 1 μl of RNAsin (1 U/ μl) and 2.5 μl of one of the diluted samples described above. These 25-μl lysates were incubated for 30 minutes at 4°C and then for 90 minutes at 30°C. 5-μl Aliquot from each lysate was mixed with 1 ml of 0.5 N sodium hydroxide/ 1.5% hydrogen peroxide for 10 minutes at 30°C. Then the samples were vortexed with 4 ml of cold 25% trichloroacetic acid with 2% casamino acids and kept at 4°C for 60 minutes. The solutions were then filtered through Whatman GF/C 2.4 cm filters. The filters were washed with 8% trichloroacetic acid and acetone and air dried. The filters were then counted in 10 ml of Hydrofluor in a Packard liquid scintillation counter. The concentration of toxin which gave 50% of maximal protein synthesis was the ID50. Toxin molarity of conjugates was derived from the average mer value of the conjugate described above. B3/25-RTA contained RTA with an ID50 of 6×10^{-11} M and the RTA prior to conjugation had an ID50 of 7×10^{-11} M. These values are indistinguishable, suggesting conjugation had no effect on the RTA enzyme activity. This was expected as the toxin had not required derivatization prior to conjugation.

F. Potency In Vitro

Tests of biologic potency were done using 4 colorectal carcinoma cell lines—WiDr, SW1116, LS174T, and HT29. These four cell lines are positive for the CEA antigen. In our laboratory WiDr was grown on Eagle's MEM with 10% fetal calf serum, 1% nonessential amino acids, 5 mM L-glutamine, 1 mM sodium pyruvate and 50 μg/ml of gentamicin. LS174T was grown on MEM with 10% fetal calf serum, 50 U/ml penicillin and 5 μg/ml streptomycin. SW1116 was grown on Leibovitz' L15 medium with 10% fetal calf serum, 50 U/ml penicillin, 5 μg/ml streptomycin, and 5 mM L-glutamine. HT29 was grown on McCoy's 5a modified medium with 10% fetal calf serum, 5 μg/ml streptomycin, and 50 U/ml penicillin. Cells were grown at 37°C in a 5% CO_2 atmosphere except SW1116 which was grown without CO_2. In a typical cytotoxicity experiment, cells at approximately 80-90% confluence were trypsinized and seeded at ten thousand cells per well into the wells of a microtiter plate. The cells were then grown for 48 hours in 100 μl of growth medium per well in order to allow them to plate and reexpress any CEA or transferrin receptor which might have been degraded during trypsinization. SW1116 were allowed to grow one week. Following the initial growth period, the cells were exposed to varying concentrations of immunotoxins during a 24-hr period. When enhancers were used, either 10 mM ammonium chloride or 50 nm monensin were added simultaneously with immunotoxin. Following this exposure to immunotoxin, cells were shifted to leucine-free MEM for one hour to deplete the endogenous leucine pools and then incubated with 1 μCi of [^{3}H]-leucine (NEN) per well in 100 μl of leucine-free MEM for 1 hour. The leucine starvation step was not required for SW1116 and WiDr. Following the pulse with [^{3}H]-leucine, the cells were washed 3 times with warmed original cell media and then solubilized with 50 μl per well of 2 M sodium hydroxide for 10 minutes at room temperature. Finally, the sodium hydroxide (Baker) was neutralized with 50 μl of 2 M hydrochloric acid (Baker), and the solution was absorbed onto methylcellulose filter cylinders (Skatron Harvesting System). Total cell incorporated radioactivity was then determined by liquid scintillation counting on a Packard 4640. The concentration of immunotoxin which gave 50% (ID50) or 90% (ID90) inhibition of protein synthesis was compared in order to estimate immunotoxin potency. For example, B3/25-RTA gave an ID50 of 1 pM on LS174T cells. B3/25-RTA in the presence of 50 nm monensin gave an ID50 of 5×10^{-14} M. In contrast, Ab2-RTA was not cytotoxic to LS174T cells in the absence of monensin. In the presence of 50 nm monensin the ID50 was 10^{-10} M (Fig. 5). Ammonium chloride at 10 mM was unable to enhance Ab2-RTA cytotoxicity on LS174T cells. Ab2-RTA was nontoxic to 3 other CEA-positive colorectal carcinoma cell lines, even in the presence of monensin. These results are similar to those reported by Watanabe and Griffin (8,27,51). Enhancers may improve potency and efficacy to varying degrees dependent on the antibody-antigen system and the particular enhancer.

Measurement of immunotoxin efficacy can be done directly by monitoring the log tumor cell kill at saturating amounts of immunotoxin in a clonogenic assay or indirectly by measuring the kinetics of protein synthesis inhibition by immunotoxin as discussed earlier. We have chosen the latter assay and have exposed LS174T cells to 10 nM immunotoxin for varying time periods followed by exposure to a [^{3}H]-leucine pulse as described above. Protein synthesis of control and immunotoxin-treated cells at each time point was measured and compared. The log percent inhibition of protein synthesis is plotted versus the time of exposure to immunotoxin to obtain the slope. The slope is the protein synthesis inactivation rate in -log fractional protein synthesis inhibition per hour. The B3/25-RTA inactivation rate on LS174T cells was .12 logs/hour in the absence of monensin and .50 logs/hour in the presence of monensin (Fig. 6). In contrast, the Ab2-RTA inactivation rate on LS174T cells in the presence of monensin was only .03 logs/hour. Compared to inactivation rates described by Neville (52), the antitransferrin receptor-RTA conjugate is a potent and efficacious immunotoxin and the anti-CEA conjugate is a weak and inefficacious im-

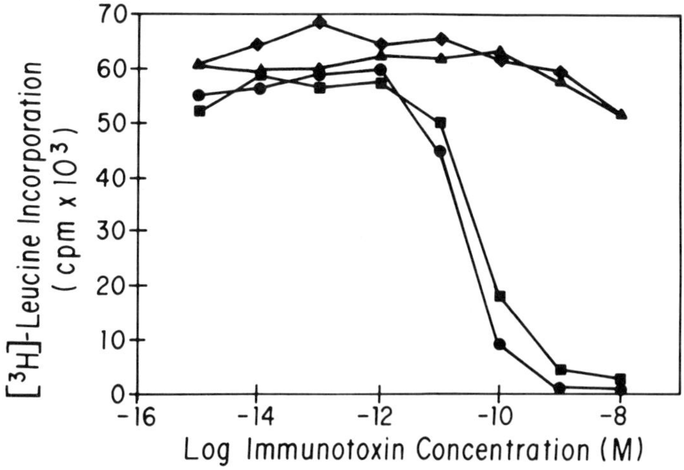

Figure 5 Protein synthesis inhibition by B3/25-RTA and Ab2-RTA on LS174T cells as described in the text. (■) B3/25-RTA alone, (●) B3/25-RTA with 50 nM monensin, (♦) Ab2-RTA alone, (▲) Ab2-RTA with 50 nM monensin.

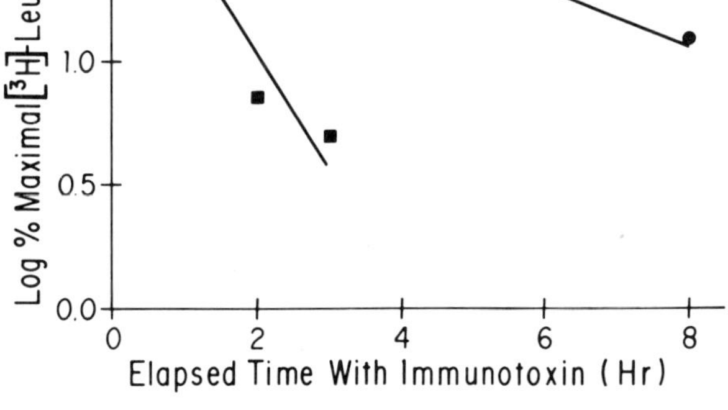

Figure 6 Kinetics of protein synthesis inhibition by B3/25-RTA as described in the text. (●) 10^{-8} M B3/25-RTA alone, (■) 10^{-8} M B3/25-RTA with 50 nM monensin.

munotoxin. Further, the transferrin receptor is found on most or all proliferating tumor cells, whereas the CEA antigen density and immunotoxin sensitivity is markedly heterogeneous.

While the B3/25-RTA is clearly the more potent and efficacious immunotoxin, the broader normal tissue reactivity of B3/25 has limited its preclinical and clinical development. However, its use in intracavitary applications, such as neoplastic meningitis, ovarian cancer, superficial bladder cancer and mesothelioma, may provide adequate therapeutic indices for using such a reagent clinically.

REFERENCES

1. Morgan, A. C., Schroff, R. W., Hwang, K. M., and Pavanasasivam, G. (1985) 1. Monoclonal antibody therapy of cancer: Parameters which affect the efficacy of immunotoxins. In *Monoclonal Antibody Therapy of Human Cancer* (K. Foon and A. Morgan, Eds.). Martinus Nijhoff Publishing, Boston, pp. 1-22.
2. Trowbridge, I., and Domingo, D. (1981) Anti-transferrin receptor monoclonal antibody and toxin-antibody conjugates affect growth of human tumour cells. *Nature 294*: 171-173.
3. Krolick, K., Yuan, D., and Vitetta, E. (1981) Specific killing of a human breast carcinoma cell line by a monoclonal antibody coupled to a A-chain of ricin. *Cancer Immunology and Immunotherapy 12*: 39-41.
4. Lambert, J., Senter, P., Yau-Young, A., Blattler, W., Ritz, J., Yetz, J., and Letvin, N. (1986) Purified immunotoxins that are reactive with lymphoid cells. *J. Biol. Chem. 260*: 12035-12041.
5. Bjorn, M., Ring, D., and Frankel, A. (1985) Evaluation of monoclonal antibodies for the development of breast cancer immunotoxins. *Cancer Research 45*: 1214-1221.
6. McIntosh, D., Edwards, D., Cumber, A., Parnell, G., Dean, C., Ross, W., and Forrester, J. (1983) Ricin B chain converts a non-cytotoxic antibody-ricin A chain conjugate into a potent and specific cytotoxic agent. *FEBS Letters 164*: 17-20.
7. Lesley, J., Domingo, D., Schulte, R., and Trowbridge, I. (1984) Effect to an anti-murine transferrin receptor-ricin A conjugate on bone marrow stem and progenitor cells treated in vitro. *Experimental Cell Research 150*: 400-407.
8. Watanabe, Y., Miyazaki, H., and Osawa, T. (1984) Effect of a monoclonal anti-carcinoembryonic antigen antibody-ricin A-chain conjugate on human carcinoembryonic antigen-producing tumor cells. *J. Pharm. Dyn. 7*: 593-603.
9. Ring, D. B., Bjorn, M. J., Hsieh-Ma, S. T., and Kassel, J. (1987) Breast cancer associated antigens that make effective immunotoxin targets. In *Second International Conference on Monoclonal Antibody Immunoconjugates for Cancer* (I. Royston, Ed.) UCSD Press, San Diego, p. 86.
10. Colombatti, W., and Bron, C. (1985) Sensitivity of target cells to immunotoxins: possible role of cell-surface antigens. *Immunology 55*: 331-337.

11. Youle, R., and Neville, D. (1987) Role of endocytosis and receptor recycling in ligand-toxin and antibody-toxin conjugate activity. In *Immunoconjugates: Antibody Conjugates in Radioimaging and Therapy of Cancer* (C. Vogel, Ed.). Oxford University Press, New York, in press.
12. Bernhard M., Foon, K., Oeltmann, T., Key, M., Hwang, K., Clarke, G., Christensen, W., Hoyer, L., Hanna, M., and Oldham, R. (1983) Guinea pig line 10 hepatocarcinoma model: characterization of monoclonal antibody and in vivo effect of unconjugated antibody and antibody conjugated to diphtheria toxin A chain. *Cancer Research 43*: 4420-4428.
13. Bourrie, B., Casellas, P., Blythman, H., and Jansen, F. (1986) Study of the plasma clearance of antibody-ricin-A-chain immunotoxins. *Eur. J. Biochem. 155*: 1-10.
14. Weil-Hillman, G., Uckun, F., Manske, J., and Vallera, D. (1987) Combined immunochemotherapy of human solid tumors in nude mice. *Cancer Research 47*: 579-585.
15. Gros, O., Gros, P., Jansen, F., and Vidal, H. (1985) Biochemical aspects of immunotoxin preparation. *Journal of Immunological Methods 81*:283-297.
16. Blakey, D., Watson, G., Knowles, P., and Thorpe, P. (1987) Effect of chemical deglycosylation of ricin A chain on the in vivo fate of cytotoxic activity of an immunotoxin composed of ricin A chain and anti-Thy 1.1 antibody. *Cancer Research 47*: 947-952.
17. Chang, T., and Neville, D. (1977) Artificial hybrid protein containing a toxic protein fragment and a cell membrane receptor-binding moiety in a disulfide conjugate. *J. of Biol. Chem. 252*: 1505-1514.
18. Gilliland, D., and Collier, R. (1980) A model system involving anti-concanavalin A for antibody targeting of diphtheria toxin fragment A. *Cancer Research 40*: 3564-3569.
19. Fitzgerald, D., Trowbridge, I., Pastan, I., and Willingham, M. (1983) Enhancement of toxicity of antitransferrin receptor antibody-Pseudomonas exotoxin conjugates by adenovirus. *Proc. Natl. Acad. Sci. USA 80*:4134-4138.
20. Foxwell, B., Ross, W., and Thorpe, P. (1984) Antibody-ricin conjugates: a method of linkage which blocks the galactose binding site of ricin. *Behring Inst. Mitt. 74*: 101-107.
21. Raso, V., and Griffin, T. (1980) Specific cytotoxicity of a human immunoglobulin-directed Fab′-ricin A chain conjugate. *J. Immunol. 125*: 2610-2615.
22. Blattler, W., Kuenzi, B., Lambert, J., and Senter, P. (1985). New heterobifunctional protein cross-linking reagent that forms an acid-labile link. *Biochem. 24*: 1517-1524.
23. Marsh, J., and Neville, D. (1987) Ricin-antibody conjugates: enhancement of toxicity by introduction of a peptide linker. *J. Biol. Chem.* in press.
24. Blakey, D., Wallace, P., and Thorpe, P. (1987) Blood clearance rates of a panel of immunotoxins. In *Second International Conference on Monoclonal Antibody Immunoconjugates for Cancer* (I. Royston, Ed.). UCSD Press, San Diego, p. 60.

25. Marsh, J., and Neville, D. (1986) Immunotoxins: chemical variables affecting cell killing efficiencies. In *Protein Tailoring for Food and Medical Uses* (R. Feeney and J. Whitaker, Eds.). Marcel Dekker, New York, pp. 291-316.
26. Masuho, Y., Umemoto, N., Hara, T., and Ohtomo, N. (1981) Cytotoxicity of a hybrid prepared by coupling diphtheria toxin A-chain with immunoglobulin Fab′ with N,N′-o-phenylenedimaleimide. *Biochem. Biophys. Res. Comm. 102*: 561-567.
27. Griffin, T., Childs, L., and Levin, L. (1984) Enhancement of the specific cytotoxicity of anti-carcinoembryonic antigen immunotoxins by adenovirus and carboxylic ionophores. *Prot. Biol. Fluids 32*: 449-453.
28. Moolten, F., Capparell, N., and Cooperband, S. (1972) Antitumor effects of antibody-diphtheria toxin conjugates: use of hapten-coated tumor cells as an antigen target. *JNCI 49*: 1057-1062.
29. Moolten, F., Cooperband, S. (1970) Selective destruction of target cells of diphtheria toxin conjugated to antibody directed against antigens on the cells. *Science 169*: 68-70.
30. Smagh, B., and Gregory, K. (1972) Antibody to lactate dehydrogenase. V. Use as a carrier for introducing diphtheria toxin into mouse tumor cells. *Biochim. Biophys. Acta 273*: 188-198.
31. Philpott, G., Bower, R., and Parker, C. (1973) Improved selective cytotoxicity with an antibody-diphtheria toxin conjugate. *Surgery 73*: 928-935.
32. Ross, W., Thorpe, P., Cumber, A., Edwards, D., Hinson, C., and Davies, A. (1980) Increased toxicity of diphtheria toxin for human lymphoblastoid cells following covalent linkage to anti- (human lymphocyte) globulin or its F(ab′)2 fragment. *Eur. J. Biochem. 104*: 381-390.
33. Paraskeva, C., Buckle, B., and Thorpe, P. (1985) Selective killing of contaminating human fibroblasts in epithelial cultures derived from colorectal tumours using an anti-Thy-1 antibody-ricin conjugate. *Br. J. Cancer 51*: 131-134.
34. Hwang, J., Fitzgerald, D., Adhya, S., and Pastan, I. (1987) Functional domains of Pseudomonas exotoxin identified by deletion analysis of the gene expressed in E. coli. *Cell 48*: 129-136.
35. Thorpe, P., Cumber, A., Williams, N., Edwards, D., Ross, W., and Davies, A. (1981) Abrogation of the non-specific toxicity of abrin conjugated to anti-lymphyocyte globulin. *Clin. Exp. Immunol. 43*: 195-200.
36. Blythman, H., Casellas, P., Gros, O., Jansen, F., Laurent, J., Richer, G., and Vidal, H. (1983) Immunotoxins. In *Monoclonal Antibodies and Cancer* (B. Boss, R. Langman, I. Trowbridge, R. Dulbecco, Eds.). Academic Press, Orlando, pp. 99–106.
37. Fitzgerald, D., Waldmann, T., Willingham, M., and Pastan, I. (1984) Pseudomonas exotoxin-anti-TAC cell specific immunotoxin active against cells expressing the human T cell growth factor receptor. *J. Clin. Invest. 74*: 966-971.
38. Hwang, K., Foon, K., Cheung, P., Pearson, J., and Oldham, R. (1984) Selective antitumor effect on L10 hepatocarcinoma cells of a potent immunocon-

jugate composed of the A chain of abrin and a monoclonal antibody to a hepatoma-associated antigen. *Cancer Research 44*: 4578-4586.
39. Thorpe, P., Blakey, D., Wawrzynczak, E., and Stirpe, F. (1986) Anti-tumor effects of immunotoxins. In *Membrane-mediated Cytotoxicity*. UCLA Symposia on Molecular and Cellular Biology, Vol. 45 (B. Bonavida, R. Collier, Eds.). Alan Liss, New York, in press.
40. Thorpe, P., Brown, A., Bremner, J., Foxwell, B., and Stirpe, F. (1985) An immunotoxin composed of monoclonal anti-Thy-1.1 antibody and a ribosome-inactivating protein from Saponaria officinalis: potent antitumor effects in vitro and in vivo. *JNCI 75*: 151-159.
41. Canevari, S., Mezzanzanica, D., Orlandi, R., Pupa, S., Conde, F., and Colnaghi, M. (1987) Optimization of immunoconjugates against human ovarian carcinoma. In *Second International Conference on Monoclonal Antibody Immunoconjugates for Cancer* (I. Royston, Ed.). UCSD Press, San Diego, pp. 62.
42. Fitzgerald, D., Bjorn, M., Ferris, R., Winkelhake, J., Frankel, A., Hamilton, T., Ozols, R., Willingham, M., and Pastan, I. (1987) Antitumor activity of an immunotoxin in a nude mouse model of ovarian cancer. *Cancer Research 47*: 1407-1410.
43. Colombatti, M., Greenfield, L., and Youle, R. (1986) Cloned fragment of diphtheria toxin linked to T cell-specific antibody identifies regions of B-chain active in cell entry. *J. Biol. Chem., 261*: 3030-3035.
44. Ramakrishnan, S., and Houston, L. L. (1984) Inhibition of human acute lymphoblastic leukemia cells by immunotoxins: Potentiation by chloroquine. *Science 223*: 58-60.
45. McIntosh, D. P., Edwards, D. C., Cumber, A. J., Parnell, G. D., Dean, C. J., Ross, W. C. j., and Forrester, J. A. (1983) Ricin B chain converts a non-cytoxic antibody-ricin A chain conjugate into a potent and specific cytoxic agent. *Federation of European Biochemical Societies 164*: 17-20.
46. Fulton, R. J., Uhr, J. W., and Vitetta, E. S. (1986) The effect of antibody valency and lysosomotrophic amines on the synergy between ricin A chain and ricin B chain containing immunotoxins. *J. Immunol. 136*: 3103-3109.
47. Akiyama, S., Seth, P., Pirker, R., Fitzgerald, D., Gottesman, M. M., and Pastan, I. (1985) Potentiation of cytotoxic activity of immunotoxins on cultured human cells. *Cancer Research 45*: 1005-1007.
48. Fitzgerald, D., Padmanabhan, R., Pastan, I., and Willingham, M. (1983) Adenovirus-induced release of epidermal growth factor and Pseudomonas toxin into the cytosol of KB cells during receptor-mediated endocytosis. *Cell 32*: 607-617.
49. Casellas, P., Bourrie, B., Gros, P., and Jansen, F. (1984) Kinetics of cytotoxicity induced by immunotoxins. *J. Biol. Chem. 259*: 9359-9364.
50. Thorpe, P. (1987) Overview of immunotoxin therapy. In *Second International Conference on Monoclonal Antibody Immunoconjugates for Cancer* (I. Royston, Ed.). UCSD Press, San Diego, p. 27.
51. Levin L, Griffin, T., Haynes, L., and Sedor, C. (1982) Selective cytotoxicity for a colorectal carcinoma cell line by a monoclonal anti-carcinoembryonic

antigen antibody coupled to the A chain of ricin. *J. Biol. Resp. Mod. 1*: 149-162.

52. Youle, R., and Neville, D. (1982) Kinetics of protein synthesis inactivation by ricin-anti-Thy-1.1 monoclonal antibody hybrids. *J. Biol. Chem. 257*: 1598-1601.
53. Siena, S., Villa, S., Bregni, M. Bonnadonna, G., and Gianni, A. (1987) Amantadine potentiates T lymphocyte killing by an anti-pan-T cell (CD5) ricin A-chain immunotoxin. *Blood 69*: 345-348.
54. Vidal, H., Casellas, P., Gros, P., and Jansen, F. (1985) Studies on components of immunotoxins: purification of ricin and its subunits and influence of unreacted antibodies. *Int. J. Cancer 36*: 705-711.
55. Murphy, J., Bishai, W., Borowski, M., Miyanohara, A., Boyd, J., and Nagle, S. (1986) Genetic construction, expression and melanoma-selective cytotoxicity of a diphtheria toxin related alpha-melanocyte stimulating hormone fusion protein. *Proc. Natl. Acad. Sci. USA 83*: 8258-8262.
56. Chaudhary, V., Fitzgerald, D., Adhya, S., and Pastan, I. (1987) Activity of a recombinant fusion protein between transforming growth factor alpha and Pseudomonas toxin. *Cell*, in press.

9

Radioiodinated Monoclonal Antibodies in the Imaging and Treatment of Human Renal Cell Carcinoma Xenografts in Nude Mice

ROBERT L. VESSELLA and PAUL H. LANGE
Veterans Administration Medical Center and University of Minnesota, Minneapolis, Minnesota

DONALD F. PALME II, REI K. CHIOU*
University of Minnesota, Minneapolis, Minnesota

MICHAEL K. ELSON
Veterans Administration Medical Center, Minneapolis, Minnesota

BARRY W. WESSELS
The George Washington University Medical Center, Washington, D.C.

I. INTRODUCTION

The concept of targeting a tumor with antibodies is attributed to Ehrlich (1), who at the turn of the century discussed the in vivo potential of "magic bullets." However, it was not until the classic studies of Pressman (2) were published in 1953 that research on tumor targeting using antibodies was documented. In recent years the ability to produce monoclonal antibodies (MAbs) has greatly advanced the field, and prospects for the development of antibody-mediated diagnosis and therapy are brighter than ever before. This chapter details some of our efforts to target and treat human renal cell cardinoma (RCC) xenografts in nude mice using radioiodinated MAbs.

Tumor targeting with MAbs involves two major areas of focus. The first is tumor detection or imaging using radiolabeled MAbs and gamma scintigraphy—often referred to as radioimmunoscintigraphy (RIS)—and the second is therapy. The therapeutic potential of a MAb is investigated if it is sufficiently specific for the tumor, over other tissues, in vivo. In this chapter, we limit our discussion to the use of ^{131}I-labeled MAbs. Other investigators have used unconju-

---

**Current affiliation*: George Washington University, Washington, D.C.

gated MAbs that invoke or participate in a host-mediated response to the tumor or MABs conjugated to cytotoxic agents, such as the toxins ricin, gelonin, diphtheria toxin, or abrin or the drugs methotrexate, adriamycin, or vinblastine. Reviews of these alternate approaches to MAb-mediated therapy have recently been published (3-5).

Renal cell carcinoma is believed to derive from cells of the proximal tubule of the kidney based on the results of electron microscopy studies and, more recently, MAb immunohistochemistry stratification schemes (6,7). Approximately 20,000 people per year are diagnosed as having RCC; there is a 3:1 male predominance. Approximately 60% of these people have known or occult metastatic disease at the first clinical presentation. There are currently no tumor markers in use for detection or monitoring of RCC. Surgical excision of the primary tumor and on occasion a solitary metastatic tumor is the only effective therapy, although some chemotherapy (i.e. vinblastine) and hormone (diethylstilbesterol) regimens have produced a temporary response in some patients. Recently, biological response modifiers, such as interferon (8) and lymphokine-activated killer (LAK) cells (9), have been used in a number of studies, and early reports suggest some benefit. Nevertheless, for the majority of patients with metastatic disease there is no effective treatment.

The biological behavior of RCC is intriguing. Spontaneous remission occurs in approximately 7% of patients with metastatic disease; this is one of the highest spontaneous remission rates among all human tumors. The interior of primary or metastatic tumors is often necrotic and laden with lymphocytes. These observations support the speculation that a host response of some magnitude may be mounted to RCC, yet that response has not been shown to significantly alter the clinical course of the disease.

For the reasons cited above, we believe RCC is an unusually attractive human tumor for MAb studies; clinical benefits would result from MAbs that aided staging of the tumor on presentation (e.g., via RIS), the lack of effective treatment for metastatic disease allows opportunities for several innovative therapeutic approaches singularly or in combination with other experimental protocols, and the generation of MAbs to RCC might result in the detection of the first serum or urine tumor marker for RCC. Our efforts to generate tumor-preferential MAbs resulted in a panel of RCC-reactive MAbs (10,11), and from these we selected those best suited for in vivo studies of RIS and MAb radiotherapy. We have conducted RIS and MAb-radiotherapy experiments using five radioiodinated MAbs and ten human tumor xenografts carried in athymic mice. We present here our in vivo preclinical experience with ^{131}I-labeled MAbs, including the imaging of several subcutaneous RCC xenografts and the detection by gamma scintigraphy of RCC xenografts weighing less than 30 mg that have been implanted under the renal capsule. In addition we detail several of our MAb-radiotherapy efforts, including the therapeutic effect of two 100-μCi doses of ^{131}I-labeled MAb A6H on established subcutaneous RCC xenografts.

II. RESULTS

The results presented here comprise a concise summary of our efforts to utilize ^{131}I as a radionuclide label for both imaging and MAb radiotherapy in the RCC preclinical model. We believe these data will be viewed as quite encouraging, as they demonstrate detection of small tumors by RIS and long-term tumor growth control by our ^{131}I-labeled RCC-reactive MAbs. However, as has been stressed in the literature, caution must be used when extrapolating from results in nude mice to the condition for man.

Radioiodination and Radioimmunoscintigraphy

Many protocols are available for labeling MAbs with a radioactive isotope of iodine (Table 1) (12,13). With a gamma energy of 360 KeV, ^{131}I is suitable, although admittedly not ideal, for detection by scintigraphy. Similarly, its beta energy of 0.608 MeV has therapeutic potential, although other isotopes might be better for therapy experiments if they were as easily coupled to a MAb. For simple in vivo biodistribution studies that do not require gamma scintigraphy, ^{125}I can be used; the coupling procedure is the same as that used for ^{131}I. Finally, of the isotopes generally considered for scintigraphy (e.g., ^{99}Tc, ^{111}In) or therapy (e.g., ^{90}Y), the iodines are relatively inexpensive, readily available commercially, and well suited to use in the moderately sophisticated research laboratory.

Table 1 Common Methods for the Radioiodination of Proteins

Method	Target	Exposure to oxidizing agent	Specific activity	Labeling efficiency	References
Chloramine T[a] and Iodo Beads	Tyrosine phenol ring	Yes–1[d]	High	High	68
Iodogen[b]	Tyrosine phenol ring	Yes–2[d]	High	High	71
Lactoperoxidase	Tyrosine phenol ring	Yes–3[d]	Medium	Medium	70
Bolton-Hunter[c]	Lysine	No	Medium	Medium	74

[a]N-Chloro-benzenesulfonamide.
[b]1,3,4,6-Tetrachloro-3, 6-diphenyl glycoluril.
[c]N-Succinimidyl 3-(4-hydroxy-5-I-iodophenyl)propionate.
[d]Organized from strongest to weakest oxidizing potential.

In our laboratory, we most commonly use the Chloramine T procedure (see Fig. 1; details of this procedure are presented in the Materials and Methods section). Single iodinations of >50 mCi can be performed with this method, although additional shielding and safety precautions are required at these levels of radioactivity. We assess the quality of the radiolabeled MAbs by a determination of specific activity, protein incorporation (TCA precipitability), presence of aggregates by HPLC and immunological reactivity using a live cell binding assay. Specific activities of from 3 to 15 mCi/mg can be routinely achieved; below 10 mCi/mg there is little adverse effect on immunological activity. Protein incorporation is typically above 98%. Aggregates should not exceed 5% of the labeled MAb or remaining protein fractions (monitor both HPLC peaks; see Fig. 2). Immunological reactivity must exceed 50% and should be from 70-95% for use in vivo. If the MAb is used more than 24 hours after labeling, the above quality assessment studies should be repeated.

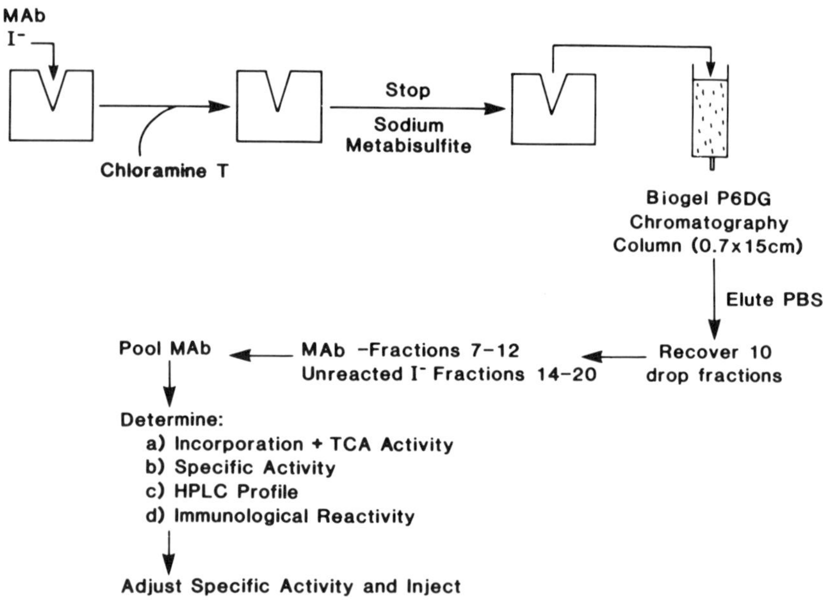

Figure 1 Schematic of the Chloramine T iodination procedure as used in our laboratory for routine labeling of MAbs. Details of this procedure are provided in the Materials and Methods section.

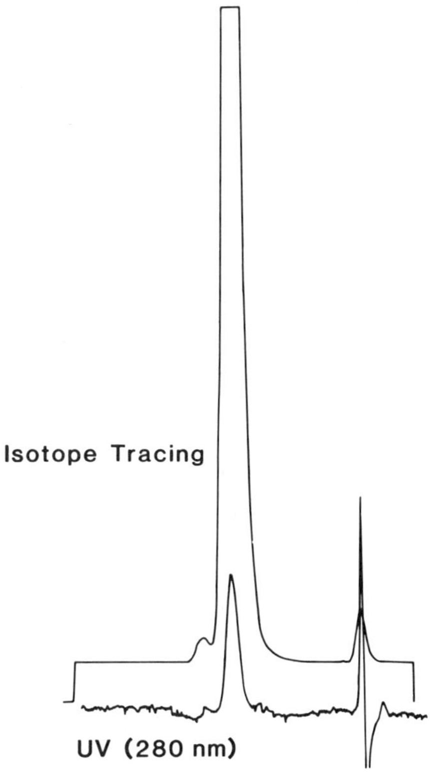

Figure 2 A dual pen tracing of HPLC fractionation of ^{131}I-labeled MAb A6H showing both protein (UV) and isotopic profiles. This graph indicates the presence of little, if any, aggregated MAbs in the radiolabeled preparation. The column, buffers, and flow rate used are explained in the Materials and Methods section.

Of the MAbs described in this chapter, those designated A6H, B4F, C5H, and AFP are relatively resistant to damage by iodination via the chloramine T method, but D5D is somewhat more susceptible, as measured by immunoreactivity. Accordingly, we aim for specific activities of from 3 to 5 μCi/μg for D5D. In experiments with $F(ab')^2$ fragments of A6H some (but not consistent) decreases in immunological reactivity were observed at the specific activities used for the entire molecule.

A factor that must be considered when iodinating MAbs is the rate of dehalogenation that occurs in the body. We do not block the thyroid of mice receiving radioiodinated MAbs; this allows the visualization of uptake of free iodine by the thyroid during scintigraphy. In our studies the rate of dehalogenization was highly variable among animals receiving the same lot and amount of radioiodinated MAb and bearing identical xenografts of similar weight: Some showed no significant dehalogenization over the course of study while others rapidly dehalogenated the MAb; there is no apparent explanation for these differences among individuals. Therefore, dehalogenization may severely limit attempts to monitor the presence or distribution of radioiodinated MAbs by tracing the radiolabel.

Radioiodinated MAbs with an acceptable level of immunological reactivity were used in our in vivo tumor-targeting studies. Immunological specificity of a MAb was often assessed in mice bearing a RCC xenograft on one shoulder and a non-RCC xenograft on the other. Biodistribution studies were conducted using a ^{131}I-labeled, RCC-specific MAb (e.g., A6H), and a ^{125}I-labeled nonspecific MAb (e.g., anti-AFP) of the same isotype. Analysis of samples of various tissues provides an estimate of the ratio of these MAbs in the tumor and in murine organs (14). The assessment of biodistribution has been the subject of numerous reports in the scientific literature (15,16), but no consensus has been reached on the most appropriate manner in which to present these data. The data we present are expressed as tumor:blood ratios (T:B), tumor:normal tissue ratios (e.g., T/liver), percent of the injected dose per gram of tissue (%ID/g), and micrograms of MAb per gram of tissue. It must be remembered that in all of these methods, it is the presence of labeled antibody at best, not the presence of total MAb at a given site, that is being measured. Considerable controversy also exists on the appropriate size for tumors used in these experiments (17,18). In our system, tumors weighing more than 500 mg are often necrotic, hemorrhagic, or fibrotic; these tendencies are often characteristic of a given xenograft (e.g., Tk-82 becomes very hemmorrhagic and develops a necrotic center, which closely resembles the histologic appearance of clinical specimens, but TK-39 is more firm and cellular). The data presented here reflects our recent change to only use tumors weighing less than or equal to 400 mg for study.

Representative RIS images for mice treated with six xenograft/MAb combinations are shown in Figure 3; post mortem biodistribution data for these animals are presented in Table 2. These tumors ranged in size from 97 to 367 mg. As shown in image A, the RCC xenograft TK-82 does not exhibit significant nonspecific binding of the control MAb anti-AFP (we rarely observe T:B ratios >2, or 10% of the ID/g). TK-82 does bind the RCC-preferential MAb A6H (image B). We have used TK-82 and A6H extensively in our in vivo studies. The MAb A6H is preferentially reactive with RCC and normal renal proximal tubules (10). In Figure 3, ^{131}I-radiolabeled A6H provides an image of the RCC xenograft TK-177C (image C) but not the control colon carcinoma xenograft HT-29 (image D). Although there was considerable variability in the biodistribution of A6H among individual mice, in general the average T:B ratios for subcutaneous RCC

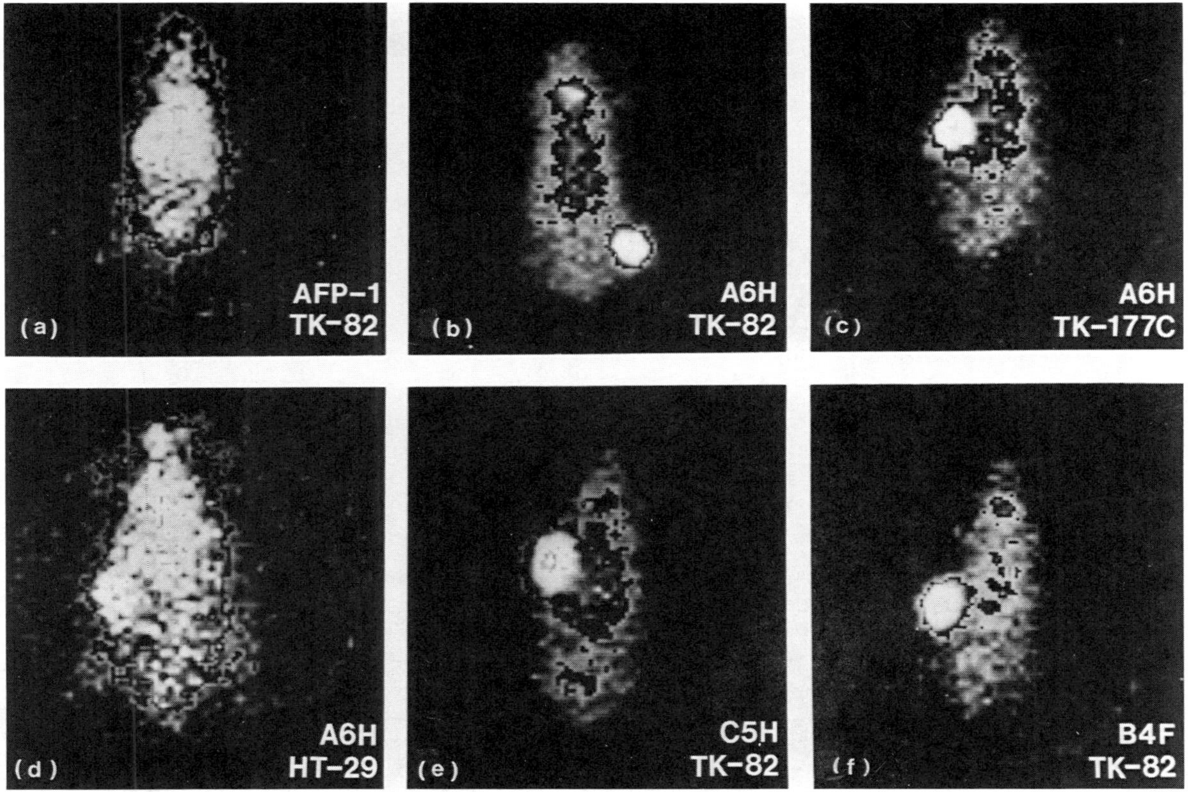

Figure 3 Radioimmunoscintigraphy of six mice carrying subcutaneous xenografts 48 hours after injection with approximately 40 μCi of ^{131}I-labeled MAbs. MAbs A6H, B4F, and C5h are preferential for the RCC xenografts TK-82 and Tk-177; MAb AFP-1 is specific for alpha-fetoprotein. The colon xenograft HT-29 was obtained from the ATCC and is used as a control for the RCC-preferential MAbs. Biodistribution data for these animals are provided in Table 2. All images were acquired on our Pho-Gamma IV gamma camera with a pinhole collimator.

Table 2 Biodistribution of Radioiodinated MAbs in Animals (represented in Figs. 3 and 4)

						Tumor: Tissue ratio			
Image	MAb	Xenografts	Wt(mg)	% ID/G	μCi/G	Blood	Liver	Spleen	Kidney
Fig. 3A[a]	AFP-1[c]	TK-82	316	4	1.6	0.4	0.7	0.1	0.2
3B	A6H	TK-82	183	65	25	10	33	44	33
3C	A6H	TK-177C	97	62	21	6	20	23	26
3D	A6H	HT-29	300	9	3.6	1.2	0.3	0.2	0.3
3E	C5H	TK-82	223	35	14	6	16	20	28
3F	B4F	TK-82	367	68	27	12	27	38	27
Fig. 4A[b]	A6H	TK-82	27	180	72	26	88	86	96
4B	A6H	TK-177C	15	187	74	15	60	47	20

[a]All xenografts implanted subcutaneously.
[b]Xenografts were implanted beneath the renal capsule.
[c]Biodistribution results obtained 48 hours postinjection (40 μCi) for all ^{131}I-radiolabeled MAbs.

xenografts TK-39, TK-82, TK-163, and TK-177C ranged from approximately 4:1 to 15:1. Another MAb that we have developed and used in in vivo studies, C5H, shows reactivity to many human tumors and the normal renal glomerulus (10). Part E of Figure 3 illustrates a typical image produced by C5H and the RCC xenograft TK-82. Finally, a relatively new MAb, designated B4F, has been isolated and partially characterized in our laboratory (19). This IgG_{2b} MAb, shown in Figure 3, image F, has a reactivity profile similar to that for A6H and has performed well in preliminary in vivo RIS studies. Biodistribution results for B4F are similar to those for A6H (see Table 2).

As is apparent from the composite of images presented in Figure 3, ^{131}I-labeled RCC-preferential MAbs did target specific tumor xenografts, providing clear scintigraphic images. In addition, it appeared that A6H had the potential to image even smaller xenografts than these subcutaneous implants (>25 mg). To determine if smaller xenografts could be imaged successfully, we adapted the method of Bogden et al. (20) for subrenal implantation. Preliminary results of the studies have been published (21,22). Figure 4 shows RIS images for two animals receiving subcapsular implants. In these animals 1-2-mg xenografts were inserted under the renal capsule and 10-14 days later (the period required for implant vascularization and growth) the mice were injected with approximately 5 μg of ^{131}I-labeled A6H. Both images in Figure 4 were obtained 48 hours after intravenous injection of approximately 40 μCi of ^{131}I-labeled A6H.

In image A of Figure 4, the TK-82 xenograft is seen as an asymmetric uptake in the region of the left kidney. This tumor weighed 27 mg and contained 0.4 μg of MAb at the time of imaging as determined by biodistribution. This represents injected dose or, when normalized to a unit weight, 180% ID/g. In image B, similar asymmetric uptake of the label is noted and tumor targeting was confirmed by the biodistribution data: tumor weight of 15 mg and 0.3 μg (1.5 μCi) of A6H detected within the tumor at sacrifice (3% of injected dose; 187% ID/g). These images and supporting biodistribution data illustrate the remarkable potential of ^{131}I-labeled MAbs to target tumors in vivo. Additional biodistribution data for these two xenografts is provided in Table 2. Figure 5 indicates the relative size of a 10-mg RCC sub renal capsule xenograft in situ.

B. Monoclonal Antibody-mediated Radiation Therapy

Our biodistribution studies indicated that A6H targeted three RCC xenografts (TK-82, TK-39, and TK-177C) unusually well: At an antibody mass dose of 10 μg and a xenograft weight of 100 mg, one could expect to achieve more than 50% ID/g. At a projected activity dose of 100 μCi, this would result in targeting 5 μCi to the tumor, a level at which a therapeutic effect might be expected. To examine this possibility we initiated a series of MAb-radiotherapy studies

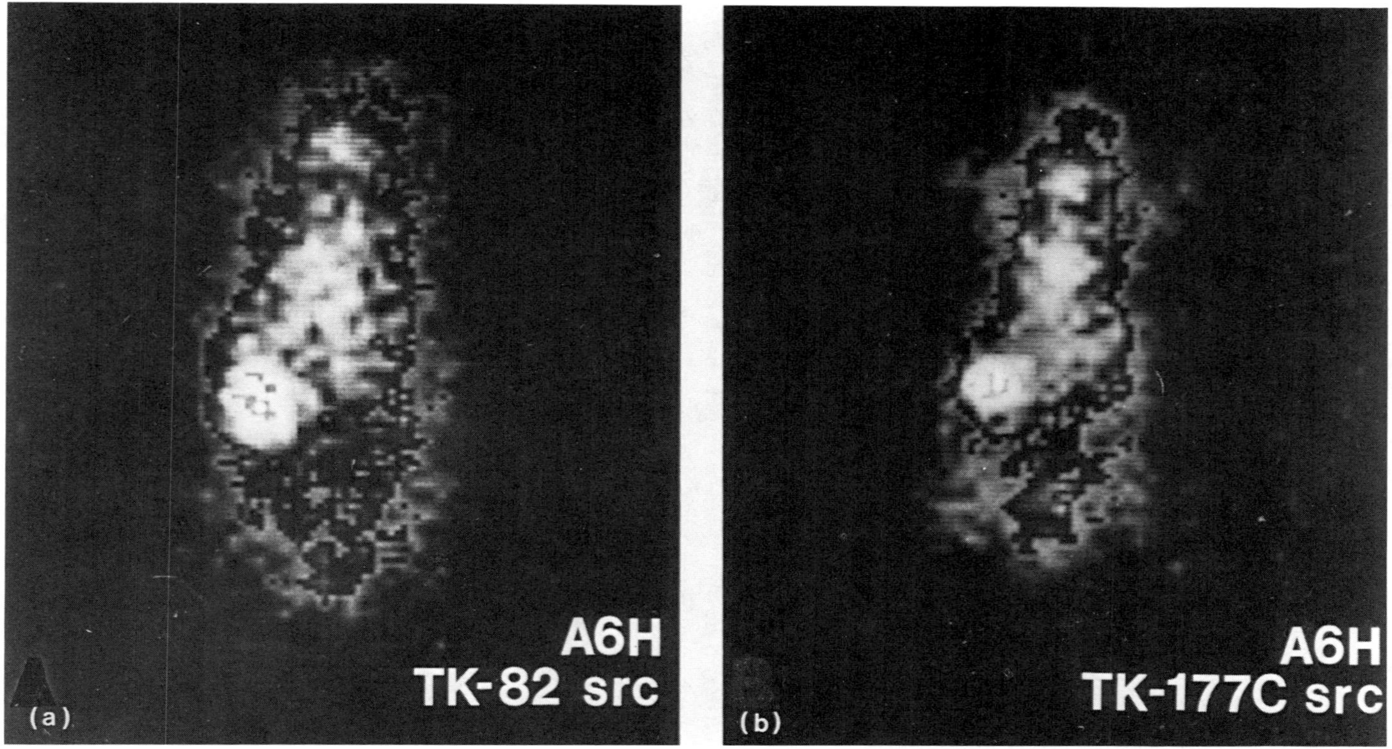

Figure 4 Radioimmunoscintigraphy of two mice 48 hours after injection with ^{131}I-labeled A6H. These mice carried a TK-82 or TK-177 xenograft beneath the renal capsule of the left kidney. The TK-82 xenograft weighed 27 mg and the TK-177 xenograft weighed 15 mg. Biodistribution data for these animals are provided in Table 2. Images acquired as in Figure 3.

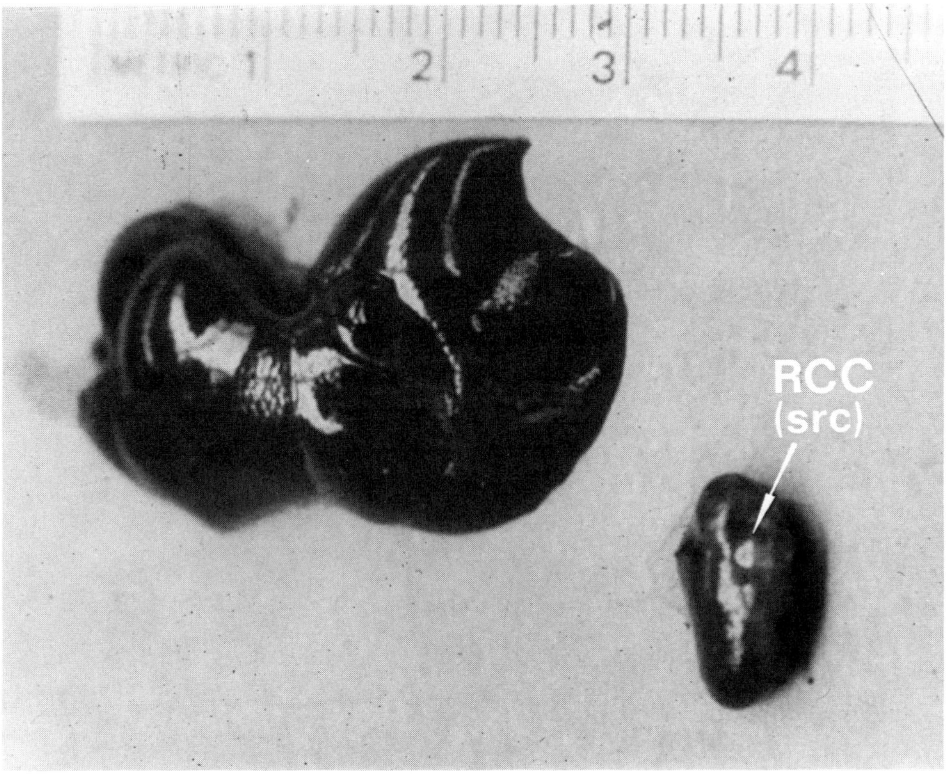

Figure 5 The relative size of a 10-mg xenograft in the upper pole of the kidney (at arrow). The liver is also shown for reference.

with ^{131}I-labeled A6H and xenografts TK-82 and TK-39. The results from some of our preliminary studies with TK-82 and more recent work with TK-39 are included here. In all of our MAb-radiotherapy studies, xenografts had grown to at least 40 mg (implanted at 25 mg) before being selected for use. At the time of MAb injection (designated day 0) xenografts ranged in size from 40 to 250 mg. We injected approximately 100 μCi per animal via tail vein infusion (actual amount determined by measuring the total body activity dose; see Materials and Methods). Since a few mice receive considerably more or less radiolabel than expected, quantitation of the injected activity dose is routine in our laboratory and strongly recommended. These data need to be taken into consideration when assessing the therapeutic effect of the radiolabeled MAb.

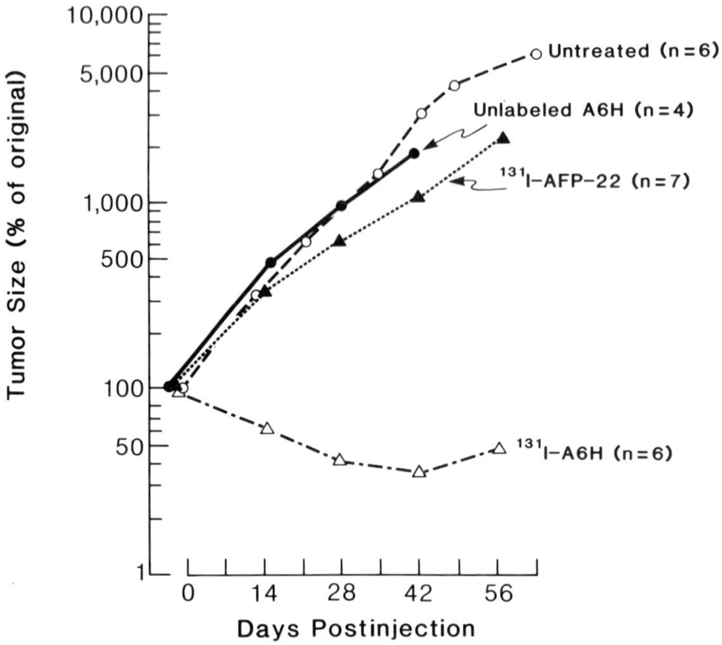

Figure 6 MAb radiotherapy with ^{131}I-labeled A6H in mice bearing TK-82 RCC xenografts. The figure illustrates tumor growth from the time of first injection. Control and treatment groups are as follows: (○- - -○) Group A, control animals that received no treatment; (●——●) Group B, received unlabeled A6H at an antibody mass (μg) dose equivalent to the MAb radiotherapy group D; (▲·······▲) Group C, received ^{131}I-radiolabeled MAb AFP at an equivalent activity μCi dose and specific activity range as group D; (△–·–·–△) Group D, the MAb radiotherapy test group received approximately 100 μCi of ^{131}I-labeled A6H with a specific activity range of 7 to 12 μCi/μg. Details of the technique used in these studies are provided in the Materials and Methods section. A comparison of radiobiological responses of TK-39 and TK-82 to external beam irradiation and MAb-radiotherapy appears in Table 3.

Figure 6 illustrates the growth rates of TK-82 in four groups of mice in our first series of MAb-radiotherapy studies. A clear therapeutic effect was associated with ^{131}I-labeled A6H; rapid tumor growth occurred in the three control groups.

In our second series of MAb-radiotherapy studies, growth rates of TK-39 were compared in another set of four groups of mice (Fig. 7). Again, it is apparent that ^{131}I-labeled A6H had a significant and long-lasting therapeutic effect on the RCC xenograft. This effect is also clearly shown in Figure 8, where a photo-

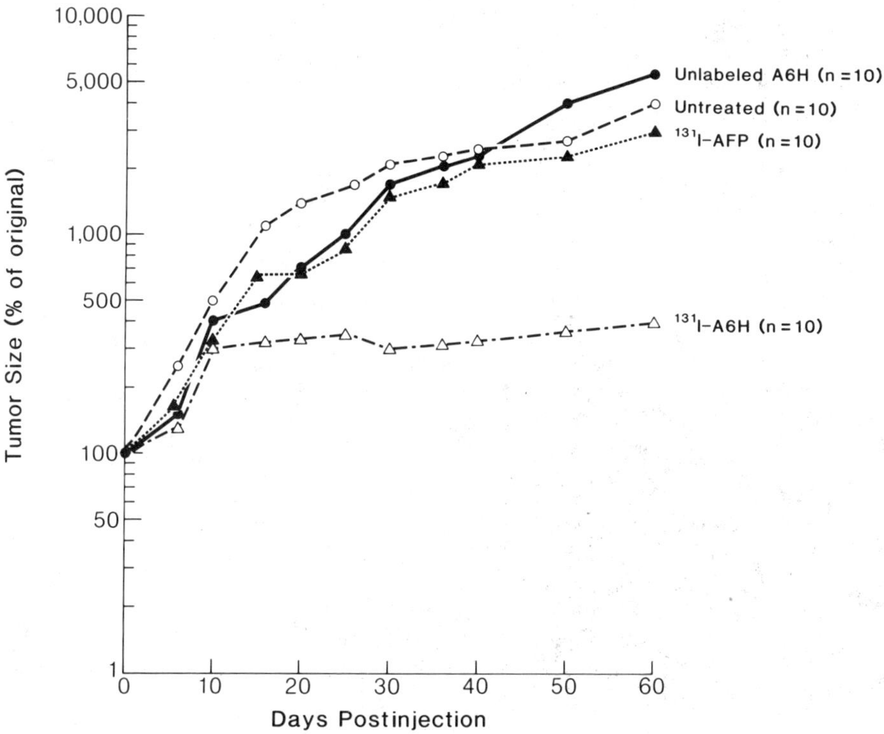

Figure 7 MAb radiotherapy with ^{131}I-labeled A6H in mice bearing TK-82 RCC xenografts. The figure illustrates tumor growth from the time of first injection. Control and treatment groups are as follows: (○- - -○) Group A, control animals that received no treatment; (●——●) Group B, received unlabeled A6H at an antibody mass (μg) dose equivalent to the MAb radiotherapy group D; (▲······▲) Group C, received ^{131}I-radiolabeled MAb AFP at an equivalent activity (μCi) dose and specific activity range as group D; (△-·-·-△) Group D, the MAb radiotherapy test group received approximately 100 μCi of ^{131}I-labeled A6H with a specific activity range of 7 to 12 μCi/μg.

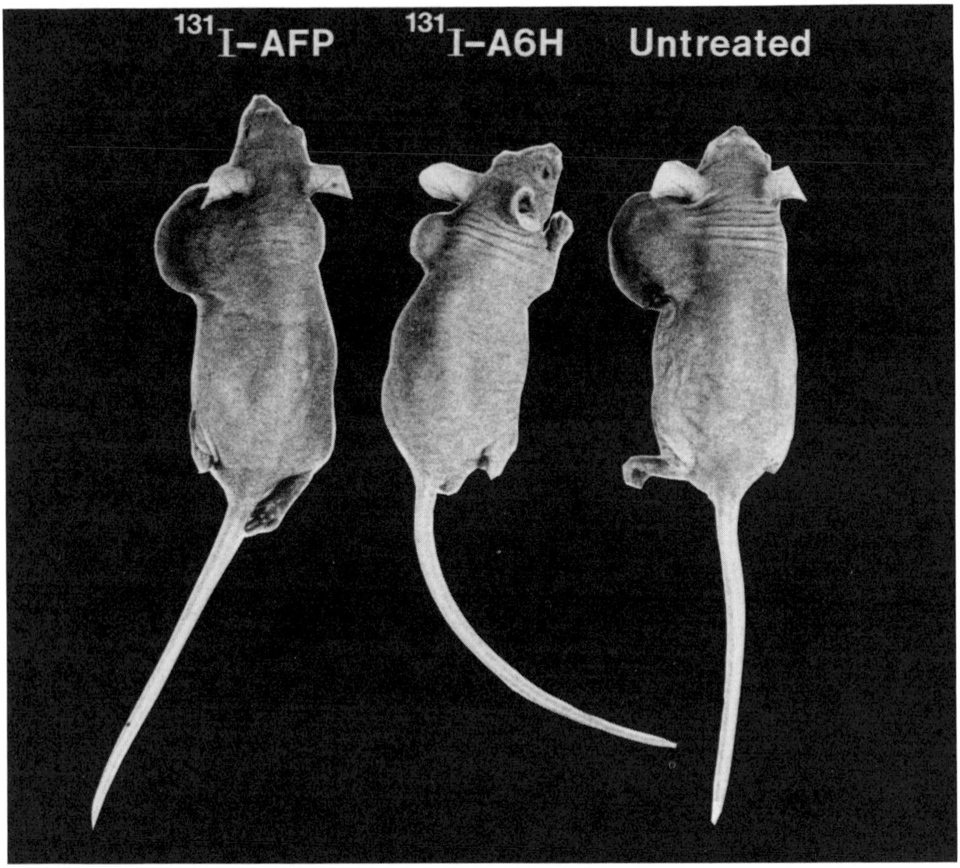

Figure 8 Three mice carrying TK-39 xenografts day 60 of the radiotherapy study. The stabilized tumor growth in the mouse treated with ^{131}I-labeled A6H is contrasted to the growth in two control mice—one that received an equivalent dose of ^{131}I-labeled AFP and one that was untreated.

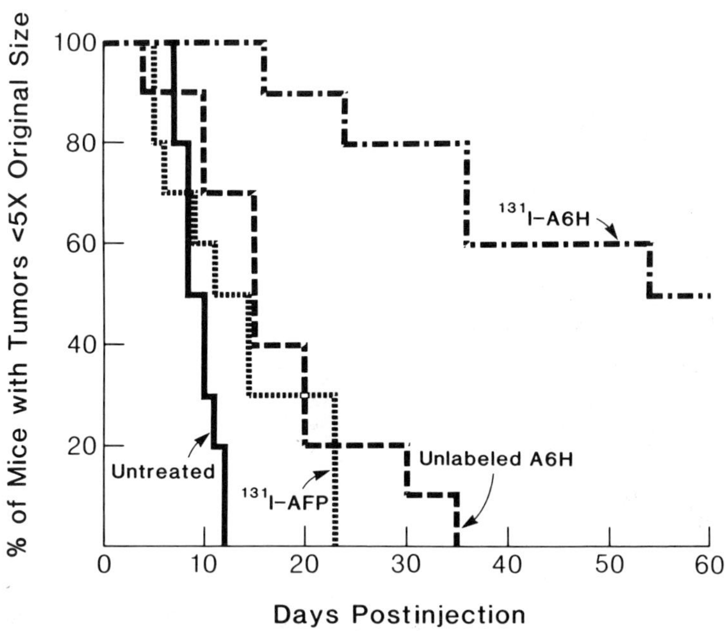

Figure 9 Plot of the percentage of mice in the TK-39 radiotherapy maintained tumor burdens <5 times the initial tumor size at the first MAb injection (day). At day 35, 60% of the mice treated with ^{131}I-labeled A6H had tumors that had not exceeded five times the initial size; in all of the control mice tumors had exceeded five times the initial size. Even at day 60, only 50% of the treated mice had tumors that exceeded this limit.

graph of three mice from this series, taken 60 days after injection, illustrates comparative tumor sizes.

An alternate means of evaluating the therapeutic effect of MAb-radiotherapy is shown in Figure 9. In this figure the percentage of animals in various groups whose TK-39 xenografts increased in size by a factor of five from the time of MAb injection are shown. Xenografts in all of the control mice increased five times in size within 35 days after injection. Only 40% of the xenografts in mice receiving ^{131}I-labeled A6H had increased to this size at 35 days, and even 60 days after injection 50% of the mice had tumors less than five times the original size.

One of the most difficult tasks in MAb-radiotherapy experiments is to quantify, even in approximate terms, the amount of locally absorbed radiation dose received by the xenograft (23), as expressed in rads or cGy (1 rad = 1 cGy). (The reasons for this are addressed in the Discussion.). In an initial effort to more accurately determine the absorbed dose, miniature thermoluminescent dosimeters (TLD), as pictured in Figure 10, were inserted into the tumors and normal tis-

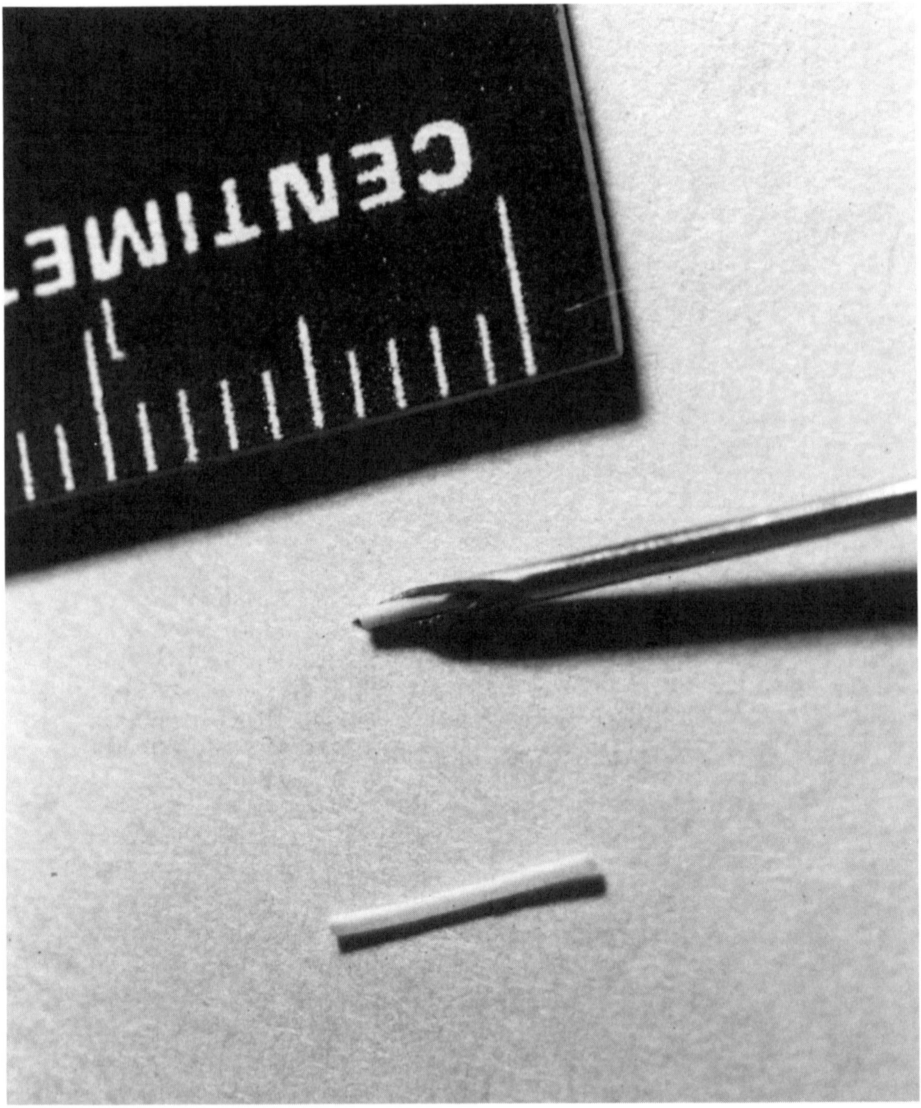

Figure 10 A TLD alongside a 20-gauge needle through which it is inserted into normal or tumor tissues. The composition and production details are provided in the text.

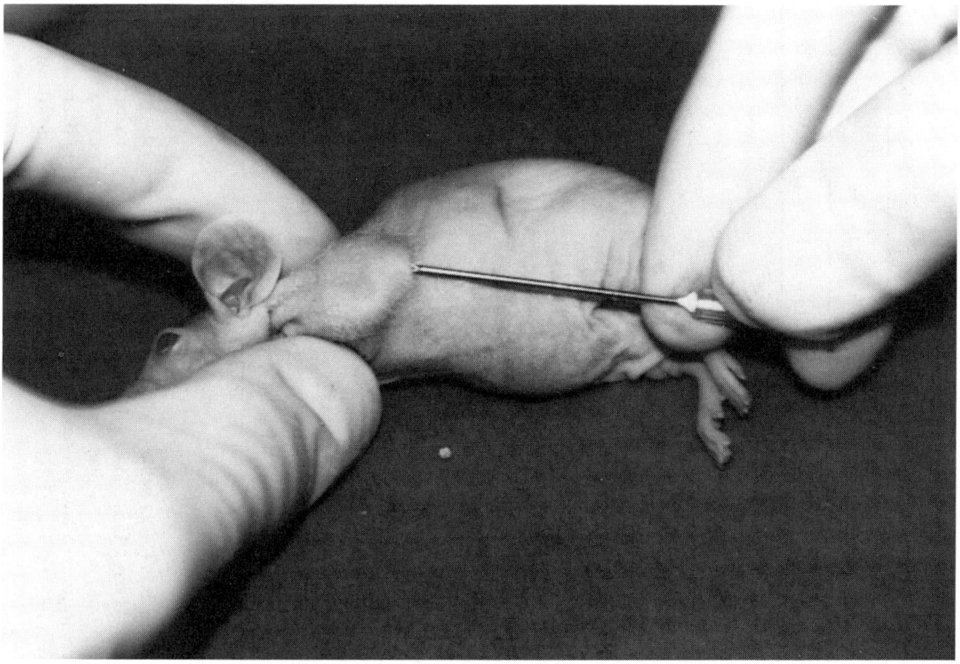

Figure 11 A TLD being implanted into a RCC xenograft.

sues (Figure 11) of mice receiving ^{131}I-labeled A6H or ^{131}I-labeled AFP injections. At sacrifice, the TLD were removed and the radioactivity they had absorbed was quantitated. Some tumors were serially sectioned, and autoradiography of the sections indicated a heterogeneous pattern of MAb distribution (>4-fold range). The data from two of these TLD studies using TK-39 and TK-82 are shown in Table 3; the ranges cited reflect only the values obtained from the TLD and do not encompass the autoradiographic data (addressed below).

Although it would appear that the TLD measurements are recording absorbed doses to organs that are less than what one would calculate through the MIRD (Medical Internal Radiation Dose committee) formalism (24) based on biodistribution data, the autoradiography patterns document a wide range of labeled MAb deposition throughout the tumor. The center of the tumor usually received a manyfold smaller absorbed dose from labeled antibody than the exterior or the perivascular areas. Since in this initial study the TLD were placed in the central region of the tumors, the TLD values presented in Table 3 do not encompass the hot spots in activity which are noted toward the periphery of

Table 3 Biodistribution Results and Thermoluminescent Dosimetry from a 50 μCi Dose of I^{131}-A6H in RCC-bearing Mice[a]

		Biodistribution of radiolabel		TLD dosimetry (cCy)[b]		
Day	Xenograft	Tumor: Liver (mean)	μCi/g Tumor (mean)	Tumor (mean)	Body (mean)	Tumor:Whole body
1	TK-39 (n = 8)	7-12(9)	3-12(9)	12-28(15)	2-3(2.3)	6-9
3	TK-39 (n = 7)	15-30 (25)	17-24(10)	50-70(53)	7-10(7.2)	7-8
5	TK-39 (n = 6)	17-23(18)	3-6(4.5)	75-112(78)	8-13(9)	8-10
10	TK-39 (n = 5)	10-17(15)	0.5-1 (0.7)	90-220(105)	6-21(11.3)	10-15
1	TK-82 (n = 7)	12-38(35)	26-45(35)	27-114(46)	2-12(6)	8-13
3	TK-82 (n = 8)	40-66(59)	20-38(30.5)	140-345(230)	8-16(10)	18-20
5	TK-82 (n = 6)	61-92(88)	7-15(12)	116-420(223)	9-19(12)	13-19
10	TK-82 (n = 8)	22-31(29)	2.1-2.8 (2.5)	140-403(170)	7-21(11)	18-20

[a]Tumors weighed from 40 to 240 mg; data presented as range followed by mean ( ).
[b]Absorbed doses are reported in cGy (1 cGy = 1 Rad).
Two TLD studies are presented with biodistribution data and absorbed dose data (cGy) being portrayed. Mice were implanted with TK-39 (n = 26) or TK-82 (n = 29) and received a single 50-μCi dose of ^{131}I-A6H. At days 1, 3, 5, and 10, representative mice were sacrificed. TLD were removed from the various tissues and sent to Dr. Wessels for a determination of the absorbed dose. Tissues were also analyzed by radiolabeled MAb content by conventional biodistribution methods and by computerized autoradiography. However, the >4-fold differences in MAb dispersion as documented by autoradiography were not incorporated into the calculations or presentation of the absorbed dose values.

the tumor. The TLD reports only a single "average" value of the absorbed dose along its length. However, as one combines TLD values with autoradiographic patterns, there will exist a more accurate portrayal of MAb dispersion within the tumor resulting in the presentation of a range or spectrum of absorbed doses.

We were not the only laboratory collaborating in studies of MAb dosimetry with TLD. In 1986, 8000 TLD were implanted in over 1000 mice bearing eight different tumor xenografts. Data were collected for 12 distinct radionuclide/antibody/mouse combinations. These data indicated that there is a good correlation between the time-dependent antibody localization indices and the integrated absorbed dose for various organ and tumor sites. Experimental model variables include use of (a) two types of antibody bound radionuclides (^{131}I, ^{30}Y), (b) five tumor types (colorectal, renal cell carcinoma, lymphoma, melanoma, and breast carcinoma), and (c) both whole IgG and fragments of two different subclasses (IgG_1 and IgG_{2a}). Dosimetry results indicated tumor:blood ratios of from 1.5:1 to 32:1 (the T:B ratio of 32:1 was obtained with TK-82 and ^{131}I-A6H at 3 days postinjection of a 50 μCi activity dose). The corresponding TLD integrated dose measurements indicated tumor:whole body ratios of 2:1 to 20:1 (the T:whole body ratio of 20:1 was achieved with A6H targeting of TK-82) (25).

In all of the collaborative TLD studies, autoradiography was routinely performed on all tumor-antibody-radionuclide combinations and was correlated with TLD measurements and the location of the TLD relative to the activity patterns in the autoradiographs. It is possible to divide the 5 mm long TLD into slices 20 μm thick while embedded in the tissue sample used for autoradiography. This allowed the absorbed dose to be measured at specific sites in the tumor. These patterns showed a heterogeneity in absorbed dose deposition for various ^{131}I-labeled MAbs: 500 to 1000 cGy for a 340-μCi injected dose of ^{131}I-labeled B72.3 in a LS174T colon carcinoma , 400 to 1600 cGy for a 500-μCi injected dose of ^{131}I-labeled Lym-1 in a Raji B lymphoma, and 700 to 2400 cGy for a 150-μCi injected dose of ^{131}I-labeled A6H in the RCC xenograft TK-82 (25,26).

The TLD method combined with autoradiographic techniques provides much needed relative and absolute direct dose measurements for the comparative assessment of efficacy for MAb-radiotherapy models. The above results indicate that, for tumor systems which are associated with strongly heterogeneous radiolabeled antibody deposition, the MIRD infinite media equilibrium (24) dose constants are not generally applicable and frequently lead to tumor-absorbed dose estimates that are relatively high. Point source function integrations based on calibrated autoradiographic activity patterns or the measurement techniques described above will provide absorbed dose data which are more in line with the in situ reality. The anticipated impact of the compilation of absorbed dose data associated with RIT by these methods is to compare the resultant radiobiological effect in animals with what is observed in the laboratory and clinical setting for standard external beam irradiation. In this way, fractionation patterns and dose rate sensitivity of both MAb radiotherapy and standard external beam therapy may be compared for radiobiological effect in similar absorbed dose delivery ranges.

III. DISCUSSION

Beginning with the pioneering studies of Pressman and colleagues, which demonstrated the ability of ^{125}I-labeled polyclonal antibodies to target normal tissue antigens and tumor antigens (2), iodinated antibodies have been used in numerous studies of tumors, e.g., the work of Bale, Spar, and Goodland (27) on ^{131}I-labeled antibodies in radiotherapy, the first successful use of RIS for the detection of a tumor reported by Quinones, Mizejewski, and Beierwaltes (28), and the initial studies of Goldenberg (29), who has continued to contribute significantly to the use of labeled antibodies for tumor targeting. After the classic work of Kohler and Milstein (30), the production of tumor-specific MAbs for use in vivo became the goal of tumor immunologists. In early tumor targeting studies, and continuing today, ^{131}I is most commonly bound to MAbs for both detection and treatment. Although other isotopes have been shown to be better suited for these tasks than ^{131}I, a substantial amount of relevant data has been and continues to be acquired using ^{125}I and ^{131}I-labeled MAbs.

When we first began our in vivo studies using several RCC xenografts established by Clayman et al. (31), we were amazed at the targeting ability of our MAbs, especially A6H and C5H. In contrast to T:B ratios of 2:1 to 5:1 that had appeared in the literature, we were consistently achieving T:B ratios of at least 4:1 and more commonly in the range of 5:1 to 15:1 using small tumors (40 to 500 mg) as targets (32). Subsequent studies of several different MAb/RCC xenograft combinations at our facility and at collaborating laboratories (22,25,33) confirmed these initial data. This excellent localization ability extended to small (<20 mg) xenografts established beneath the renal capsule. We are uncertain as to the reasons for these unusually good in vivo performances of our MAbs, but one contributing factor is our policy to inject only radiolabeled MAbs with >50% immunoreactivity; several other groups that have reported low targeting ability either did not test for immunoreactivity prior to injection or used preparations with immunoreactivities considerably less than 50%. Finally, it is possible that our RCC xenografts are better suited than some other preclinical models. Although several other groups (34-38) have developed MAbs to RCC, there have been only two recent preliminary reports (39,40) of studies in which MAbs were successfully used to image RCC xenografts. No potentially unique feature of the RCC xenografts were reported.

To eliminate the possibility that uptake by our RCC xenografts was due to Fc receptor binding, studies similar to those described by Mosakis (14) were performed using ^{125}I-labeled control IgG_1 MAbs and ^{131}I-labeled A6H or ^{131}I-labeled C5H. Consistently, the control MAbs failed to localize to the tumors; the ratio of nonspecific to specific binding was often greater than 20:1. This good targeting of A6H and C5H was not limited to one or two RCC xenografts, but was observed in at least six xenografts.

One of the primary reasons for performing biodistribution studies is to assess the potential for MAb-based therapy. However, biodistribution data can be reported in several ways, some of which may be somewhat misleading, and a direct extrapolation to therapeutic potential should not be assumed. For example, the T:B ratio is useful in evaluating imaging studies because it reflects the degree of differentiation, in counts per minute, between the tumor and the vascular pool. This ratio may not be useful in predicting the therapeutic potential of the MAb because it often is not indicative of the MAb concentration within the tumor. There are several approaches that can be taken to increase the T:B ratio. One approach is to use Ig fragments, which produce higher T:B ratios than whole molecules because the fragments are cleared from the circulation faster (41,42). Recent studies by us (data not shown) indicate that the amount of MAb $F(ab')_2$ within the tumor two days after injection is actually less than the amount of whole molecule. Increased T:B ratios can also be achieved by using a second antibody that clears the labeled MAb from the circulation before imaging (43).

Another method for measuring biodistribution that can lead to erroneous therapeutic expectations is the reporting of data solely as %ID/g. Especially for small tumors, such as those we implanted under the renal capsule, this value becomes quite high as one normalizes to one gram (see data in Table 2). This value is also strongly influenced by dose and equilibrium kinetics. An antibody that may be excellent for therapy might easily be overlooked if the tumor with which it is tested is small and the dose injected greater than that needed to saturate all the available antigenic sites. Other variables affecting the %ID/g include the site of implantation, the vascularity of the tumor, and the Ig subclass of MAb. These variables also influence the time of maximum accumulation within the tumor, which can vary from day 1 to day 7 after injection. Of course, these factors also play a role in other biodistribution measurements.

We prefer to assess the therapeutic potential of a MAb in terms of micrograms of MAb per gram of tumor. This value allows one to roughly estimate the extrapolated and theoretical absorbed dose of radioactivities, provided the distribution is homogeneous throughout the tumor and the xenograft is relatively large (see TLD discussion which follows). Also, it is easy to convert micrograms of MAb to the number of MAb molecules within the vicinity of the tumor. Also, as in any study using radiolabels, it must be remembered that what is being followed is the label, not the actual MAb. A MAb that undergoes dehalogenation at the tumor site might still be bound to the tumor yet be undetectable by imaging or biodistribution analysis. Catabolism of radiolabeled MAbs has been evaluated and current knowledge of this area was recently reviewed by Sands and Jones (44). Various factors influence the rate of MAb dehalogenation; among the most critical of these is the endogenous enzymes in the circulation and the tumor, as well as conformational aspects of the iodinated tyrosine residues. Protein dehalogenation has been discussed in a number of key articles (45,46). For critical studies that require very accurate quantitation of MAb, it might be better to use internally labeled antibodies using the tracers ^{35}S, ^{75}Se, ^{3}H, or ^{14}C (47). However, none of these tracers are suited for imaging or therapeutic applications.

As previously mentioned, the gamma energy profiles of other radionuclides, such as ^{111}In and ^{99}Tc, are better detected by the cameras used for imaging than is the profile of ^{131}I. This difference is especially important for clinical trials. Carrasquillo has recently reported the results of a study comparing ^{131}I and ^{111}In-labeled T-101 in a series of patients; he concluded that the clinical information provided by the ^{111}In-labeled MAb was decisively better than for the ^{131}I-labeled MAb (48). In a previous publication (22), we described our success with ^{111}In-labeled A6H using site-specific conjugation to the carbohydrate moieties on the MAb (50). The immunoreactivity was excellent, and imaging and biodistribution results were at least as good as those obtained with ^{131}I. However, recent attempts to label A6H with ^{99}Tc using more classic methodologies (51) resulted in an unstable product that was not suitable for injection. Although we have attempted to address some common considerations in the selection of an appropriate radionuclide for scintigraphy, we refer the reader to several excellent reviews on this topic (52-55).

Results from both the TK-82 and TK-39 radiotherapy studies using an injected activity dose of approximately 100 μCi (15 μg) ^{131}I-A6H suggested that $>$30 μCi/g was achieved and maintained in these RCC xenografts for a period of several days. The selected activity dose was, for the most part, arbitrary and is below that required for saturation of a 50 mg TK-82 xenograft. The TK-82 MAb-radiotherapy data presented in Figure 6 were compiled from two early studies. The results clearly indicate a cessation of tumor growth for a period exceeding 60 days in mice carrying TK-82 xenografts and receiving two 100-μCi doses of ^{131}I-labeled A6H on days 0 and 20. This delay in tumor growth contrasts sharply with the progressive growth observed in the three control groups, which were not treated, received an equal microgram quantity of A6H or received an equal microcurie injection of the control MAb. The analysis of these radiobiological data in terms of tumor growth delay (TGD) and tumor control dose (TCD) is in progress.

Although delay in growth was also achieved in xenograft TK-39, it appears that TK-82 is the more sensitive of the two xenografts to 2 × 100 μCi doses of ^{131}I-labeled A6H. Studies are underway to determine the optimal activity dose and injection schedule for the RCC xenografts TK-82, TK-39, and TK-177C. Other reported ^{131}I MAb-radiotherapy studies using colon carcinoma (56) and neuroblastoma (57) xenografts have achieved significant tumor growth delay using doses of 1.1 mCi (35 to 220 mg MAb) and 0.125 to 1.0 mCi (100 to 200 μg MAb), respectively.

The selection of ^{131}I as a radiolabel for radiotherapy studies is influenced by many of the same factors considered in its selection for RIS—ease of use, good immunoreactivity of the MAb after labeling, inexpensive cost per millicurie, imaging concurrent with therapy, and a reasonably good beta and gamma energy profile. When considering ^{131}I for therapy, the issue of dehalogenation is a more important consideration than in RIS, since the tumor-absorbed dose is cumulative. If the microcurie per gram of tumor is initially high but rapidly diminishes due to dehalogenation, the absorbed dose received by the tumor would be much less than anticipated from day 1 or 2 biodistribution studies. An encouraging preliminary report has recently discussed a modified iodination procedure that results in a more stable, dehalogenation-resistant product for in vivo use (58). Although the ability to concurrently acquire images while delivering radiotherapy is often considered an advantage of ^{131}I, the presence of gamma irradiation also possess a risk of damage to tissues quite distant from the tumor. While probably insignificant at the activity doses used for imaging, at those currently being contemplated for clinical studies (>100 mCi) this gamma energy warrants consideration. For this and other reasons reviewed in depth by a number of authors (52-55,59,60), radionuclides other than ^{131}I are often cited as being more appropriate for MAb radiotherapy.

In general, the selection process for a radionuclide should by necessity consider the type and size of the tumor (solid or lymphoid histology), location (e.g., proximity to a radiation-sensitive critical organ), and, if a solid tumor, the distribution of MAb within the mass (homogeneous or heterogeneous). For example, although alpha emitters such as ^{212}Bi or ^{211}At have a tremendous cytotoxic effect when targeted to single cells, the notorious heterogeneity that exists in some solid tumor xenografts could significantly diminish the effectiveness of these limited range radionuclides. However, where the effort is to eliminate micrometastases, these isotopes might work much better than ^{90}Y or ^{131}I, where the major portion of the isotopic energy is delivered outside several cell diameters.

As initially discussed by Pimm et al. (61) there are two considerations which have tremendous impact on the potential of MAb therapy—that is, accessibility of the tumor cells to the antibody and the concentration of the MAb in antigen-rich areas. We recently conducted a collaborative study with Sands et al. (33) to compare tumor blood flow, vascular volume, vascular permeability, and actual MAb distribution within an RCC xenograft (7860) using MAb A6H and a breast carcinoma xenograft (Clouser) using MAb B6.2. The vascular permeability of the RCC xenograft significantly exceeded that of the Clouser xenograft. The distribution of A6H within xenograft 7860 was heterogeneous; many "pockets" of concentration MAb were observed. Extrapolation from these data leads to several possible conclusions about therapy: (a) Multiple areas within the tumor may contain higher concentrations of MAb than previously envisioned because simple analysis of radiolabel content by tissue counting as routinely performed during biodistribution studies has a tumor-averaging "artifact," (b) accessibility to these pockets of concentrated MAb is enhanced by a tumor vasculature that is unusually permeable to immunoglobulins, (c) due to the interspersing of MAb-dense and MAb-sparse areas throughout the tumor, a beta-emitting isotope showing a good dose range (e.g., ^{90}Y or ^{131}I) would be required to irradiate unaccessible cells, and (d) with extremely high concentrations of MAb throughout the vasculature, perhaps an alternate or combined approach would be the use of alpha-emitting radionuclides to destroy the vascular bed. An obvious question under study is whether the MAb-sparse regions are antigen-sparse and, if so, whether other RCC-reactive MAbs should be used to target these areas (e.g., a cocktail approach).

The determination of the absorbed dose of radioactivity from radionuclides bound to antibodies is a challenge to conventional dosimetry techniques. The MIRD formalism (24), which uses quantities such as compartmental mean residence times, effective half-lives, and "S" factors, may not be an accurate method for assessing this dose. Nonlinear uptake of antibody and differential shedding rates in all compartments render the above quantities of limited value. Direct incorporation of measured biodistribution data to obtain cumulated activities per organ offers first-order accuracy in calculating dose through equilibrium dose constants (53). However, this method is not predictive when examining particulate radiation in the subcentimeter range for tumor heterogeneities and at tumor/organ boundaries. In particular, highly heterogeneous deposition of radiolabeled antibody in the millimeter range, as occurs with A6H and other MAbs, will not meet the build-up criteria necessary to apply the MIRD equilibrium dose constant. For these reasons we sought a method for directly measuring radiolabeled antibody absorbed dose on the submillimeter scale to serve as an integrating dosimeter.

The TLD provides a quantitative measurement of absorbed dose; it may demonstrate a 20-fold differential between the dose delivered to the tumor and that delivered to normal body tissues (Table 3). However, we now know that MAb distribtuion within at least two RCC xenografts (7860 and TK-82) is variable. There are intense areas of MAb accumulation in some regions and little accumulation in others. Under such biological conditions we recommend that both an average dose value be given based on TLD measurements and that a range of values be quoted based on calibrated autoradiographic results (62). The preliminary results quoted in Table 3 represent the range in dose values as determined by TLD values alone. Determining a range of doses by autoradiography would necessitate serial sectioning and analysis of each section in relation to placement of the TLD. Although this will hopefully not need to be performed on each and every tumor, it is conceivably the best and most accurate manner in which to assess the absorbed dose delivered by MAb-radionuclide conjugates.

In summary, radioiodination is an easy and inexpensive method for labeling MAbs to be used for the in vivo detection and treatment of tumors in animals and in man. We have imaged tumors smaller than 20 mg using ^{131}I-labeled A6H and have presented here the successful growth arrest of established tumor xenografts for more than 60 days with two 100-μCi doses of ^{131}I-labeled A6H. Although not directly discussed, it must be remembered that the performance of MAbs in athymic mice cannot be directly extrapolated to performance in man. Nevertheless, the mouse model offers us excellent opportunities to define at least some of the variables that exist in tumor targeting and therapy. Finally, we view the near future as an tremendously exciting period in which the opportunities for collaboration among investigators of various disciplines are great and will be critical to the eventual clinical success of MAb conjugates in tumor scintigraphy and adjuvant therapy.

IV. MATERIALS AND METHODS

A. Monoclonal Antibodies

We have previously described (10,11) our methods for generating and selecting IgG_1 MAbs preferential for RCC and the control anti-AFP MAbs used in the present studies. We used standard methods for immunization and fusion, with the exception that A6H was generated by immunization with human fetal kidney homogenates. We hypothesized that fetal kidney might express an oncodevelopmental antigen in common with one expressed by RCC. MAb B4F (19), an IgG_{2b} MAb, was recently generated from Robersonian mice immunized in tandem (63) with a series of different RCC cell lines. The fusion partner was the Taggart cell line (64). Screening of MAbs for reactivity was assessed to cell lines of various origins, and to frozen and paraffin-embedded tissues (fetal, normal adult, and tumor). Details of these methods are provided in the references cited.

B. Purification of MAbs

Purification of MAbs begins with the precipitation of immunoglobulin from clarified (100,000 *g* for 25 minutes) ascites fluid; neutral salts of divalent ions (e.g., Na_2SO_4 or $(NH_2SO_4)SO_4$), which are soluble at high concentrations in water, are commonly used (65). The ionic strength of the solution increases as the neutral salt is added and protein solubility decreases, presumably as a result of dehydration. Proteins of a specific class precipitate at known salt concentrations. Nearly complete precipitation of a selected protein class can be achieved using this method. In our laboratory, anhydrous sodium sulfate is slowly added over a period of 1 to 2 hours at room temperature to a final concentration of 20% (wt/v). This results in the relatively clean precipitation of the IgG immunoglobulin (i.e., 75% of total precipitated protein). The mixture is then stirred for an additional 45 minutes and allowed to stand at room temperature overnight. The precipitate is collected by centrifugation, resuspended in 0.02 M phosphate buffer (pH 8.0), and dialyzed overnight at 4°C against this same buffer. The dialysate is applied to a CM Affi-Gel Blue (Bio-Rad Laboratories, Richmond, CA) chromatography column to remove albumin and proteases, the major contaminants of the sodium sulfate precipitate. The immunoglobulin IgG-enriched fractions are then concentrated and dialyzed against 0.02 M Tris-HCl buffer at pH 7.2.

In our initital studies, the immunoglobulin-enriched dialysate was applied to a DEAE Affi-Gel Blue (Bio-Rad Laboratories) chromatography column. Nonimmunoglobulin proteins were eluted with 0.02 M Tris-HCl buffer, pH 7.2, containing 0.008 M NaCl. The monoclonal IgG_1 fractions were typically eluted isocratically with the Tris-HCl buffer containing 0.018 to 0.040 M NaCl (concentration depends on the MAb). The MAb fractions were collected, pooled, concentrated, and dialyzed against phosphate-buffered saline. Purity of the MAbs was assessed by sodium dodecyl sulfate-polyacrylamide gel electrophoresis (66) and silver staining (67) using Pierce reagents. The final preparation was tested for immunological reactivity by comparing results from a cell-binding ELISA and an endpoint titration for a standard MAb preparation. Typically, our procedure gave MAb yields from ascitic fluid of 50-70% with a final MAb purity of >90%.

An alternate procedure now currently in use involves Protein A chromatography to purify immunoglobulin-enriched fraction. Early attempts to use Protein A chromatography were unsuccessful; IgG_1 MAbs were not sufficiently purified. However, within the past two years, newer approaches have been introduced for protein A purification of mouse IgG_1. We have adopted one of these protocols that uses the MAPS II buffer system (Bio-Rad Laboratories). Following Affi-Gel Blue chromatography, the immunoglobulin-enriched fraction is dialyzed against 0.01 M phosphate buffer (pH 7.2). The dialysate is then diluted 1:2 with Bio-Rad Affinity Gel Protein A binding buffer and applied to a Protein A chromatography column that has been equilibrated with this buffer. The flow rate is adjusted to approximately 4 ml/hour, which results in excellent binding of the MAb to the Protein A. The system is flushed with buffer until a stable base line monitored by absorbance of UV radiation is achieved. The elution buffer (supplied as part of the MAPS II buffering system) is applied to the column at a flow rate of 8 ml/hour and the protein peak is collected. The protein (immunoglobulin)-containing fractions are collected and dialyzed against PBS (pH 7.2), and the protein concentration is quantitated with the Pierce BCA protein assay using bovine serum albumen as the standard. Using this protocol, MAb purity averages greater than 95% as assessed by SDS-PAGE and silver staining as described above.

C. Iodination of MAbs

Iodination of MAbs is accomplished by the reaction of I_2 with the phenolic ring of tyrosine and, to a lesser degree, with the imidazole ring of histidine moieties (Fig. 12). The methods for iodination of MAbs vary primarily in the manner in which the reactive species I_2 is generated. A summary of some common iodination procedures is presented in Table 1, and a comprehensive review of iodination has recently been published (13). Radioactive iodine, either ^{123}I, ^{125}I, or ^{131}I is purchased as the sodium salt in a solution of high pH. To label protein, it is necessary to oxidize two I^- to I_2. It is possible to equilibrate an I_2 solution with radioactive iodine and use I_2 as the oxidizing agent, but this approach results in very low specific activity because of the large amount of unlabeled I_2 in the reaction mixture. The oxidizing agents generally considered for the radioination of proteins include Chloramine T (68), ICl (69), lactoperoxidase (70), and Iodogen (71).

The most common oxidizing agent used in the iodination of proteins is Chloramine T (n-chloro-p-toluenesulfonamide sodium salt) (68). An excess of an agent such as Chloramine reoxidizes the I^- produced by the labeling reaction to I_2, and incorporation of 70-90% of the added radiolabel is easily achieved. Al-

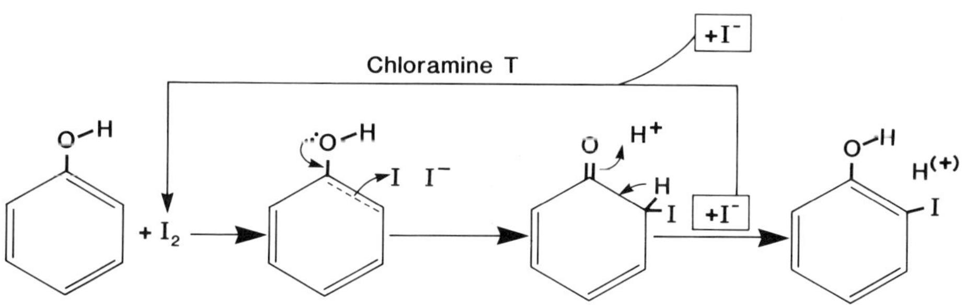

Figure 12 A schematic description of the Chloramine T reaction and the iodination of the tyrosine phenolic ring.

though Chloramine T oxidizes the MAb as well as the I^-, which may compromise immunoreactivity, adjusting the concentration of Chloramine T and limiting the time of exposure to oxidizing conditions produces a good compromise between labeleing efficiency and immunoreactivity. The labeling reaction is stopped by the addition of a reducing agent, such as sodium metabisulfite, which destroys the Chloramine T and reduces any reactive I_2 to I^-. The labeled MAb can be separated from the reaction mixture on a gel permeation column. Unfortunately, a reducing agent may be as damaging as an oxidizing agent to the MAb. An alternative to the use of a reducing agent is flooding the reaction vessel with tyramine (10 mg/ml or 100 μl), which scavenges unreacted I_2. The tyramine is used in such an excess that it consumes all of the I_2 not reacted with the MAb. Again, the labeled MAb can be separated from the reaction mixture on a gel permeation column.

Approximately 100 to 1000 μg of purified MAb in 100 to 200 μl PBS (no protein carrier) is added to 500 μCi to 5 mCi of ^{131}I or ^{125}I obtained as sodium iodide in V-reaction vials from DuPont-NEN (Boston, MA). The labeling procedure is depicted in Figure 11. Chloramine T at a concentration of 1 mg/ml phosphate buffer (pH 7.2) is added to the reaction vial in a volume equal to 0.2 times the volume of the MAb solution. After 60 seconds, the reaction is stopped by the addition of sodium metabisulfite at a concentration of 1.2 mg/ml in dH_2O (volume added equal to that of the Chloramine T solution). The contents of the vial are transferred to the bed of a 0.7 × 15 cm Bio-Gel P-6DG column. Ten drop fractions are collected as the column is flushed with PBS. The iodinated MAb is in fractions 7-12 and the unreacted I^- is in fractions 14-20. Specific activity generally ranges from 3 to 5 μCi/μg. Higher specific activity can be achieved by increasing the amount of sodium iodide while keeping the amounts of the other reactants constant.

Assessment of the quality of the labeled MAb includes a determination of the radioactivity bound to protein compared to that in the supernatant fractions. This is usually accomplished by a simple TCA (trichloroacetic acid) precipitation of proteins from solution and a determination of counts in the pellet versus that in the starting material. Briefly, a 10% TCA (wt/vol) stock solution is prepared with saline. A volume of labeled MAb containing approximately 10^4 to 10^6 cpm (remove 20 μl from the pooled fractions, perform several 1:10 dilutions, and then use a 50-μl aliquot of the appropriate dilution) is added to a 12 mm × 75 mm glass tube. This is followed by 500 μl of a 0.1% protein carrier solution (BSA in saline works well) and then 500 μl of the 10% TCA solution; at this point the proteins begin to precipitate (opaque color). After 30 minutes the radioactivity in the solution is counted (total counts). The tube is then centrifuged at 100 × *g*. The supernatant is discarded in the manner prescribed by the radiation safety procedures at the facility and the radioactivity in the semisolid pellet is counted. We do not use a preparation if the pellet contains less than

95% of the total radioactivity (this is extremely rare) because this situation signifies that an unusually large amount of free iodine is contaminating the MAb fraction. Passing such a MAb fraction over another Bio-Gel P-6DG might allow the fraction to be used.

The possible presence of aggregated antibody in the final MAb preparation is assessed by HPLC. A Gilson HPLC with a Bio-Rad Bio-Sil TSK-250 column (7.5 × 300 mm), a Beckman radioisotope detector (Model #170), and a LKB UVICORD S (Model #2138) are used. Twenty-microliter samples are injected. The mobile phase is 10 mM $NaPO_4$, 300 mM NaCl, 10% DMSO, and 0.05% NaN_3 (pH 6.8) with a flow rate of 1 ml/min. By monitoring retention times for both UV (280 nM) and isotopic profiles we are able to determine if the preparation contains aggregated MAbs. Typically, >97% of the MAb is monomeric. An acceptable scan is illustrated in Figure 2.

The final, highly critical step in determining the quality of the labeled MAb is an assessment of immunoreactivity. Labeled MAb (100-μl sample); 10×10^3 cpm is incubated with 5×10^5 antigen-positive cells for 1 hour at room temperature. For most of our studies we use RCC cells removed from the culture flask by shaking, not by treatment with trypsin, which can damage or remove MAb-reactive antigens. These cells are then washed, resuspended in PBS, and counted. A final cell suspension of 5×10^5 viable cells/ml is prepared, and a 1-ml aliquot in duplicate is used for each determination. After incubation, the total amount of radioactivity in the tubes is counted. A pellet of cells is then obtained by centrifugation (100 × *g*, 10 minutes), the supernatant is discarded as previously described, and the radioactivity in the cell pellet is recounted. The percent of counts associated with the pellet as compared to the counts for the total amount of radioactivity represents the immunoreactivity. We do not use iodinated MAbs for any in vivo experiments if the immunoreactivity is less than 50%. Typically, immunoreactivities in the range of 65 to 85% are achieved. Because some MAbs are clearly more susceptible to iodination damage than others, lower specific activities might be necessary to produce a usable product (fewer iodines per MAb molecule and fewer MAbs being iodinated). If the immunoreactivity assay is to provide meaningful information, the test cells must provide sufficient antigen for the theoretical complete binding of all immunoreactive MAbs. Also, the incubation time must be long enough to allow for complete reaction—low affinity antibodies may require longer periods to bind. Finally, in some MAb/cell systems (e.g., lymphocyte-reactive MAbs), the reaction should proceed on ice to inhibit the capping and subsequent shedding of bound antibody.

D. Human Tumor Xenografts

The RCC xenografts used in our studies and their reactivities with various MAbs have been previously described (10,31). Xenografts are established from freshly implanted surgical specimens and are serially passaged in BALB/c nu/nu male mice. For subcutaneous implantation, an established xenograft is removed from a donor mouse and cut into small (approximately 25 mg) pieces within the confines of a laminar flow hood (keep pieces moist). An incision is made in the subcostal flank region of the recipient mouse and a subcutaneous "tunnel" is made to the shoulder region using a mosquito clamp. A piece of tumor is then maneuvered through the tunnel to the shoulder using a fine-tipped forceps. The incision is closed by using 9-mm surgical staples. For implantation beneath the renal capsule, an incision approximately 1 cm long is made through the loin muscle and peritoneal lining in the lumbar region above the renal area. This process exposes the kidney, which is gently pulled through the incision and stabilized with a Halsted mosquito hemostat. A 2-mm incision is made through the renal capsule, a 1-mm^3 piece of tumor is inserted with an 18-gauge trocar, and the tumor is maneuvered to a stable position under the capsule. The kidney is released and the skin incision is closed with sterile surgical staples.

E. Radioimmunoscintigraphy

Established xenografts are used for imaging studies. Mice are injected with MAbs when subcutaneous xenografts are between 50 and 400 mg in size. We attempt to use xenografts under the renal capsule that are approximately 15 mg, but it is difficult to estimate the time needed for the xenograft to grow to this size, a size much too small to palpate. Unfortunately, since the take rate of subcapsular xenografts is often 70-90%, depending on the technican and tumor, some mice are injected and it is later discovered by biodistribution studies that they did not have an established tumor. Careful palpation can reveal subcapsular tumors 25 to 40 mg in size.

Mice selected for study receive 30 to 50 μCi of radiolabeled MAb (RCC-preferential MAb or the control IgG_1 anti-AFP-1). A 100-μl MAb in 0.02 M PBS aliquot is injected into the tail vein with a w8-gauge needle and, with practice, success in injecting the tail vein can exceed 95%. The activity dose actually delivered to each mouse is quantitated using a customized remote 2" gamma counter crystal attached to an LKB model #1282 Compugamma counter. Although this information is not critical for routine scintigraphy, it is important for biodistribution studies if biodistribution is being calculated as the percent of the injected dose per gram of tissue. For many investigations we use a double-label approach (^{131}I MAb #1 and ^{125}I MAb #2), which allows a more precise direct comparison of MAb performance in each mouse.

Scintigraphy is performed from one to seven days after injection; most of the images shown in this report were acquired two days after injection. Images are acquired on a Siemens Pho Gamma IV camera (gift of Siemens Medical Systems, Inc.; Schaumburg, IL) equipped with a pinhole collimator. The camera is interfaced to a customized image acquisition IBM AT computer (Cardiac Medical Systems, Chicago, IL). Usually, 10,000 counts are obtained for each image, and background subtraction is not performed.

All mice are sacrificed immediately after the final scintigraphy image for analysis of MAb biodistribution. Blood, which is obtained by cardiac puncture, as well as normal tissues, such as the liver, lung, spleen, kidney, muscle, skin, intestine, and thyroid region, and tumorous tissues are weighed and placed in tubes, and the amount of radioactivity in each is determined by the LKB gamma counter. If a urine sample is obtainable it is treated similarly. Using a biodistribution software program we calculate the tumor to blood ratio, tumor to tissue ratio, %ID/gram, μCi/gram, μg MAb/gram, μg MAb/organ, and, where applicable, the ratio of tumor 1 to tumor 2 radioactivity (if an RCC tumor and a non-RCC tumor have been implanted subcutaneously) and the ratio of ^{131}I MAb to ^{125}I MAb in each tumor.

F. MAb Radiotherapy

We selected mice bearing a single established subcutaneous xenograft (40 to 250 mg) for MAb radiotherapy studies. All MAbs met the established criteria for in vivo use as described previously. Mice were divided into the following four groups: (1) untreated; (2) 100 μCi (15 μg) of ^{131}I anti-AFP-1; (3) 15 μg of unlabeled A6H; and (4) 100 μCg (15 μg) of ^{131}I A6H. These activity and antibody mass doses correspond to a specific activity of approximately 6.4 μCi/μg (specific activities for MAb radiotherapy range from 5-10 μCi/μg). If the specific activities of the ^{131}I A6H and ^{131}I AFP are dissimilar in a given study, groups (2) and (4) receive the same activity dose (μCi), whereas groups (3) and (4) receive the same antibody mass dose (μg). The MAbs were injected into the tail vein and the activity dose was determined as described for RIS. Because of variations in tumor growth among individual mice, we now start each experiment with at least seven mice per group. The day of the first injection is considered day 0. In the studies presented here, mice also received a second injection of freshly labeled MAbs at day 20.

We monitor therapeutic effectiveness by measuring the tumor (width × depth × length) weekly using precision calipers. By measurements taken at the time of biodistribution studies, we have established that for TK-82, the tumor size divided by 2.4 approximates the tumor weight. (This conversion factor varies among tumors and among individuals measuring the tumors.) For tumor growth curves, we plot the percentage change in tumor size over time using the tumor's size at day 0 as the starting point. Animals that expire during the course of the study are classified into two groups: death due to tumor burden and death from other causes such as the effects of anesthesia or an infection. When a tumor becomes overbearing for an animal (often >2000 mg), the mouse is sacrificed, and its death is classified as due to tumor burden.

F. Thermoluminescent Dosimeter (TLD) Technique

In an attempt to quantitate the radiation dose actually delivered to the tumor, we have initiated a series of studies using miniature thermoluminescent dosimeter(s) (TLD). Dosimeters were fabricated from ultra-thin disc dosimeters available from Teledyne, Inc. Precise cutting and sizing of the TLD were peforemd with a microtome using a micrometer under a low-power magnification microscope. TLD may be implanted directly into animals to assess the absorbed dose of radioactivity (72,73). TLD are rods containing chemically inert Teflon-embedded $CaSO_4$:Dy crystals measuring 0.2 × 0.4 × 5 mm^3 or smaller (a TLD before implantation shown in Fig. 10). These rods store energy in the crystal lattice upon irradiation. The energy is released as light when the TLD is heated to between 120 and 270°C. A TLD reader automatically heats the dosimeter to the correct temperature and records the light output with a photomultiplier tube. The intensity of the emitted light is proportional to the radiation exposure of the TLD. The TLD have been shown to be linear in response (+/−5%) from 10 to 5000 cGy for ^{131}I, ^{186}Re, ^{32}P, and ^{90}Y. The TLD have been calibrated in a thin-wall tumor phantom comparing measured value with ion chambers and MIRD formalism for 4 MeV X-ray radiation and radionuclide irradiation, respectively.

TLD may be sterilized by autoclaving at 250°C for 1 hour or soaking for 10 minutes in 90% methanol. Sterilized TLD may be implanted using a 20-gauge needle (Figs. 10 and 11). Typical implant sites include subcutaneously in the left hind flank, left shoulder, right shoulder, and two TLD in the tumor–intraperitoneal cavity, the liver, subcutaneously 1 cm above the tumor, and subcutaneously 1 cm toward the midline from the tumor. Twelve to two hundred and forty hours after implantation, mice are sacrificed and the dosimeters are carefully recovered; their exact anatomical location is noted. The recovered dosimeters are washed in dilute Radiac wash to remove animal matter and surface contamination. Before the TLD are measured for light output, a health physics survey is performed to ensure that all contaminating radioactivity has been removed from the TLD. At the time of TLD recovery, we also perform the standard biodistribution studies as previously described. In the studies presented here in which TLD were used, we injected ^{131}I MAb A6H (50-μCi activity dose) into mice bearing TK-39 or TK-82 xenografts.

ACKNOWLEDGMENTS

The authors would like to acknowledge our dedicated support staff: the numerous technicians who participated in these studies and expended every effort to assure that the projects were carried out as proposed, Doris Knettle, who prepared the manuscript, and Karla Gunsolus, our medical editor. In addition, we wish to thank those whose financial support made possible this research: the Veterans Administration, Abbott Laboratories, and the Minnesota Medical Foundation. Finally, significant equipment donations were made by Siemens Medical Systems, Inc. (nuclear medicine camera) and Quest Research (computer hardware and software).

REFERENCES

1. Ehrlich, P., Herta, C. A., and Shiga, K. (1904) über einige Verwendungen der Naphtochinonsulfosaure. *Z. Physiol. Chem. 61*: 379-392.
2. Pressman, D., and Korngold, L. (1953) The in vivo localization of anti-wagner-osteogenic-sarcoma antibodies. *Cancer 6*: 619-623.
3. Kaminski, M. S., Kitamura, K., Maloney, D. G., Campbell, M. J., and Levy, R. (1986) Importance of antibody isotype in monoclonal anti-idiotype therapy of a murine B cell lymphoma. A study of hybridoma class switch variants. *J. Immunology 136;3*: 1123-1130.
4. Ghose, T., and Blair, A. H. (1987) The design of cytotoxic-agent-antibody conjugates. In *Critical Reviews in Therapeutic Drug Carrier Systems* (Bruck, S. D., Ed.). CRC Press, Boca Raton.
5. Pastan, I., Willingham, M. C., and FitzGerald, D. J. P. (1986) Immunotoxins. *Cell 47*: 641-648.
6. Cordon-Cardo, C., Bander, N. H., Fradet, Y., Finstand, C., Whitmore, W. F., Oettgen, H. F., Melamed, M., and Old, L. J. (1984) Immunoanatomic dissection of the human urinary system with mouse monoclonal antibodies. *J. Histchem. Cytochem. 32*: 1035-1040.
7. Oosterwijk, E., Ruiter, D. J., Wakka, J. C., Huiskens, J. W., Meij, V. D., Jonas, U., Fleuren, G. J., Zwartendijk, J., Hoedemaeker, and Warnaar, S. O. (1986) Immunohistochemical analysis of monoclonal antibodies to renal antigens. *American J. Pathology 123;2*: 301-309.
8. Umeda T., and Niijima, T. (1986) Phase II study of alpha interferon on renal cell carcinoma. *Cancer 58*: 1231-1235.
9. Rosenberg, S. A. (1984) Immunotherapy of cancer by the systemic administration of lymphoid cells plus interleukin-2. *J. Biol. Resp. Modifiers 3*: 501-511.
10. Vessella, R., Moon, T., Chiou, R., Nowak, J., Arfman, E., Palme, D., Peterson, G., and Lange, P. (1985) Monoclonal antibodies to human renal cell carcinoma: Recognition of shared and restricted antigens. *Cancer Res. 45*: 6131-6139.
11. Moon, T., Vessella, R., Palme, D., Nowak, J., and Lange, P. (1985) A highly restricted antigen for renal cell carcinoma defined by a monoclonal antibody. *Hybridoma 4*: 163-171.
12. Powe, J. (1986) Radiolabeling of monoclonal antibodies. *Hybridoma 5;1*: S39-S42.
13. Dewansee, and Marinal K. (Eds.). (1987) *Radioiodination: Theory and Practice*. (Submitted for publication.)

14. Moshakis, V., McKhinney, R., Raghavan, D., and Neville, A. (1981) Localization of human tumor xenografts after i.v. administration of radiolabeled monoclonal antibodies. *Br. J. Cancer 44*: 91-99.
15. Pimm, M. V., and Baldwin, R. W. (1984) Quantitative evaluation of the localization of a monoclonal antibody (791T/36) in human osteogenic sarcoma xenografts. *Eur. J. Cancer Clin. Oncol. 20*: 515-524.
16. Halpern, S. E., and Hagan, P. L. (1986) Reply to Nuclear Med. (Ref. #117-#118). *Nuclear Medicine 27;11*: 1790.
17. Pimm, M. V., and Baldwin, R. W. (1986) Effect of tumor size on monoclonal antibody uptake in tumor models. *Nuclear Medicine 27;11*: 1788-1789.
18. Cohen, M. B., Saxton, R. E., and Mann, B. (1986) Effect of tumor size on monoclonal antibody uptake in tumor models. *Nuclear Medicine 27;11*: 1789-1790.
19. Vessella, R. L., et al. Generation of a new monoclonal antibody (B4F) that is reactive to a unique epitope on the antigen defined by monoclonal antibody A6H. Manuscript in prep.
20. Bogden, A. E., Kelton, D. E., Cobb, W. R., and Esber, H. J. (1978) A rapid screening method for testing chemotherapeutic agents against human tumor xenografts. In *Proceedings of the Symposium on the Use of Athymic (Nude) Mice in Cancer Research*. Gustav Fisher, New York.
21. Palme, D. F., Arfman, E. D., Elson, M. K., Klicka, M. J., Lange, P. H., and Vessella, R. L. (1986) Human renal cell carcinoma xenografts implanted sub renal capsule: radioimmunoscintigraphy with monoclonal antibody A6H and tumor growth kinetics. *FASEB 45(4)*: Abstract #4821.
22. Vessella, R., Alvarez, V., Chiou, R., Rodwell, J., Elson, M., Palme, D., Shafer, R., and Lange, P. (1987) Radioimmunoscinitigraphy and radioimmunotherapy of renal cell carcinoma xenografts. *NCI Monographs 3*: 159-167.
23. Wessels, B. W., Griffith, M. H., Bradley, E. W., and Skibinski, B. (1986) Dosimetric measurements and radiobiological consequences of radioimmunotherapy in tumor bearing mice. Fourth Int. Rad. Dosemetry Sym. Conf-851113-de86010102. Oak Ridge Associated Univ., Tenn. pp. 446-457.
24. Halpern, S. E., Stern, P. H., Hagan, P. L., et al. (1983) The labeling of monoclonal antibodies with 111-In technique and advantages to radioiodine labeling. In *Radioimmunoimaging and Radioimmunotherapy* (Burchiel, S. and Rhodes, B., Eds.). Elsevier North-Holland Biomedical Press, New York.
25. Wessels, B. W., Vessella, R. L., Neacy, W. P., DeNardo, G. L., and Frinke, J. M. (1987) Correlation of biodistribution data with TLD absorbed dose measurements for radioimmunotherapy in mice. In *International Conference on Monoclonal Antibody Immunoconjugates for Cancer.* March 12-14, p. 48.
26. Palme, D. F., Berkopec, J. M., Elson, M. K., Bono, M. D., Wessels, B. W., Lange, P. H., and Vessella, R. L. (1987) Immunoradiotherapy of renal cell

carcinoma xenografts by I-131 monoclonal antibody A6H compared to single fraction external beam irradiation. *Society of Nuclear Med.* Abstract Ref. No. 394.

27. Bale, W. F., Spar, I. L., and Goodland, R. L. (1960) Experimental radiation therapy of tumors with I-131 carrying antibodies to Fibrin*. *Cancer Res. 20*: 1488-1494.
28. Quinones, J., Mizejewski, G., and Beierwaltes, W. H. (1971) Choriocarcinoma scanning using radiolabeled antibody to chorionic gonadotrophin. *Nuclear Medicine 12;2*: 69-75.
29. Goldenberg, D. M. (1978) Immunodiagnosis and immunodetection of colorectal cancer. *Cancer Bull. 30*: 213-218.
30. Kohler, G., and Milstein, C. (1975) Continuous cultures of fused cells secreting antibodies of predefined specificity. *Nature 256*: 495.
31. Clayman, R. V., Figenshau, R. S., Bear, A., Limas, C. (1985) Transplantation of human renal cell carcinoma into athymic mice. *Cancer Res. 45*: 2650-2653.
32. Chiou, R. K., Vessella, R. L., Elson, M. K., Clayman, R. V., Gonzalez-Campoy, J., Klicka, M. J., Shafer, R. B., and Lange, P. H. (1985) Localization of human renal cell carcinoma xenografts with a tumor-preferential monoclonal antibody. *Cancer Res. 45*: 6140-6146.
33. Sands, H., Jones, P. L., Shah, S. A., Palme, D. F., Vessella, R. L., and Gallagher, B. M. (1988) Correlation of vascular permeability and blood flow with monoclonal antibody uptake by Clouser and renal cell carcinoma. *Cancer Res., 48*: 188-193.
34. Ueda, R., Ogata, S., Morrissey, D. M., Finstad, C. L., Szkudlarek, J., Whitmore, W. F., Oettgen, H. F., Lloyd, K. O., and Old, L. J. (1981) Cell surface antigens of human renal cancer defined by mouse monoclonal antibodies: identification of tissue-specific kidney glycoproteins. *Proc. National Acad. Sciences 78;8*: 5122-5126.
35. Luner, S. J., Ghose, T., Chatterjee, S., Cruz, H. N., and Belitsky, P. (1986) Monoclonal antibodies to kidney and tumor associated surface antigens of human renal cell carcinoma. *Cancer Res. 46*: 5816-5820.
36. Muller, G. A., and Muller, C. (1983) Characterization of renal antigens on distinct parts of the human nephron by monoclonal antibodies. *Klin. Wochenschr. 61*: 893.
37. Scharfe, T., Becht, E., Kaltwasser, R., Thuroff, J. W., Jacobi, G. H., and Hohenfellner, R. (1985) Tumor specific monoclonal antibodies for renal cell carcinoma. *Eur. Urol. 11*: 117.
38. Oosterwijk, E., Ruiter, D. J., Hoedemaeker, Ph. J., Pauwels, E. K. J., Jonas, U., Zwartenbijk, J., and Warnaar, S. O. (1986) Monoclonal antibody G-250 recognizes a determinate present in renal cell carcinoma and absent in normal kidney. *Int. J. Cancer 38*: 489-494.
39. Alvarez, V. L., Lopes, A. D., Lee, C., Rodwell, J. D., and McKearn, T. J. (1986) Radioimmunoimaging of human tumor xenografts in nude mice using site-specifically labelled monoclonal antibodies. *AACR Proceedings 27*: abstract 1346.

40. Oosterwijk, E. (1987) Renal cell carcinoma: diagnostic procedures with monoclonal antibodies. Doctorial dissertation, from the Department of Pathology and Urology, University of Leiden, The Netherlands, 107-128.
41. Colcher, D., Zalutsky, M., Kaplan, W., et al. (1983) Radioloalization of human mammary tumors in athymic mice by a monoclonal antibody. *Cancer Res. 43*: 736-742.
42. Moldfsky, P. J., Powe, J., Mulhern, C. B., et al. (1983) Metastatic colon carcinoma detected with radiolabeled F(ab′)2 monoclonal antibody fragments. *Radiology 149*: 549-555.
43. Begent, R. H., Green, A. J., Bagshawe, K. D., et al. (1982) Liposomally entrapped second antibody improves tumour imaging with first antitumour antibody. *Lancet 2*: 739.
44. Sands, H., and Jones, P. L. (1987) Methods for the study of metabolism of radiolabeled monoclonal antibodies by liver and tumor. *J. Nuc. Med. 28*: 390-398.
45. Sullivan, D. C., Silva, J. S., Cox, C. E., et al. (1982) Localization of I-131 labeled goat and primate anti-carcinoembryonic antigen (cea) antibodies in patients with cancer. *Invest. Radiol. 17*: 350-355.
46. Halpern, S. E., Hagan, P. L., Garver, P. R., Koziol, J. A., Chen, A. W. N., Frincke, J. M., Bartholomew, R. M., David, G. S., and Adams, T. H. (1983) Stability, characterization and kinetics of 111IN-labeled monoclonal antitumor antibodies in normal animals and nude mouse-human tumor models. *Cancer Res. 43*: 5347-4355.
47. Bradwell, A. R., Fairweather, D. S., Dykes, P. W., Keeling, A., Vaughan, A., Taylor, J. (1985) Limiting factors in the localization of tumours with radiolabeled antibodies. *Immunology Today 6;5*: 163-170.
48. Carrasquillo, J. A., Mulshine, J. L., Bunn, P. A., Jr., Reynolds, J. C., Foon, K. A., Schroff, R. W., Perentesis, P., Steis, R. G., Keenan, A. M., Horowitz, M., and Larson, S. M. (1987) Indium-111 T101 monoclonal antibody is superior to iodine-131 T101 in imaging of cutaneous T-cell lymphoma. *Nuclear Medicine 28*: 281-287.
49. Rodwell, J. D., Alvarez, V. L., Lee, C., Lopes, A. D., Goers, J. W., King, H. D., Powsner, H. J., McKearn, P. J. (1986) Site specific covalent modification of monoclonal antibodies: in vitro and in vivo evaluations. *Proc. Natl. Acad. Sci. 83;8*: 2632-2636.
50. Paik, C. H., Ebbert, P. R., Murphy, P. R., et al. (1983) Factors influencing DTPA conjugation with antibodies by cyclic DTPA anhydride. *J. Nuc. Med. 24*: 1158-1163.
51. Urdal, D. L., and Hakomori, S. I. (1980) Tumor-associated ganglio-N-triosylceramide. Target for antibody-dependent, avidin-mediated drug killing of tumor cells. *Cancer Investigation 255;21*: 10509-10515.
52. Wessels, B. W., and Rogus, R. P. (1984) Radionuclide selection and model absorbed dose calculations for radiolabeled tumor associated antibodies. *Med. Phys. 11*: 638-645.
53. Lyster, D. M., and Alcorn, L. N. (1986) Antibody imaging and therapy in human cancer. *Radiopharmaceuticals: Prog. & Clin. Perspectives 1*: 41-59.

54. Humm, J. L. (1986) Dosimetric aspects of radiolabeled antibodies for tumor therapy. *J. Nuc. Med. 27*: 1490-1497.
55. Zalcberg, J. R., Thompson, C. H., Lichtenstein, M., and McKenzie, I. F. C. (1984) Tumor immunotherapy in the mouse with the use of I-131 labeled monoclonal antibodies. *JNCI 71*: 697-704.
56. Cheung, N. K. V., Landmeier, B., Neely, J., Nelson, A. D., Abramowsky, C., Ellery, S., Adams, R. B., and Miraldi, F. (1986) Complete tumor ablation with Iodine 131-radiolabeled disialoganglioside Gd2-specific monoclonal antibody against human neuroblastoma xenografted in nude mice. *JNCI 77;3*: 739-745.
57. Wilbur, S., Hadley, S., Grant, L., Seubert, J., Morgan, A. C., Fritzberg, A. R. (1987) Evaluation of radioiodination monoclonal antibody conjugates which are resistant to in vivo deiodination. *Int. Conf. on Monoclonal Antibody Immunoconjugates for Cancer*, Abstract #45, p. 102.
58. DeNardo, G. L., Raventos, A., Hines, H. H., Scheibe, P. O., Macey, D. J., Hays, M. T., and DeNardo, S. J. (1985) Requirements for a treatment planning system for radioimmunotherapy. *International Journal of Radiation Oncology Biology Physics 11*: 335-348.
59. Dillman, R. O. (1984) Monoclonl antibodies in the treatment of cancer. *Critical Reviews in Oncology/Hematology 1;4*: 357-384.
60. Pimm, M. V., Embleton, M. J., Perkins, A. C., Price, M. R., Robins, R. A., and Robinson, G. R. (1982) In vivo localization of anti-osteogenic sarcoma 791T monoclonal antibody in osteogenic sarcoma xenografts. *Int. J. Cancer 30*: 75-85.
61. Snyder, W. S., Ford, M. R., Warner, G. C., et al. (1975) "S" absorbed dose per unit accumulated activity for selected radionuclides and organs. MIRD phamplet No. 11. The Society of Nuclear Medicine, New York.
62. Yorke, E. D., Griffith, M. H., and Wessels, B. W. (1987) Quantitative autoradiography and micro-TLD measurements for radioimmunotherapy. *J. Nuc. Med. 28*: 617.
63. Vessella, R., Moon, T., and Lange, P. (1983) Monoclonal antibodies reactive with renal cell carcinoma. *Fed. Proc. 42*: 401.
64. Taggart, R., and Samloff, I. (1983) Stable antibody-producing murine hybridomas. *Science 219*: 1228-1230.
65. Fudenberg, H. (1967) Purification of antibodies. In *Methods in Immunology and Immunochemistry* (Williams, C. A., and Chase, M. W., Eds.). Academic Press, New York.
66. Lacmmli, V. (1970) Cleavage of structural proteins during the assembly of the head of bacteriophage T4. *Nature 227*: 680-685.
67. Sammons, D., Adams, L., and Nishizawa, E. (1981) Ultrasensitive silver based color staining of poly peptides in polyacrylamide gels. *Electrophoresis 2*: 135-141.
68. Greenwood, F. C., Hunter, W. M., and Glover, J. S. (1963) The preparation of 131-I labeled human growth hormone of high specific activity. *Biochem. J. 89*: 114-123.

69. McFarlane, A. S. (1956) Labeling of plasma proteins with radioactive iodine. *Biochem. J. 62*: 135-143.
70. Marchawnis, J. J. (1969) An enzymatic method for the trace iodination of immunoglobulins and other proteins. *Biochem. J. 113*: 299-305.
71. Fraker, P. J., and Speck, J. C. (1978) Protein and cell membrane iodinations with a sparingly soluble chloroamide 1,3,4,6-tetrachloro-3&,6&-diphenylglycoluril. *Biochem. Biophys. Res. Comm. 80*: 849-857.
72. Wessels, B. W., Griffith, M. H. (1986) Miniature thermoluminescent dosimeter absorbed dose measurements in tumor phantom models. *Nuclear Medicine 27*:1308-1314.
73. Neacy, W. P., Wessels, B. W., Bradley, E., Kovandi, S., Justice, T., Danskin, S., and Sands, H. (1986) Comparison of radioimmunotherapy (RIT) and 4 MV external beam radiotherapy of human tumor xenografts in athymic mice. *J. Nuc. Med. 27*: 902 (Abstract #109).
74. Bolton, A. E., Hunter, W. M. (1973) The labeling of protein to high specific radioactivity by conjugation to a 125 I-containing a cyclating agent. *Biochem. J. 133*: 529-539.

10

Site-Specific Modification of Monoclonal Antibodies

Studies of ^{111}Indium-Labeled Antibodies Using Nude Mouse Xenograft Systems

VERNON L. ALVAREZ, A. DWIGHT LOPES, CHYI LEE, DANIEL J. COUGHLIN, JOHN D. RODWELL, and THOMAS J. McKEARN
CYTOGEN Corporation, Princeton, New Jersey

I. INTRODUCTION

The concept of a "magic bullet," which could be used to selectively destroy tumor cells, dates from the early studies and concepts of Paul Ehrlich (1) and the elegant work of David Pressman, who, using antibodies labeled with isotopes of iodine (2), gave a practical demonstration of this technology. The pioneering clinical studies of investigators such as Beierwaltes (3), who in 1956 documented a cure using ^{131}I-labeled antibodies raised to a patient's own cancer, further emphasized the promise of such an approach.

For more than two decades after the work of Pressman and Beierwaltes, studies in the area of "directed delivery" were hampered by the use of cross-reactive polyclonal antisera raised in multiple animal types. The discovery of monoclonal antibodies by Köhler and Milstein (4) led to production of homogeneous reagents, which prompted careful, controlled studies of in vivo localization of tumors and other targets, such as thrombi. Since the early 1980s the uses of monoclonal antibodies to deliver radioisotopes, toxins, and drug conjugates has grown to the sophistication of clinical trials throughout the world.

One key issue in the use of monoclonal antibodies is the need for covalent modification, either by direct labeling with isotopes or conjugation to drugs, chelators, or toxins. It is now recognized (5) that such modification can severely hamper the immunoreactivity of the antibody and that, in general (6), increasing the "loading" of a substance on the antibody will cause a decrease in the immunoreactivity. This issue was directly addressed in a novel approach to modification of monoclonal antibodies by Rodwell et al. (7), who demonstrated that the carbohydrate moieties on antibodies could be used to attach various substances at specific positions away from the antibody combining site. This method was shown to preserve the immunoreactivity even with relatively high loadings and to provide excellent in vivo results in animal models.

Recent studies in our laboratory have been directed toward further characterization of monoclonal antibodies modified at their carbohydrate, with specific emphasis on their function as imaging agents, using nude mouse xenograft models. We chose to do this using antibodies coupled to a derivative of the chelator diethylenetriaminepentaacetic acid (DTPA), which is then complexed with ^{111}In. This analysis provides a direct and quantitative monitor of the performance of an antibody and is also useful for choosing which antibodies should be used in other applications, such as delivery of therapeutic isotopes or cytotoxic drugs.

In this chapter we will detail the site-specific chemical modification of antibodies and their labeling with ^{111}In. We will then present imaging and biodistribution data from two antibody/xenograft systems that illustrate the results we achieve. All experiments were performed with site-specifically modified antibodies. However, the methodology described herein for ^{111}In chelation should work for other chelator conjugates (8) as well.

II. RESULTS

A. Choice of Monoclonal Antibodies and Xenograft Systems

Initial experiments performed in our laboratories demonstrated that mouse, rat, and human monoclonal antibodies of various Ig classes could be modified by the techniques described below. Because we were interested primarily in antibodies that could be used in clinical applications, we sought to use appropriate model systems for these antibodies. It therefore was necessary to have target tumor cells reactive with the antibodies being studied and which would form xenografts in a reasonably reproducible and rapid fashion. We will discuss two antibody/xenograft systems, one using a renal cell xenograft and the other a colon xenograft, each chosen to illustrate specific differences in localization kinetics and saturation of tumor target.

1. Anti-Renal Cell Carcinoma: Antibody S4, Xenograft 7860

The antibody S4 is an IgG_{2a} and was made against a human renal cell carcinoma (9). It is reactive with many different human renal cell carcinoma cell lines, including SK-RC-1 (10) and 7860 (11). Data will be presented using xenografts of the cell line 7860.

2. Anti-Colon Carcinoma: Antibody B72.3, Xenograft LS174T

B72.3 is an IgG_1 antibody made using an antigen preparation from a human breast metastasis (12), which was shown to react extensively with colon, breast, ovarian, and other adenocarcinomas. It is also reactive with many cell lines of these types, and data will be presented using the human colon carcinoma cell line LS174T (13).

B. Site-Specific Modification of Monoclonal Antibodies

Site-specific modification refers to covalent chemical modifications at a specific site on an antibody molecule, in contrast to general methods, which result in modification of a certain class of sites on antibodies. "Class-specific" modification can lead to decreased immunoreactivity. For example, modification of amino acids, such as tyrosine, lysine, or aspartic or glutamic acid side chains, could affect the immunoreactivity of the antibody, since these residues are typically present in the antigen-binding region.

We have recently described an alternate approach, called "site-specific" modification of monoclonal antibodies (7), which makes use of the complex carbohydrate found on the heavy chains, normally at sites far from the antigen combining site (9). This provides an alternate strategy for modification of antibodies by oxidation of the sugar residues to aldehydes, followed by reaction with appropriate aldehyde-reactive groups, such as amines, hydrazides, or hydrazines. Earlier results (7) clearly demonstrated that this type of site-specific modification gave improved results over standard techniques and have prompted us to continue this work with other monoclonal antibodies in order to determine the general applicability of this method.

1. Oxidation of Antibodies

While oligosaccharides on antibodies can be converted to aldehydes either chemically or enzymatically, only chemical methods will be discussed in this chapter. Chemical oxidation was accomplished by incubating the antibodies with 10–30 mM $NaIO_4$ in PBS at pH 6.0 on ice, in the dark, for 1 hour. After this oxidation, the antibodies were either dialyzed extensively or passed through a Sephadex G-25 or Bio-Gel P-50 column. At this point the antibodies contain aldehyde residues that are reactive with many different compounds, including amines, hydrazides, and hydrazines. Although it is possible to freeze oxidized antibodies after this step for modification at a later time, they were generally reacted immediately with a chelator-linker. The chelator-linker used in these studies is a derivative of the tripeptide glycyl-tyrosyl-lysine and the chelator diethylenetriaminepentaacetic acid, abbreviated GYK-DTPA. The chelator DTPA is attached to the ϵ-amino of the lysine residue of the tripeptide, and the amino terminal glycyl residue attaches to the reactive aldehydes on the antibody.

2. Preparation of Chelator-Linker GYK-DTPA

The method of preparation of GYK-DTPA is detailed in the Appendix. Briefly, this synthesis consisted of a four-step process beginning with a synthesis of N-Fmoc-glycyl-tyrosine followed by attachment of the lysine (N-ϵ-Z) methyl ester. This was then converted to HBr salt and finally attached to diethylenetriaminepentaacetic acid (DTPA) to form the Fmoc-glycyl-tyrosyl-lysine methyl ester-DTPA. This was finally converted to GYK-DTPA by treatment with base, and the final pure product was purified by reverse phase HPLC.

3. Coupling of GYK-DTPA to Antibody

One advantage of this technique for modification of monoclonal antibodies is that it is extremely general, the following brief description having been used for more than 100 different monoclonal antibodies. After the antibody has been oxidized and either dialyzed or passed through a Sephadex G-25 column, it is incubated overnight at 4°C with a 2000-fold molar excess of GYK-DTPA. The antibody is finally purified using Sephadex G-50, Superose 12, or some other gel filtration method. It should also be noted that it is possible to recycle the chelator, if desired, by collecting the salt fraction containing the unreacted chelator and repurifying using reverse-phase chromatography.

4. Extent of Derivitization of Antibody

The number of chelator-linkers attached to the antibody via the carbohydrate can be determined by either of two methods: (a) preparation of a known specific activity mixture of "cold" and "hot" indium followed by evaluation of specific activity on the antibody after chelation, and (b) direct iodination of the tyrosine residue on the GYK-DTPA to a known specific activity before coupling to antibody and evaluation of the final antibody-GYK-DTPA conjugate. Both of these techniques require careful calculation of initial specific activity.

These analyses have been performed on the two monoclonal antibodies described here, and the results are shown in Table 1.

It is very important to emphasize that both of these antibodies, as well as approximately 100 others (see Refs. 7 and 15 for other examples), have been modified using exactly the same protocol. This method appears to be universal for most types of monoclonal antibodies (although IgG_3 isotypes require minor

Table 1 Derivitazation of Monoclonal Antibodies S4 and B72.3 with GYK-DTPA

	Number of GYK-DTPA groups (mol/mol Ab)	
Antibody	Indium method	Iodine method
S4	5.5	4.5
B72.3	5.1	4.3

modification), and the resulting conjugates contain 3-7 chelators per antibody. As described below, this degree of modification appears to have little or no effect on the immunoreactivity of the antibody.

5. Immunoreactivity Assays

Several reports (6,7,16) have shown that standard techniques involving lysine modification to attach derivatives of DTPA onto antibodies result in severe loss of immunoreactivity when the derivitization ratio is greater than 1 mole of DTPA/mole of antibody. As mentioned above, the technique of modifying via the carbohydrate allows much higher loading with little loss of immunoreactivity. Specific data on the antibodies S4 and B72.3 will be discussed below.

The immunoreactivity of the GYK-DTPA-modified S4 was assayed using live SK-RC-1 cells as the source of antigen. The assay used was a classical direct-binding type of assay using ^{111}In-labeled S4-GYK-DTPA. The results, shown in

Table 2 Immunoreactivity of ^{111}In-labeled S4-GYK-DTPA: Direct Cell Binding Assay with Multiple Cell Pellets

Pellet	Percent counts bound[a]	Control[b]
1	59	8
2	14	5
3	5	0
4	0	0
Total	78	13

[a]10^6 cells per binding; supernatant from first pellet incubated with second, etc.
[b]Binding to nontarget cells.

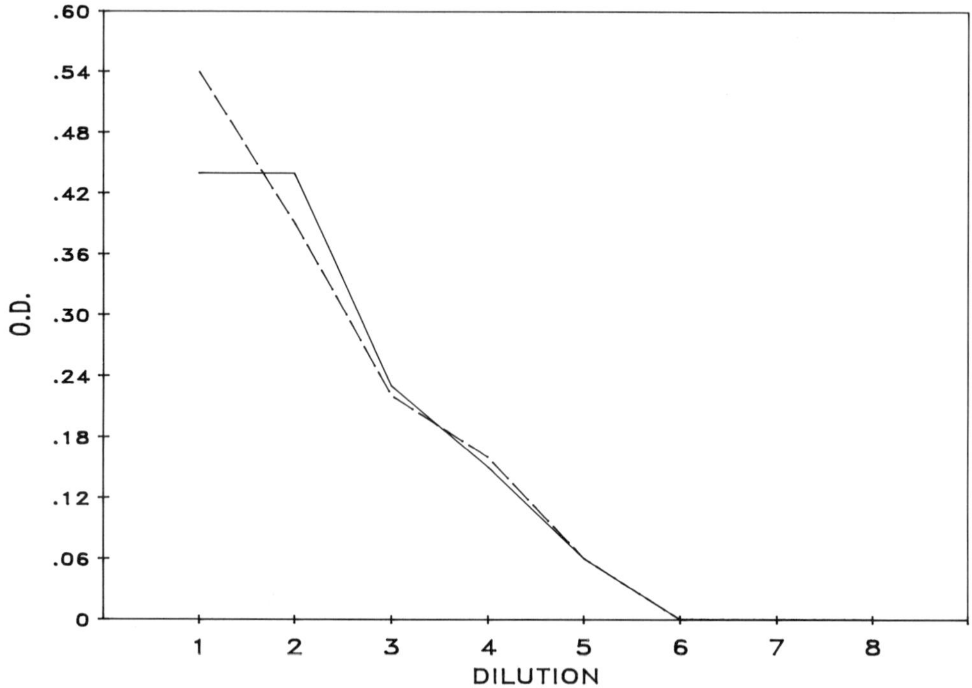

Figure 1 ELISA assay of S4 and S4–GYK-DTPA on fixed cell plates using 7860 cells. Dashed line (– –), native S4; solid line (–), S4–GYK-DTPA.

Table 2 demonstrate that after modification of this antibody and labeling with ^{111}In, it is possible to bind approximately 80% of the counts to the target cells. Note that although this direct-binding experiment adequately measures the immunoreactivity of the labeled conjugate, it is not possible to directly compare the reactivity of the initial native antibody with the derivatized species.

S4–GYK-DTPA was also assayed in an ELISA-type assay using fixed 7860 cells. In this type of assay it is possible to compare the native antibody with modified antibody. Serial dilutions of native S4 and S4-GYK-DTPA were made and antibody binding assayed by horseradish peroxidase–labeled goat-antimouse antibody (e.g., Kirkegaard & Perry #14.18.07). Orthophenyl diamine was added and after incubation the optical density read on a 96-well plate reader. The results of this assay are shown in Figure 1, which compares native, nonconjugated S4 with S4–GYK-DTPA. It is clear from this figure that there is no loss of immunoreactivity after modification.

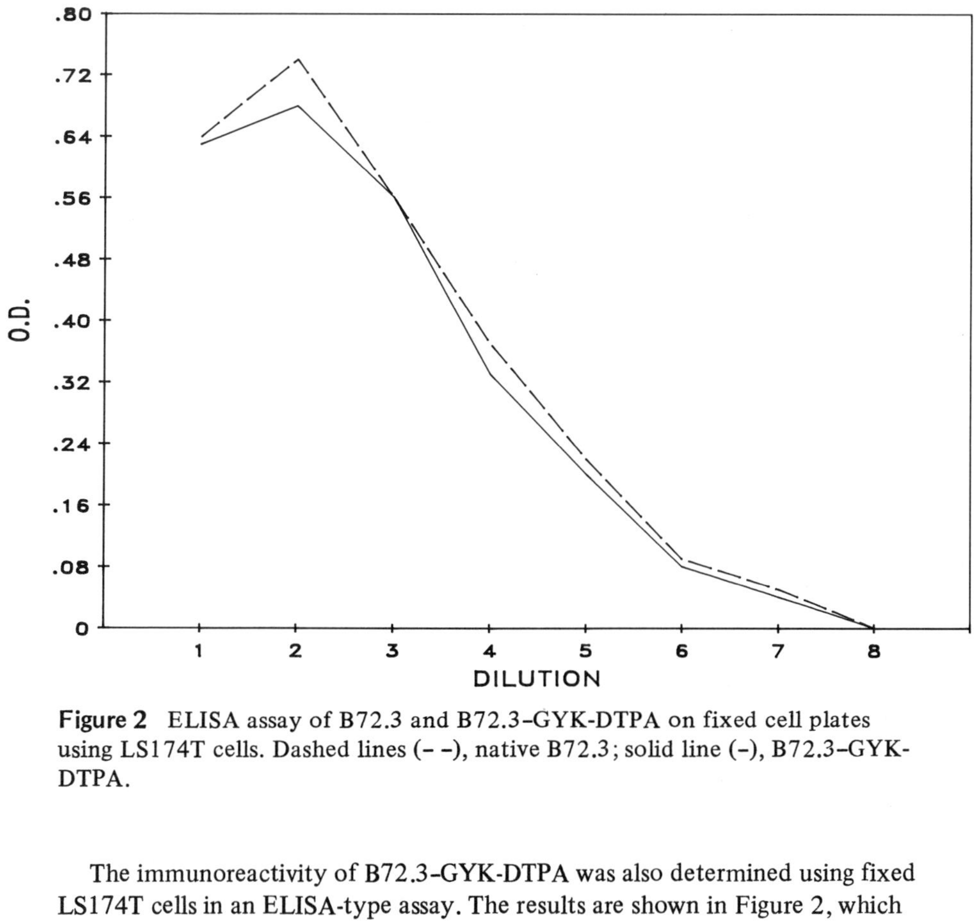

Figure 2 ELISA assay of B72.3 and B72.3-GYK-DTPA on fixed cell plates using LS174T cells. Dashed lines (- -), native B72.3; solid line (-), B72.3-GYK-DTPA.

The immunoreactivity of B72.3-GYK-DTPA was also determined using fixed LS174T cells in an ELISA-type assay. The results are shown in Figure 2, which illustrates the results with the native and the GYK-DTPA derivative of B72.3. It is evident from this figure that this type of modification results in very little or no loss of immunoreactivity, as measured by this assay.

C. Labeling with ^{111}In

One of the goals of the studies with chelator antibodies was to develop a reproducible technique for labeling with ^{111}In. In the course of many experiments, it became apparent that several factors were important for this labeling reaction. In this section these various factors will be discussed.

1. Source and Quality of ^{111}In Chloride

^{111}In chloride is available from DuPont-New England Nuclear (NEN), Amersham, Medi-Physics, and the Atomic Energy of Canada, Ltd. Although we have used ^{111}In from each of these sources, most of the experiments have been done with ^{111}In from NEN or Amersham. Each of these suppliers typically send out decay-corrected amounts of ^{111}In. For example, the isotope received on a Monday will have excess activity to account for decay until Wednesday, when the activity is certified.

A principal quality requirement for ^{111}In is that it is "carrier-free," since any nonradioactive indium metal ions would compete for the chelation sites and reduce the specific activity. The presence of trace metal contaminants must also be controlled, since this would also lead to competition for chelation sites with reduction in specific activity.

An additional observation in this laboratory was that the age of the ^{111}In appeared to affect the chelation. Specifically, ^{111}In over a week old (from the time the activity was certified) would not chelate as well as fresh ^{111}In. Although the methods of ^{111}In labeling are still somewhat of an art, the technique described in the Appendix work well in this laboratory and give uniform labeling from week to week.

2. Evaluation of Labeling

After the antibody–chelator conjugate is labeled with ^{111}In, it is evaluated in order to determine the efficiency of labeling.

In this laboratory, we have developed a system using a TSK G-3000SW gel filtration HPLC column and two detectors, one a UV monitor at 280 nm and the other a radiation detector. These are coupled with a Nelson Chromatography System to quantitate both the radioactivity and the protein concentration. After the ^{111}In labeling (see Appendix), the antibody is injected into the HPLC column and fractions collected. An example of a typical print-out from the computer is seen in Figure 3, showing both the radioactivity (upper trace) and the absorbance at 280 nm (lower trace).

This analysis is useful for several reasons. First, it is possible to assess the degree of labeling by comparing the ratio of radioactivity to protein concentration. Since the area under the peaks is quantitated by the integrator, accurate values for both radioactivity and protein concentration can be achieved. This method is used to obtain protein concentration, but μCi of ^{111}In are quantitated by counting aliquots on a gamma-counter.

A second important feature of this analysis is that it also gives an indication of the presence of aggregates, fragments of the antibody, or low molecular weight material. This is useful to assess the effect of the conjugation, the ^{111}In labeling, and subsequent stability of the antibody, as well as an aid in interpretation of the in vivo studies.

3. Quantitation of Specific Activity

The specific activity of the labeled antibody is determined by the HPLC analysis described above and by collecting and counting fractions in a gamma-counter.

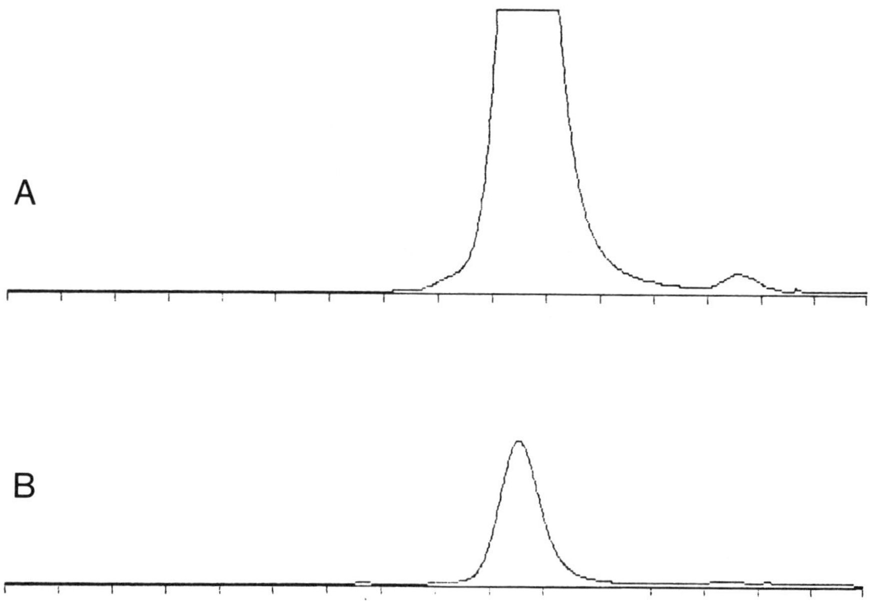

Figure 3 Dual channel computer display of TSK3000SW chromatography of ^{111}In-labeled B72.3-GYK-DTPA. A, radiation monitor; B, absorbance at 280 nm.

The HPLC detector is calibrated to convert the area to micrograms (μg), and the counts per minute are converted to microcuries (μCi). The specific activity is then the ratio of microcuries to micrograms. Typical specific activities obtained in our laboratory vary from 1 to 5 μCi/μg.

Variations in specific activity may be due to the variations in ^{111}In discussed above, to metal contamination from any source, or to the degree of modification with GYK-DTPA. In our experience, it is very important to use metal-free water and evaluate the containers in which the conjugates are stored in order to maintain reproducible labeling. Due to these problems, it is difficult to use specific activities to compare different antibodies unless they have been prepared in parallel experiments and stored for the same length of time.

4. Immunoreactivity of Labeled Conjugates

It is important to assess the immunoreactivity of the labeled conjugate in order to evaluate the effect of the labeling protocol on this important parameter. Although it is possible to use any of the assay methods described in Sec. IV.B.5, it should be pointed out that some methods may not be sensitive enough to detect small changes in immunoreactivity. Since only a small fraction of the conjugates are actually labeled with the isotope (our calculations indicate that a specific activity of 1 μCi/μg means that only about 1 out of 1000, or 0.1%, of the DTPAs has an ^{111}In atom), the assay must be capable of detecting immunoreactivity of this fraction. This means that assays such as the ELISA described above, although excellent for analyzing the bulk conjugate, are not sensitive enough to detect variations in the labeled antibody.

Obviously, these considerations imply that it is much better to use a direct cell binding or competition-inhibition assay using the ^{111}In counts to determine the percent binding. These type of assays are common using ^{125}Io-labeled antibodies, and it is simple to convert them to the ^{111}In isotope. An example of a direct cell binding assay was discussed above for the antibody S4, where it was shown that 78% of the counts could be bound to multiple cell pellets. It is important to do the assay with multiple cell pellets because the antigen density on cells varies extensively and the activity may be underestimated.

In the case of B72.3, the antigen that this antibody recognizes is not an integral cell membrane antigen, but an intracellular mucin. This complicates the cell binding assay, although it is possible to use a fixed-cell assay to determine the percent of counts bound to a 96-well plate.

D. Nude Mouse Xenograft Models

1. 7860 Xenografts

When 1×10^7 7860 cells from culture are subcutaneously injected into nude mice, 20-50% of the animals will develop palpable tumors. Some will spontaneously regress, but tumors that regress will often reappear and grow progressively. Prior treatment with Cyclophosphamide, 100 mg/kg injected i.p. the day before tumor cells are injected, does not increase the number of animals that develop tumors, nor does it affect the number that regress.

More reproducible tumor growth is seen when the tumors are started by implanting chunks. Palpable tumors develop in some animals by two weeks after implantation. Loss of antigen was seen after three serial in vivo passages of the tumor.

2. LS174T Xenografts

Measurable tumors (approximately 5 mm diameter) are present in 50% of the mice by day 7 after injection of 1×10^6 LS174T cells from culture. By day 14 they grow to approximately 11 mm diameter (about 0.4 g). The tumors grow quickly and progressively and will eventually kill the mice.

E. Imaging and Biodistribution

After conjugation of the antibody with the chelator GYK-DTPA and labeling with ^{111}In, the next step in the analysis is to inject the labeled antibody into xenograft-bearing mice and to evaluate its localization and distribution.

Table 3 Quantitation Parameters for Biodistribution Parameters

Variable	B72.3-GYK-DTPA-111-Indium
Antibody conc. (μg/ml)	35.0
Specific Act. (cpm/μg)	2.3×10^6
Wt. syringe	
before injection	2.98 g
after injection	2.77 g
Volume injected	0.22 ml
Mass injected	7.7 μg
μCi Syringe	
before injection	52.6 μCi
after injection	3.7 μCi
μCi injected	48.9 μCi
μCi/mouse	43.2 μCi
cpm of 10-μl aliquots	
1	835,240 cpm
2	865,644 cpm
3	723,041 cpm
Average	810,975 cpm
Injected dose[a]	17,841,450 cpm

[a]Injected dose calculated as follows: [(average cpm of 10-μl aliquot) $\times$ (ml injected)] $\times$ 100.
Data from ^{111}In-labeled B72.3-GYK-DTPA.

1. Injection Protocol

Any generalizations made from in vivo experiments with monoclonal antibody conjugates require careful quantitations of the injected dose. As described in the Appendix, we have developed an imaging biodistribution worksheet that allows careful quantitation of the injection and biodistribution of the ^{111}In-labeled antibody conjugate. Table 3 lists the data parameters and calculated results used in the biodistribution worksheet, with actual examples from a study involving ^{111}In-labeled B72.3-GYK-DTPA. This list of variables was developed in order to ensure that the dose was actually injected into the animal and to provide the numbers necessary for subsequent quantitation.

2. Imaging and Biodistribution Protocol

After injection of the ^{111}In-labeled conjugate, animals were imaged at various times and then dissected. Imaging was done using a General Electric StarCam

Table 4 Explanation of Biodistribution Ratios

Ratio	Explanation
cpm/g	counts per minute per gram; ratio of counts per minute divided by weight of organ in grams
tissue/blood	tissue-to-blood ratio; ratio of cpm/g organ divided by cpm/g blood
% I.D./g	% injected dose per gram; ratio of cpm/g divided by injected dose
% I.D./organ	% injected dose per organ; product of % I.D./g times weight of organ
μg Ab/g organ	micrograms antibody per gram organ; ratio of micrograms antibody[a] divided by weight of organ

[a]Micrograms antibody calculated as follows: micrograms antibody = (cpm)/(cpm/μg). See Table 3 for calculation of cpm/μg.

300, without collimation. Animals were anesthetized, placed in a restrainer, and then laid directly on the head of the camera. Typically, images were made by acquiring constant counts in order to compare images directly.

Upon completion of the imaging, mice were dissected and organs were weighed and counted. In some cases, the entire organ was counted; in others, it was necessary to take a smaller representative sample, which was also weighed and counted. The values of the weights and counts were then used in the biodistribution worksheet, along with the injection data discussed above, and the ratios (described in Table 4) calculated.

Among the issues addressed in our imaging/biodistribution experiments were the following: degree of localization to tumors in xenograft-bearing mice, differences between non–tumor-bearing and xenografted mice; kinetics of localization, effect of dose on localization, and saturation of xenograft with antibodies.

3. Anti–Renal Cell Carcinoma: Antibody S4, Xenograft 7860

Our experiments with the renal cell carcinoma system using S4, an IgG_{2a}, and the cell line 7860 have demonstrated that this system is unique in several respects, most notably the rapid and high degree of localization seen in the xenograft models. Images obtained with this antibody show exquisite localization, as demonstrated in Figure 4. The biodistribution numbers obtained corroborate these images as shown in Tables 5 and 6.

Table 5 compares the tissue-to-blood ratios obtained one day after injection of ^{111}In-labeled S4-GYK-DTPA animals bearing 7860 xenografts and in normal, non–tumor-bearing animals. Several features are evident from this table. First,

Table 5 Tissue-to-Blood Ratios Obtained 24 Hours Postinjection of 10 μg (35 μCi) ^{111}In-labeled S4–GYK-DTPA

Organ	Average tissue-to-blood ratio: 7860 Xenograft n = 5 (S.D.)	Average tissue-to-blood ratio: Non–tumor-bearing n = 4 (S.D.)
Blood	1.00 (0)	1.00 (0)
Lung	0.70 (0.01)	0.78 (0.01)
Spleen	1.56 (0.110	0.79 (0.05)
Liver	0.78 (0.58)	0.67 (0.08)
Kidney	0.92 (0.05)	0.55 (0.05)
Muscle	0.89 (0.05)	0.11 (0.05)
Tumor	19.50 (1.90)	–

the site-specifically modified S4–GYK-DTPA localizes extremely well to this xenograft, with tumor-to-blood ratios of 19.5:1. Accumulation in other organs, most notably the liver and spleen, is very low, with T:B ratios just above 1. We have previously shown (15) that non-tumor-bearing animals are valuable controls and that the tissue-to-blood ratios in such animals are all less than 1.0.

Table 6 presents the same data in a slightly different form, the percent injected dose per gram. This form indicates the degree of accumulation into each organ on a weight basis and can be very useful for subsequent calculations involving therapeutic delivery of isotopes or drugs. S4–GYK-DTPA again shows a high degree of specificity, with 117.5% I.D./g tumor, clearly much higher than into other organs. The amount in the blood of 7860-bearing mice compared with the non–tumor-bearing controls shows that much more of the antibody is present in the blood of controls than in the xenografted mice. This is due to the localization into the tumors of the 7860-bearing mice, which has the effect of removing the antibody from the circulation.

As we have previously shown (13), the use of normal, non–tumor-bearing mice as controls aids interpretation of in vivo results. This is because in a non–tumor-bearing animal there is no complication due to the presence of the xenograft, which may be shedding antigen or metastasizing into other organs. In this case, comparing the 7860-bearing mice with the normal controls, it appears that there is a slight localization into the spleen and possibly liver of the xenograft-bearing mice.

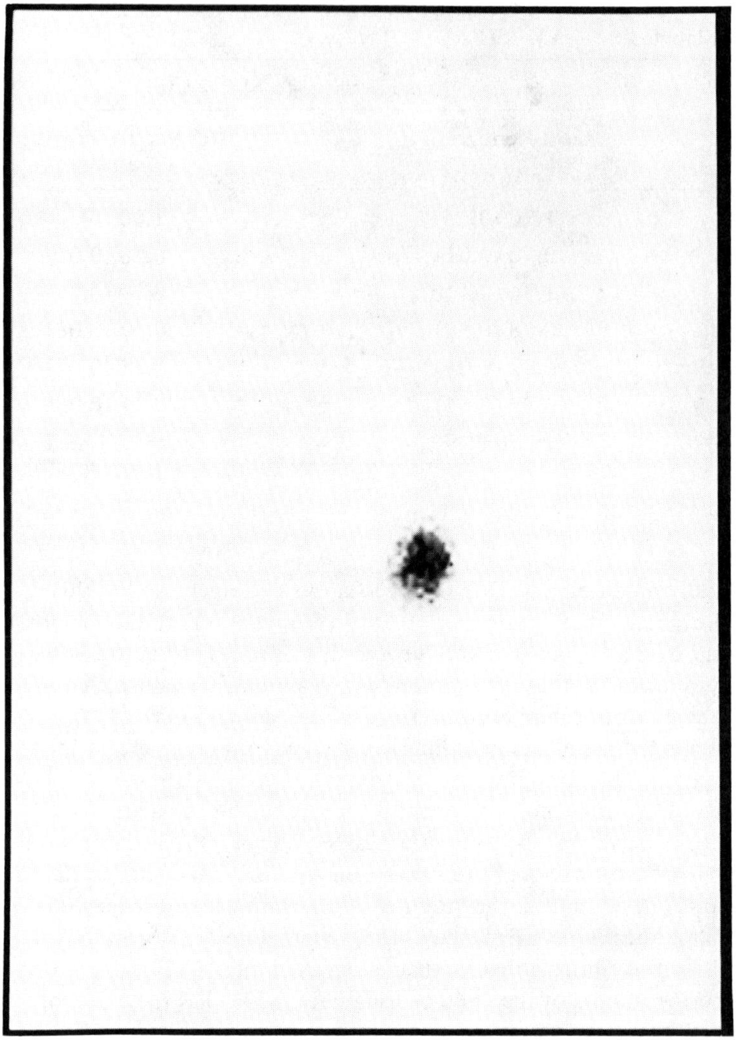

A

Figure 4 Images of ^{111}In-labeled S4-GYK-DTPA obtained 24 hours postinjection. A, 7860 xenograft-bearing mouse; B, normal, non–tumor-bearing mouse.

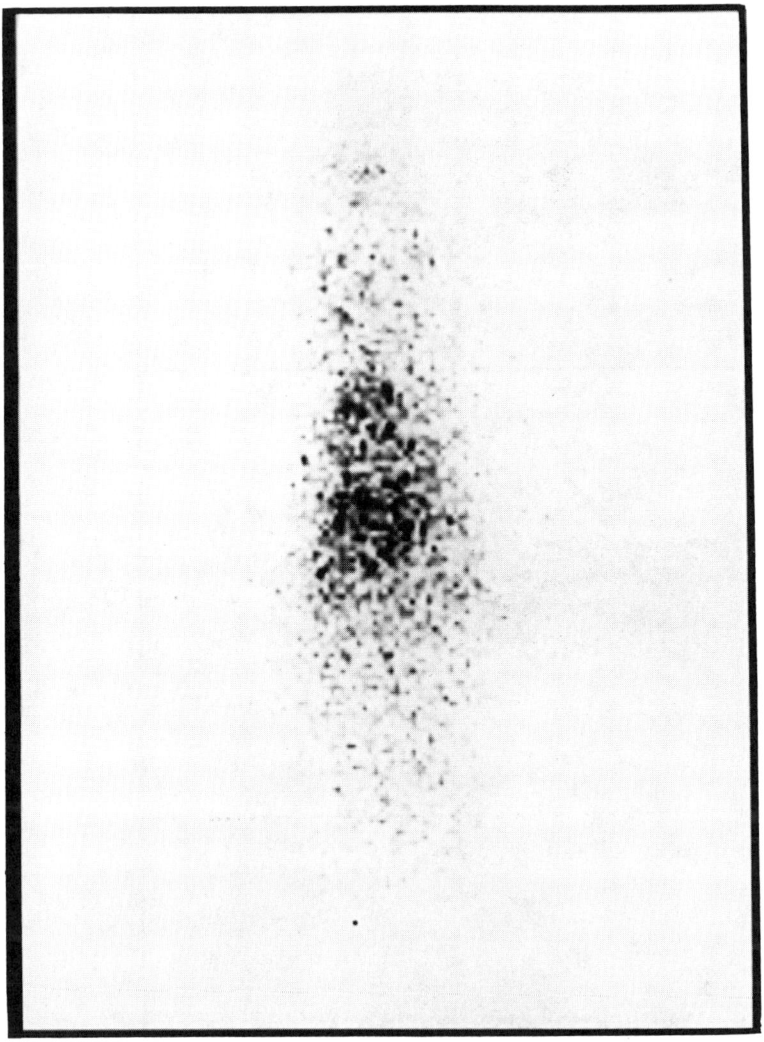

B

Figure 4 (continued)

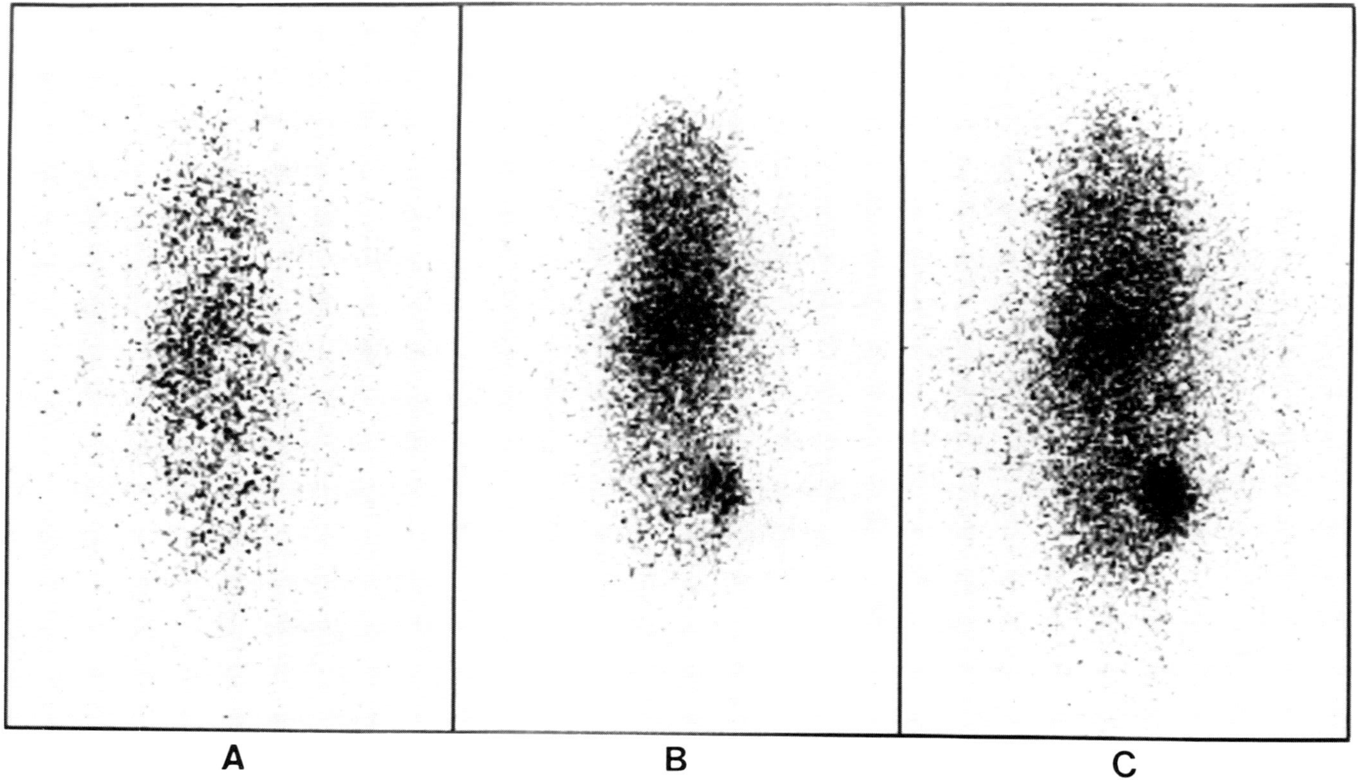
A
B
C

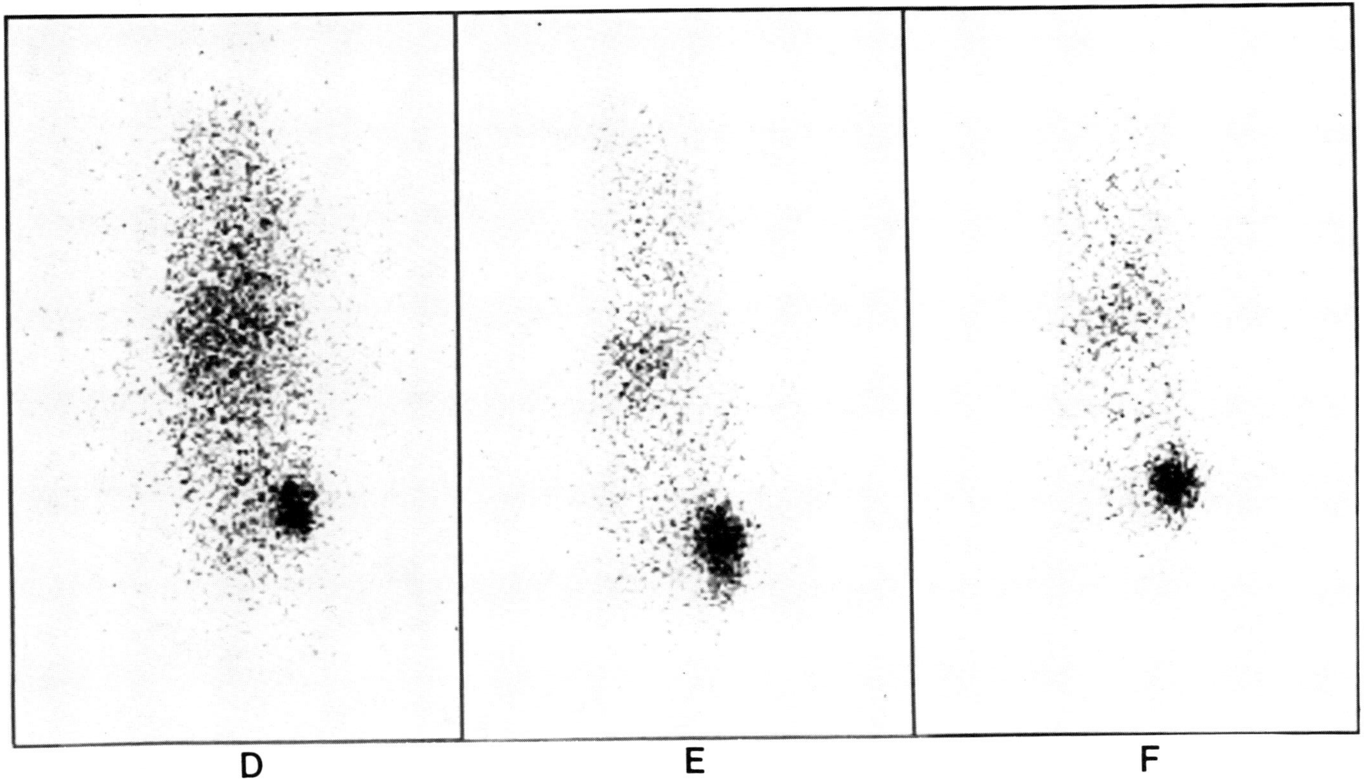

Figure 5 Images of ^{111}In-labeled antibodies in LS174T xenograft-bearing mice. A, image obtained 4 days postinjection of 500 μg of an irrelevant ^{111}In-labeled antibody conjugate. All other images obtained after injection of ^{111}In-labeled B72.3–GYK-DTPA. B, 1-day image, 5 μg injected; C, 1-day image, 50 μg injected; D, 4-day image, 5 μg injected; E, 4-day image, 50 μg injected; F, 4-day image, 1000 μg injected.

Table 6 Percent Injected Dose per Gram Values Obtained 24 Hours Postinjection of 10 μg (35 μCi) ^{111}In-labeled S4-GYK-DTPA

	Average % I.D./g	
Organ	7860 xenograft n = 5 (S.D.)	Non-tumor-bearing n = 4 (S.D.)
Blood	6.24 (0.92)	16.20 (0.20)
Lung	4.40 (0.70)	12.60 (0.30)
Spleen	9.65 (0.75)	12.75 (0.30)
Liver	8.85 (0.85)	11.05 (0.40)
Kidney	5.70 (0.50)	8.05 (0.40)
Muscle	0.73 (0.09)	1.60 (0.20)
Tumor	117.55 (5.55)	–

4. Anti-Colon Carcinoma: Antibody B72.3 and Xenograft LS174T

The antibody/xenograft system of B72.3 and LS174T illustrates a second type of localization, one which is much slower than the S4/7860 system and which can localize much more antibody. Typical images obtained with this antibody/xenograft system are shown in Figure 5, which shows images obtained with varying doses and times after injection. Biodistribution results are shown in Tables 7, 8, and 9.

The images shown in Figure 5 demonstrate that the antibody B72.3-GYK-DTPA localizes well to the xenograft LS174T and that this localization is immunospecific. Figure 5A shows the image obtained with a normal, non-tumor-bearing animal, and Figure 5D is the image obtained after injection of an irrelevant antibody (R9.75, a rat IgG_{2c} monoclonal). Figures 5B and 5C compare the localization after 24 hours of different doses (5 and 50 μg), indicating that localization is seen at this day and with both amounts of antibody. Figures 5E and 5F indicate that this localization persists at day 4 and that it is possible to obtain an image with an injection as large as 1 mg.

The kinetics of biodistribution of ^{111}In-labeled B72.3-GYK-DTPA into mice bearing the xenograft LS174T and into the non-tumor-bearing mice is shown in Table 7. This table compares the localization of 5 μg of the ^{111}In-labeled conjugate at 24 hours vs. 96 hours. It is clear that this antibody had not localized to any normal tissue at either point. Also, the degree of localization into the tumor increased dramatically, from a T:B ratio of 2.37 at 24 hours to 6.52 at 96 hours.

This uptake is slow compared to that observed for the S4 conjugate (see Table 5) and is thought to be due to slower diffusion into the tumor mass (17,

Table 7 Human Colon Carcinoma Model, Kinetics of Localization of 5 μg (15 μCi) of ^{111}In-labeled B72.3-GYK-DTPA in Mice Bearing LS147T Xenograft and Control, Non-tumor-bearing Nude Mice

	Average Tissue-to-Blood Ratio			
	24 hours		96 hours	
Organ	LS174T[a]	Control[b]	LS174T[a]	Control[b]
Blood	1.00	1.00	1.00	1.00
Lung	0.61 (0.05)[c]	0.50 (0.04)	0.53 (0.02)	0.47 (0.02)
Spleen	0.51 (0.11)	0.42 (0.03)	0.77 (0.08)	0.65 (0.08)
Liver	0.70 (0.11)	0.54 (0.05)	1.13 (0.20)	0.85 (0.06)
Kidney	0.42 (0.02)	0.43 (0.03)	0.95 (0.08)	0.57 (0.02)
Muscle	0.12 (0.02)	0.07 (0.01)	0.14 (0.02)	0.09 (0.02)
Tumor	2.37 (0.35)	–	6.52 (0.8)	–

[a]n = 6 animals per group.
[b]n = 3 animals per group.
[c]Standard deviation in parentheses.

Table 8 Human Colon Carcinoma Model, Effect of Antibody Dose on Localization of ^{111}In-labeled B72.3-GYK-STPA in LS174T Xenografted Mice

	Average Tissue-to-Blood Ratio[a]			
Organ	5 μg	50 μg	500 μg	1000 μg
Blood	1.00	1.00	1.00	1.00
Lung	0.53 (0.02)	0.49 (0.10)	0.59 (0.05)	0.50 (0.05)
Spleen	0.77 (0.08)	0.81 (0.17)	0.66 (0.08)	0.67 (0.04)
Liver	1.13 (0.20)	1.26 (0.55)	0.89 (0.08)	0.86 (0.04)
Kidney	0.95 (0.08)	0.95 (0.20)	0.78 (0.07)	0.75 (0.97)
Muscle	0.14 (0.02)	0.16 (0.04)	0.14 (0.02)	0.15 (0.06)
Tumor	6.52 (0.77)	7.17 (1.21)	5.89 (0.78)	5.59 (0.61)

[a]n = 5 animals for each group.
Standard deviation in parentheses.
Tissue-to-blood ratios 96 hours after injection.

Table 9 Human Colon Carcinoma Model, Effect of Antibody Dose on μg Ab/Organ Values Obtained 96 Hours Postinjection of ^{111}In-labeled B72.3–GYK-DTPA

	Average μg Ab/organ[a]			
Organ	5 μg	10 μg	500 μg	1000 μg
Blood[b]	0.22 (0.03)	3.39 (0.80)	32.45 (4.43)	71.14 (7.87)
Lung	0.12 (0.02)	1.94 (0.28)	12.12 (3.04)	35.44 (2.81)
Spleen	0.17 (0.02)	2.63 (0.44)	21.39 (2.92)	47.36 (3.01)
Liver	0.25 (0.02)	3.84 (0.28)	28.56 (1.62)	60.66 (5.28)
Kidney	0.22 (0.03)	3.07 (0.40)	23.63 (2.27)	52.97 (2.39)
Tumor	1.37 (0.13)	23.56 (2.36)	187.91 (10.18)	394.57 (41.45)

[a]n = 5 animals for each; standard deviation in parentheses.
[b]Blood value vased on estimate of 2 g of blood. Other average organ weights: lung = 0.186 g; spleen = 0.123g, liver = 1.640 g, kidney = 0.178 g, tumor = 0.363 g.

18). Other ratios also increase slightly with time, especially the spleen- and liver-to-blood ratios. These ratios were obtained with mice whose tumors were approximately 200 mg. In other groups of mice, in which the LS174T xenografts are larger (500 mg), spleen- and liver-to-blood ratios become as large as 3:1 (data not shown). Since the ratios in non–tumor-bearing mice remain low, these values are considered to be due to tumor-associated events, most likely reflecting the direct or indirect effects of shed antigen.

Preliminary experiments had shown that LS174T xenografts contain a great deal of antigen. Table 8 compares the tissue-to-blood ratios obtained 96 hours after injection of 5 μg, 50 μg, 500 μg, and 1000 μg of ^{111}In-labeled B72.3–GYK-DTPA into LS174T xenograft-bearing mice. All of the ratios are very similar, even comparing the low dose of 5 μg with the high dose of 100 μg, a 200-fold increase in injected dose. In other systems, such as the S4/7860 xenograft discussed above, such a large dose would saturate the tumor, leave the excess antibody in the blood, and result in a very low tumor-to-blood ratio (data not shown).

When the data is calculated as microgram antibody per organ (μg Ab/organ), the degree of accumulation into the tumor is seen more dramatically. As shown in Table 9, injected doses increasing from 5 μg to 1000 μg result in an increase of the micrograms of the antibody delivered to the tumor from 1.4 μg to almost 400 μg. This data indicates that large amounts of antibody are necessary to saturate this tumor, presumably due to the amount of antigen present.

III. DISCUSSION

The two antibody/xenograft systems discussed above were chosen to illustrate the results achieved using site-specific methodology for modification of monoclonal antibodies, the variation seen with mouse xenograft models, and the utility of ^{111}In as an isotope for in vivo imaging.

At the present time, more than 100 monoclonal antibodies of various IgG and IgM subclasses have been modified using the same protocol. Clearly, one of the strongest advantages of this technique is its universal applicability to all types of antibodies. S4 and B72.3 are examples of two different isotypes, one an IgG_{2a} and the other an IgG_1, with different specificities. After site-specific conjugation, both of these antibodies were derivatized with similar levels of the chelator GYK-DTPA (5.5 moles per mole antibody for S4, 5.1 for B72.3), and both retained their immunoreactivity (Figs. 1 and 2). Similar levels of derivatization using standard protocols are not possible for most other antibodies without severe loss of immunoreactivity (5,6,16).

In vivo studies with both antibodies and with many others (data not shown) have shown some similarities and some differences. One uniform finding with ^{111}In-labeled, site-specifically modified monoclonal antibodies is their behavior in non-tumor-bearing animals. As discussed elsewhere (15), biodistribution analyses in normal animals are very useful because they allow interpretation of results without any complications due to the presence of tumors. It is clear from the tissue-to-blood ratios (Tables 5 and 7) that there is no selective localization to any normal organ. The low liver-to-blood ratios are especially notable because uptake into the liver and spleen has been reported to be a major problem with ^{111}In-labeled monoclonal antibodies (5,8,16,19-21). As mentioned, the low liver-to-blood ratios in non-tumor-bearing mice clearly indicates no specific uptake. The percent injected dose per gram gives a more quantitative comparison. In this case, comparison of the behavior of ^{111}In-labeled S4-GYK-DTPA in normal mice with the 7860 xenograft animals (see Table 6) indicates that the amount in the liver drops substantially when there is a tumor to provide a "sink." This data supports the conclusion that the amount in the liver is primarily due to the blood pool and is still available to localize to an appropriate target.

In many ways, the results with S4-GYK-DTPA and B72.3-BYK-DTPA represent two extremes seen in our studies with site-specifically labeled monoclonal antibodies. Anti-renal cell antibody/xenograft systems appear to be unique in terms of their rapid kinetics of localization. Another antibody reactive with renal cell carcinoma, A6H (23), was shown to have similar kinetics when evaluated by one of our collaborators (24).

It is important to understand the reasons for the rapid uptake into the renal cell xenograft models. Several hypotheses have been proposed (24,25), and it appears that one of the main reasons for this rapid uptake is a high degree of vascular permeability. In other words, the antibody appears to be able to enter the extravascular space more readily than in other xenograft models, with the consequence that antibody binding is rapid. This may be a general feature of renal cell xenograft models, since other cell lines (such as SK-RC-1) and other antibodies (such as A6H) give similar results. Once the basic mechanism(s) responsible for such enhancers of permeability are known, it may be possible to utilize these mechanisms to increase the kinetics of localization in other systems.

The anticolorectal antibody system B72.3/LS174T exhibits slow localization kinetics but an extremely high antigen content, which results in the possibility of localizing large amounts of antibody to the xenografts. One intriguing use of this system would be to deliver large amounts of antibody conjugates for therapy. As evident from Tables 7–9, the percent delivery of B72.3-GYK-DTPA to the tumor is linear for doses as large as 1 mg, with about 400 μg of antibody delivered to a 300-mg tumor mass. Table 9 also indicates that such a large injected dose gives much smaller amounts to other organs; the entire liver, for example, which weighs an average of 1.6 g, receives only about 60 μg of the antibody. It should be possible to utilize data such as this to develop xenograft models for therapeutic delivery of both isotopes and drugs.

In conclusion, site-specific modification of monoclonal antibodies present a very attractive alternative for preparing antibody conjugates. We have shown that these conjugates of a chelator-linker attached to two different monoclonal antibodies are excellent for in vivo biodistribution studies. The conjugates retain immunoreactivity, label with ^{111}In readily, do not bind normal mouse tissue in non–tumor-bearing mice, and localize well to tumor targets in xenograft-bearing mice.

IV. APPENDIX

A. Materials

1. Chemicals and Suppliers

All chemicals used were reagent grade, except where noted. All were available from common suppliers such as the J. T. Baker Co., Sigma, Aldrich, etc.

The quality of water is especially important and must be as metal-free as possible, since even trace amounts of metals could "poison" the chelator. We have used two methods to solve this problem.

a. Chelex-Treated Water This treatment makes use of Chelex 100 (Bio-Rad, Richmond, CA), a metal-chelating resin. A large (2–5 liter) column is packed with this resin, and deionized water passed over this and collected for use in making buffers for the antibody–chelator conjugate preparation. This is a simple and straightforward method to prepare water of adequate quality. It is important to allow several column volumes to pass through the column and then to monitor the pH periodically. When the pH begins to rise, another column should be used; typically, a single column lasts 4-6 months and can be used to prepare up to 100 liters of water.

b. Water for Injection An alternate source of excellent water is Sterile Water for Injection, USP (Travenol Laboratories, Deerfield, IL). This water is prepared by distillation, and we find that it is also a good source of metal-free water. This is especially convenient, since it can be stored easily and is readily available for buffer preparation.

2. Monoclonal Antibodies

The antibody S4 (9) was the generous gift of Dr. Lloyd Old and was provided purified by his laboratory. The hybridoma B72.3 (11) was originally produced by Schlom and co-workers and was grown either as ascites or in tissue culture and purified using standard techniques (26).

3. Tumor Cell Lines

The human renal cell carcinoma line 7860 (11) was the generous gift of Dr. Robert Vessella. The cells are grown as a monolayer cultures in Eagles minimum essential medium (MEM), antibiotic-free, supplemented with 20% fetal bovine serum (FBS), essential and nonessential amino acids and glutamine, at 37°C in an atmosphere of 5% CO_2.

The human colon adenocarcinoma cell line LS174T (13) was obtained from the American Type Culture Collection (ATCC CL 188) and is cultured as above but with 10% FBS.

4. Mice

Female athymic nude mice (nu/nu, Swiss) were obtained from Taconic Farms (Germantown, NY) at four weeks of age. They are housed in sterile microisolators (Lab Products) and provided with autoclaved food (Purina Autoclavable Rodent Chow #5010) and sterile filtered tap water ad libitum. They are maintained at 68-72°F, 40-60% relative humidity, under fluorescent lighting on a 12-hour light/dark cycle.

B. Methods

1. Oxidation of Antibodies

The following protocol was used to prepare an oxidized monoclonal antibody:

a. Prepare 10x PBS, pH 6 Weight 87.5 g of NaCl, 12.1 g of $NaH_2PO_4 \cdot H_2O$, and 3.3 g of $Na_2PO_4 \cdot 7H_2O$, and dissolve in chelex-treated H_2O. Bring the final volume to 1 liter. Make a 1:10 dilution in chelex-treated water for injection.

b. Oxidation of Antibody

1. Prepare 1 ml of 1 mg/ml antibody in PBS buffer, pH 6.
2. Prepare 1 ml of 100 mM $NaIO_4$ in PBS. Weigh 21.4 mg of $NaIO_4$, and dissolve in 1 ml of PBS or water for injection.
3. Add 100 μl of 100 mM $NaIO_4$ into 1 ml of antibody, the final concentration of $NaIO_4$ is 10 mM.
4. Adjust the pH to 6 with 0.1 M NaOH.
5. Incubate on ice for one hour; keep in dark.
6. Two different methods are used to remove free $NaIO_4$:
   i. G-50 column
      Pack a 10 cc G-50 column, prewash with 1 ml of 10% BSA.
      Equilibrate column in PBS, pH 6. Load oxidized antibody into the column.
      Collect 1 ml fraction.
      Determine antibody concentration.
   ii. FPLC Superose 12 column
      Inject 1 ml of oxidized antibody into a 20 ml Superose 12 column
      Collect 1 ml fraction.
      Determine antibody concentration.

At this point, the antibody is oxidized and can be coupled to an appropriate amine, hydrazide, or hydrazine. It can be stored (frozen at -70°C) but is usually reacted immediately with the chelator GYK-DTPA (see Sec. IV.B.3).

2. Synthesis of Chelator-linker GYK-DTPA

The synthetic scheme for preparation of GYK-DTPA is shown in Figure 6.

a. Synthesis of N-Fmoc-Glycyl-Tyrosine (27,28) Glycyl-tyrosine (10 g, 42.0 mmol) and 9-fluorenylmethyl succinimidyl carbonate (12.95 g, 38.4 mmol) were added to a 0.1 M solution of sodium bicarbonate in 400 ml acetone/water mixture (50:50). The mixture was stirred at room temperature overnight, then acidified to pH 2 with concentrated hydrochloric acid. After removing acetone from reaction solution by rotary evaporation, the remaining aqueous solution was extracted three times with ethyl acetate. The combined organic extract was then dried with anhydrous sodium sulfate, filtered, and evaporated to dryness on a Rotavapor. The oily residue was triturated with methylene chloride to yield white solid product. The final product was collected on a filter and dried in a vacuum dessicator.

b. Synthesis of N-Fmoc-Glycyl-Tyrosyl-Lysine (N-ε-Z) Methyl Ester A solution of N-ε-Z-L-lysine methyl ester–HCl (12.57g, 37.8 mmol) and N,N-diisopropylethylamine (6.6 ml), in dry dimethylformamide (750 ml) was stirred in an

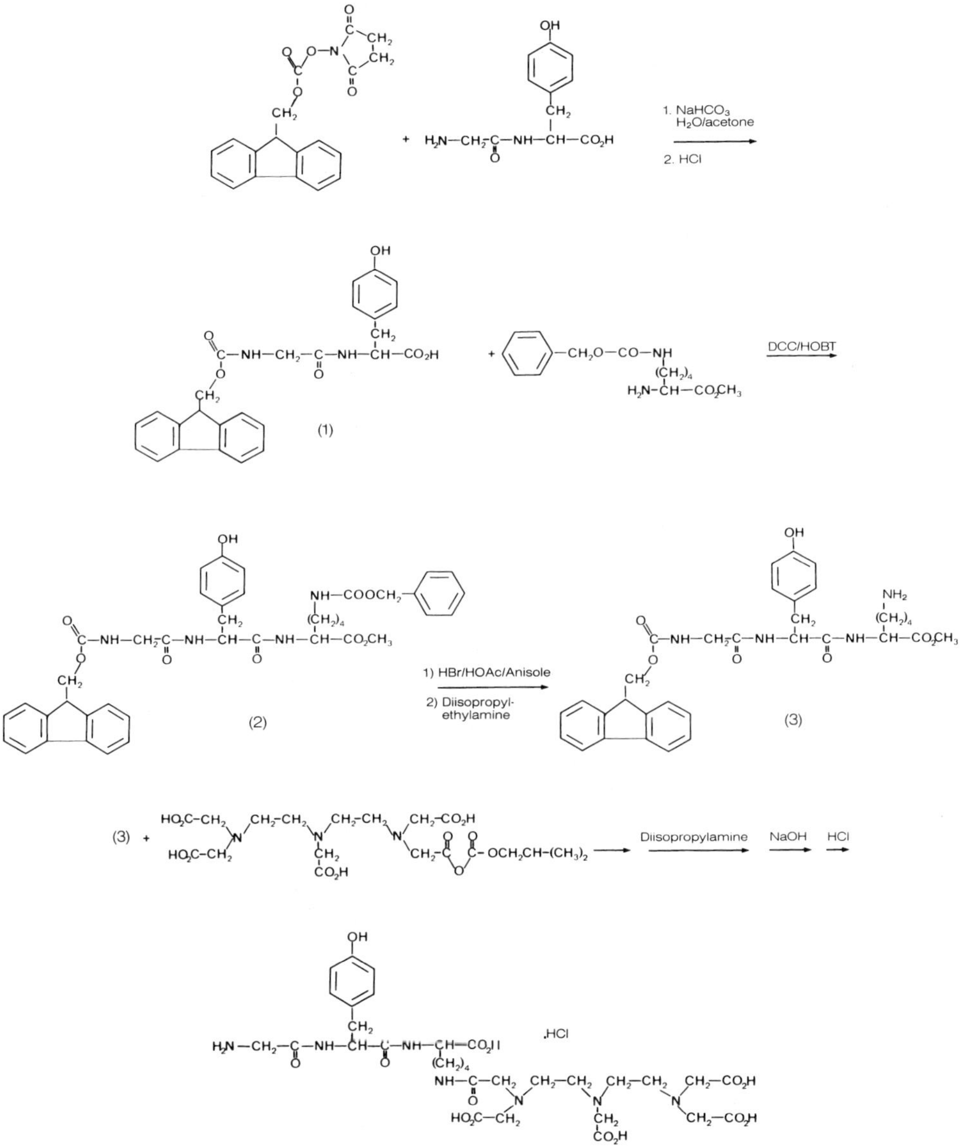

Figure 6 Scheme for synthesis of GYK-DTPA.

ice-water bath under nitrogen gas. Fifteen minutes later N-Fmoc-glycyl-tyrosine (17.23 g, 37.5 mmole), 1-hydroxygenzotriazole (5.14 g, 38 mmol), and 1,3-dicyclohexylcarbodiimide (9.40 g, 45.6 mmol) were added. The solution was stirred at 0°C for 2 hours under nitrogen gas and then overnight at room temperature. Fifty milliliters of 1.0 N HCl solution was then added and the reaction mixture stirred for 20 hours. After removal of the insoluble 1,3-dicyclohexylurea by filtration, the solvent was evaporated in vacuo. The residue was dissolved in ethyl acetate, washed with 5% $NaHCO_3$ solution (5 times), dried over anhydrous sodium sulfate, and evaporated to dryness in vacuo. The solid was then crushed and dried in a vacuum dessicator.

c. Synthesis of N-Fmoc-Glycyl-Tyrosyl-Lysine(OMe)-HBr A 30-35% solution of HBr in acetic acid (63 ml) was mixed with glacial acetic acid (63 ml) and anisole (290 ml) in a 1000-ml single-neck round-bottom flask connected to a Drierite-filled drying tube, and N-Fmoc-glycyl-tyrosyl-lysine (N-ϵ-Z) methyl ester (23.60 g, 31.8 mole) was then added. The reaction mixture was stirred for 1.5 hours at room temperature. Next, dry ether was added stirring to form a precipitate. The precipitate was collected on a filter, washed with ether, and dried in a vacuum dessicator over phosphorus pentoxide.

d. Synthesis of Glycyl-Tyrosyl-Lysine-(N-ϵ)-Diethylene Triaminepentaacetic Acid DTPA mixed anhydride was prepared by modifying the procedure of Krejcarek and Tucker (3). Diethylenetriaminepentaacetic acid (16.7 g, 43 mmol) and N,N-diisopropylethylamine (37 ml, 215 mmol) were dissolved in 300 ml of water with stirring. The solution was evaporated to dryness, and 240 ml dry DMF was added. The solution was then cooled to 0°C in an ice-water bath under nitrogen gas, and isobutyl chloroformate (5.6 ml, 43 mmol) was added. The reaction mixture was stirred at 0°C for 1/2 hour. At that time a solution of Fmoc-glycyl-tyrosyl-lysine methyl ester hydrobromide (4.45 g, 6.50 mmol) and diisopropylethylamine (6 ml) in dry DMF was cooled to 0°C and added to the reaction mixture. The reaction was stirred for 1 hour at 0°C and then an additional hour at room temperature.

The reaction mixture was then evaporated in vacuo to yield an oily residue. The oil was triturated with 1.0 mM HCl solution, and the solid was collected by filtration. This crude Fmoc-glycyl-tyrosyl-lysine(OMe)-DTPA solid was dissolved in a mixture of DMF (60 ml) and 40% dimethylamine in water (60 ml), and the solution was stirred for one hour at room temperature. The crude glycyl-tyrosyl-lysine(OMe)-DTPA solution was evaporated to dryness. The residue was then dissolved in water and the aqueous solution was extracted with ethyl acetate three times. The ethyl acetate dissolved in the aqueous layer was removed in vacuo, and the glycyl-tyrosyl-lysine(OMe)-DTPA in the aqueous solution was saponified by adjusting solution to pH 12.0 with 1 N NaOH solution. The final pure product, GYK-DTPA, was isolated from the solution by using preparative

C-18 reverse phase HPLC. Elution was accomplished using a gradient of 0.1% trifluoroacetic acid and acetonitrile.

3. Preparation of Conjugate

The GYK-DTPA conjugate was prepared using the following protocol:

a. Coupling of Oxidized Antibody to GYK-DTPA Use 200 × molar excess of GYK-DTPA to antibody for coupling reaction. Use 10 mg of GYK-DTPA for 1 mg of antibody.

Calculation

1 mg Ab = 6.67×10^{-3} μmol
2000x = 13.3 μmol
13.3 μmol GYK-DTPA = 10.6 mg
GYK-DTPA MW = 795

1. Dissolve 10 mg of GYK-DTPA in 500 μl of PBS. Adjust pH to 6 with 5 N NaOH.
2. Prepare 1 ml of 100 mM $NaCHBH_3$ in PBS. Weigh 6.3 mg of $NaCNBH_3$. Dissolve both in 1 ml PBS.
3. Add GYK-DTPA solution into oxidized antibody, mix well.
4. Add 167λ of 100 mM $NaCHNB_3$ to each 1.5 ml of Ab-GYK-DTPA. Make the final concentration of $NaCNBH_3$ 10 mM.
5. Incubate the sample at room temperature overnight. Keep in dark.
6. Next morning, concentrate the sample to 1 ml.
7. Two different methods are used to remove free GYK-DTPA:
   i. G-50 column
      Prepare a 10 mM DTPA. Weigh 3.93 mg of DTPA. Add 1 ml of chelex H_2O into DTPA. Boil the tube to dissolve DTPA in H_2O.
      Prewash column with 1 ml each 10% BSA and 10 mM DTPA.
      Equilibrate column in PBS buffer, pH 6. Load sample into column.
      Collect 1 ml fraction.
      Determine antibody concentration.
   ii. FPLC-Superose 12 column
      Inject 1 ml of sample into a 20 ml Superose column.
      Collect 1 ml fraction.
      Determine antibody concentration.

After this procedure, the GYK-DTPA conjugate of the antibody can be stored at various temperatures. Although we routinely use -70°C, we have demonstrated adequate stability at 4°C. The conjugate should be sterile filtered to prevent bacterial growth.

4. ^{111}In Labeling

The GYK-DTPA conjugates are labeled using the following protocol:

1. Prepare 0.5 M sodium acetate buffer, pH 6. Weight 410 mg of sodium acetate, dissolve in 10 ml of chelex-treated H_2O. Adjust the pH to 6 with 5 μl to 10 μl of glacial acetic acid.
2. Mix equal volumes of ^{111}In and sodium acetate buffer. Different suppliers of ^{111}In provide different concentrations, and the volume of sodium acetate should be adjusted accordingly. For our initial studies we typically use 1 mCi of ^{111}In with 100–200 μg of antibody conjugate.
3. Incubate 100 μg of Ab-GYK-DTPA with ^{111}In mixture at 37°C for one hour.
4. Make a suspension of Chelex 100 in PBS buffer. Transfer 1 ml of Chelex suspension into a 1.5-ml Centrex microfilter. Spin on a table top centrifuge. Discard effluent.
5. Load In-111-Ab-GYK-DTPA into Chelex-centrex tube. Spin. Count effluent and Chelex with dose calibrator.
6. Inject 500 μl of sample into HPLC TSK-G3000SW column. Collect 1 ml fraction.
7. Count 10 μl for each fraction.
8. Calculate specific activity.
9. Prepare syringes for injection.

The injected dose can be varied depending on the experimental design; typical values are 5–10 μg of antibody and 25–50 μCi of ^{111}In.

5. Immunoreactivity Measurements

Immunoreactivity measurements were done using standard techniques (31). In general, the techniques involving direct cell binding using ^{111}In require more cells than are typically used in RIA-type assays using ^{125}I, since the antibody is at a somewhat lower specific assay. As noted in Sec. II.C.4, this can be solved by using multiple cell pellets to determine the full amount of immunoreactive fraction.

Also, it should be re-emphasized here that assays such as ELISAs tend to measure the activity of the bulk antibody preparation and may not be sensitive enough to measure the immunoreactivity of the radiolabeled conjugate. Both of these measurements are important, since if the bulk conjugate is less reactive than the native antibody, the radiolabeled preparation would also be less reactive. However, the radiolabeling itself might have an additional deleterious effect on immunoreactivity, and this should be tested if possible.

6. Preparation of Xenografts

a. 7860 Xenografts Renal cell carcinoma xenografts can be established in nude mice by the subcutaneous injection of 1×10^7 cells from culture in 0.2 ml. Up to two additional in vivo passages can be made by transplantation of tumor chunks. A donor mouse with a viable tumor of approximately 1 cm diameter is killed by cervical dislocation and the tumor is removed aseptically. The tumor is cut into 2-mm cubes. The cubes are implanted subcutaneously into anesthetized recipient mice with a trochar placed through a small incision made in the skin.

b. LS174T Xenografts Colon adenocarcinoma xenografts can be established in nude mice by the subcutaneous injection of 1×10^6 cells from culture in 0.2 ml.

7. Imaging Protocol

The imaging protocol developed in our laboratories involves the following general steps:

a. Preparation of ^{111}In-Labeled Antibody The antibody is labeled as described above to a specific activity of 1-5 μCi/μg. Typically, 5–10 μg are injected per mouse for initial studies. The antibody is loaded in syringes at a concentration of about 5 μg/ml, so that about 200 μl is injected into the mouse. Certain studies, as described in this chapter, utilize much larger doses of antibody or radioactivity.

For the biodistribution protocol described below, it is very important to take small aliquots of the injection solution for further calculations. These samples (usually triplicate 10-μl aliquots) are placed in 12 × 75 glass tubes, which are saved for counting with the dissected organs.

b. Injection into Mice The syringe containing ^{111}In labeled are injected into the mice i.v., either via tail vein or via the retroorbital venous plexus. If the latter route is used, the mice are anesthetized. It is also possible to inject the labeled conjugate intraperitoneally.

We have found it very important to quantify carefully the dose or radioactivity that is injected into the mice. The dose delivered to the animal is controlled and quantified by the following data:

1. weight of syringe before injection
2. weight of syringe after injection
3. radioactivity in syringe before injection (determined by using a dose calibrator: e.g., Capintec Model CRC-7)
4. radioactivity in syringe after injection
5. radioactivity in mouse after injection (the mouse can be placed in a small bag and put directly in the dose calibrator)

All of this data can be used to verify that the dose was injected into the mouse, and subsequent calculations can be made with confidence.

c. Imaging Images are taken at some time postinjection of the labeled antibody conjugate. Typical imaging times are 24, 48, 72, and 96 hours postinjection. The gamma camera used is a General Electric StarCam 300.

Images are taken by anesthetizing the animlas, placing them on a restrainer board, and then laying them upon the upturned head of the gamma camera. No collimation is used. Usually mice are imaged individually, although sometimes two mice are imaged together. Various imaging times have been used, but most commonly the image is obtained by collecting a standard, fixed number of counts—usually 25,000 or 50,000 counts per mouse. The image is then recorded on X-ray film using the Film Imager, and a Polaroid picture taken from the color monitor of the StarCam 300.

8. Biodistribution Protocol

After all images are taken, animals are sacrificed by cervical dislocation, and various organs dissected. The specific organs dissected from the mouse vary somewhat, depending of the nature of the experiment, but in general the typical organs are the lungs, the spleen, the liver, the kidneys, the lymph nodes, the ovaries, the stomach, the bladder, and the tumor (if appropriate). In addition, a sample of blood and muscle are taken.

The organs are dissected out of the mouse and extraneous tissue removed, and then the organs are placed in a tared 12 X 75 glass tube and weighed and the weights recorded. Some organs, because of their size (livers, for example), are weighed separately, and then a representative sample cut out, placed in a tared 12 X 75 tube, and weighed.

After all the organs have been placed in tubes and weighed, the tubes are placed in a gamma-counter and counted. The counter we use in our laboratory is an LKB Model 1274, although any calibrated counter could be used. The counts per minute (cpm) are recorded, and various ratios are calculated from these data (see Table 4). We use Lotus 1-2-3 software to store the data and to perform the calculations.

ACKNOWLEDGMENTS

The authors would like to acknowledge the excellent technical skills of Mei-Li Wen, Kurt Richau, and Jeanette Heinert, without whom this work could not have been done. We would also like to thank Carol Peevey for her excellent secretarial skills and Bev Poole for her help with the manuscript.

REFERENCES

1. Ehrlich, P. (1906) *Collected Studies on Immunity*, translated by C. Balduon. Wiley, New York.
2. Pressman, D., and Keighley, G. (1948) The zone of activity of antibodies as determined by the use of radioactive tracers; the zone of activity of nephritoxic anti-kidney serum. *J. Immunol. 59*:141.
3. Beierwaltes, W. H. (1979) The history of the use of radioactive iodine. *Sem. Nucl. Med. 9*:151.
4. Kohler, G., and Milstein, C. (1975) Continuous cultures of fused cells secreting antibody of predefined specificity. *Nature 256*:495–457.
5. Gobuty, A. H., Kim, E. E., and Weiner, R. E. (1985) Radiolabeled monoclonal antibodies: Radiochemical pharmacokinetic and clinical challenges. *J. Nucl. Med. 26*:546–547.
6. Paik, C. H., Hong, J. J., Ebbert, M. A., Heald, S. C., Reba, R. C., and Eckelman, W. C. (1985) Relative reactivity of DTPA, immunoreactive antibody-DTPA conjugates, and nonimmunoreactive antibody-DTPA conjugates toward indium-111. *J. Nucl. Med. 26*:482–487.
7. Rodwell, J. D., Alvarez, V. L., Lee, C., Lopes, A. D., Goers, J. W. F., King, H. D., Powsner, H. J., and McKearn, T. J. (1986) Site-specific covalent modification of monoclonal antibodies: *in vitro* and *in vivo* evaluations. *Proc. Natl. Acad. Sci. USA 83*:2632–2626.
8. Hnatowich, D., Layne, W., Childs, R., Lanteigne, D., Davis, M., Griffin, T., and Doherty, P. (1983) Radioactive labeling of antibody: A simple and efficient method. *Science 220*:613–615.
9. Moon, T. D., Vessella, R. L., and Lange, P. H. (1983) Monoclonal antibodies in urology. *J. Urol. 130*:584.
10. Ueda, R., Ogata, S., Morrissey, D. M., Finstad, C. L., Szudlarek, J., Whitmore, W. F., Oettgen, H. F., Lloyd, K. O., and Old, L. J. (1981) Cell surface antigens of human renal cancer defined by mouse monoclonal antibodies. Identification of tissue specific kindey glycoproteins. *Proc. Natl. Acad. Sci. USA 78*:5122–5126.
11. Williams, R. D., Elliot, A. Y., Stein, N., and Fraley, E. E. (1978) In vitro cultivation of human renal cell cancer. *In Vitro 14*:779–786.
12. Colcher, D., Hand, P., Nuti, M., and Schlom, J. A. (1981) A spectrum of monoclonal antibodies reactive with human mammary tumor cells. *Proc. Nutl. Acad. Sci. USA 78*:3199–3203.
13. Tom, B. H., Rutzky, L. P., and Jakstys, M. M. (1976) Human colonic adenocarcinoma cells I. Establishment and description of a new line. *In Vitro 12*: 180–191.
14. Beale, D., and Feinstein, A. (1976) Structure and function of the constant regions of immunoglobulins. *Q. Rev. Biophys. 9*:135–180.
15. Alvarez, V. L., Wen, M.-L., Lee, C., Lopes, A. D., Rodwell, J. D., and McKearn, T. J. (1986) Site-specifically modified 11-In labeled antibodies give low liver backgrounds and improved radioimmunoscintigraphy. *Nucl. Med. Biol. 13*:347–352.

16. Goodwin, D. A., Meares, C. F., McCall, M. J., Haseman, M. K., McTigue, M., Diamanti, C. I., and Chaovapong, W. (1985) Chelate conjugates of monoclonal antibodies for imaging lymphoid structures in the mouse. *J. Nucl. Med. 26*:493–502.
17. Colcher, D., Zalutsky, M., Kaplan, W., Kufe, D., Austin, F., and Schlom, J. (1983) Radiolocalization of human mammary tumors in athymic mice by a monoclonal antibody. *Cancer Res. 43*:736–742.
18. Colcher, D., Keenan, A. M., Larson, S. M., and Schlom, J. (1984) Prolonged binding of a radiolabeled monoclonal (B72.3) used for the in situ radioimmunodetection of human colon carcinoma xenografts. *Cancer Res. 44*: 5744–5751.
19. Halpern, S. E., Hagan, P. L., and Garver, P. R. (1983) Stability, characterization, and kinetics of 111-In-labeled monoclonal antitumor antibodies in normal animals and nude mouse-human tumor models. *Cancer Res. 43*: 5347–5355.
20. Perkins, A. C., Pimor, M. V., and Birch, M. K. (1985) The preparation and characterization of 111-In-labeled 7915/36 monoclonal antibody for tumour immunoscintigraphy. *Eur. J. Nucl. Med. 10*:296.
21. Rosenblum, M. B., Murray, J. L., Haynie, T. P., Glenn, H. J., Jahns, M. E., Benjamin, R. S., Frinke, J. M., Carlo, D. J., and Hersh, E. M. (1985) Pharmacokinetics of 111-In-labeled anti-p97 monoclonal antibody in patients with metastatic malignant melanoma. *Cancer Res. 45*:2382.
22. Bander, N. H., Welt, S., Houghton, A. N., Lloyd, K. O., Grando, R., Yeh, S., Whitmore, W. F., Vaughan, E. D., and Old, L. J. (1983) Radionuclide imaging of human renal cancer with labeled monoclonal antibodies. *Surgical Forum Urology*:652–655.
23. Vessella, R. L., Moon, T. D., Chiou, R.-K., Lange, P. H., Elson, M. K., and Shafer, R. (1984) Monoclonal antibodies to human renal cell carcinoma: Recognition of shared and restricted tissue antigens. *Can. Res. 45*:6131–6139.
24. Vessella, R. L., Alvarez, V., Chiou, R.-K., Rodwell, J., Elson, M., Palme, D., Shafer, R., and Lange, P. (1987) Radioimmunoscintigraphy and radioimmunotherapy of renal cell carcinoma xenografts. *NCI Monographs 3*:159–167.
25. Sands, H., Jones, P. L., Shah, S. A., Palme, D., Chiou, R., Vessella, R., Lange, P. H., and Gallagher, B. M. (1986) Factors affecting the uptake of monoclonal "tumor-associated" antibodies by human xenografts grown in athymic mice. *J. Nucl. Med. 27*:922.
26. Goding, J. W. (1978) *Monoclonal Antibodies: Principles and Practice.* Academic Press, London, New York.
27. Paquet, A. (1982) Introduction of 9-fluorenylmethyloxycarbonyl, trichloroethoxycarbonyl, and benzyloxycarbonyl amine protecting groups into O-unprotected hydroxy amino acids using succinimidyl carbonates. *Can. J. Chem. 60*:976–980.

28. Olah, G., and Meidar, G. (1978) Heterogenous catalysis by solid superacids: 10′ mercury impregnated nafion-H perfluorinated resinsulfonic acid catalyzed hydration of alkynes. *Synthesis*:671-672.
29. Krejcarek, G. E., and Tucker, K. L. (1977) Covalent attachment of chelating groups to macromolecules. *Biochem. Biophys. Res. Comm.* 77:581-585.
30. Kennett, R. H., McKearn, T. J., and Bechtol, K. B., Eds. (1980) *Monoclonal Antibodies*, Plenum, New York.

11

The Development of Copper-67-Labeled Porphyrin-Antibody Conjugates

JANET A. MERCER-SMITH, JEANETTE C. ROBERTS, and STEVE D. FIGARD*
Los Alamos National Laboratory, Los Alamos, New Mexico
DAVID K. LAVALLEE
Hunter College of The City University of New York, New York, New York

I. INTRODUCTION

Radiolabeled monoclonal antibodies and antibody fragments have received much attention in recent years because of their potential for utilization in tumor imaging and internal radiation therapy. Monoclonal antibodies and their fragments enable the selective targeting of tumors. The labeled antibodies could be employed as carrier to transport radioisotopes to tumors (1), thus minimizing the total body radiation dose and radiation damage to normal tissue. Since the time required for labeled antibodies to localize at their antigenic sites and deliver the dose to the tumor is estimated to be of the order of one to three days (2), radionuclides with a one- to three-day half-life would be optimum for this purpose (2,3).

Current research efforts in radiolabeling antibodies frequently use bifunctional metal chelating agents. The bifunctional chelating agents serve two purposes: (1) formation of a covalent bond to link the chelating agent to the antibody, and (2) complexation of a radiometal. The bifunctional chelating agents should (1)

**Current Affiliation:* Abbot Laboratories, Abbot Park, Illinois have functional group(s) suitable for conjugation to the antibody to form a covalent bond that will be stable in vivo, (2) complex the desired radiometal readily, (3) retain the metal radionuclide with minimal loss in vivo, (4) be relatively nontoxic, and (5) have little or no effect on the immunologic competence of the antibody. Two chelating agents, ethylenediaminetetraacetic acid (EDTA) and diethylenetriaminepentaacetic acid (DTPA), and their derivatives, are often used as bifunctional chelating agents because they readily form chelates with a large variety of metal ions. However, many of the radiometal chelates formed from these chelating agents are not stable enough to prevent transcomplexation to serum proteins, such as transferrin or conalbumin. For example, ^{111}InDTPA-labeled antibodies have been reported to have 9% per day in vivo transcomplexation to transferrin (4,5), and ^{67}CuDTPA-antibody conjugates had a 95% loss during 24 hours in vitro in human serum (6). Thus bifunctional chelating agents which form extremely stable chelates with radiometals are needed.

We have developed new bifunctional chelating agents to label antibodies with copper-67 (^{67}Cu), a potentially useful medical radioisotope. Copper-67 has a suitable half-life (62 hours) and nuclear decay properties (7,8) for use in tumor imaging and therapy. Table 1 lists the nuclear decay properties of ^{67}Cu. This radioisotope is produced in high specific activity (15,000 Ci/g) at the Los Alamos Meson Physics Facility (LAMPF).

We selected porphyrins as ^{67}Cu chelating agents to be conjugated to antibodies for two reasons: (1) Metalloporphyrins, which are ubiquitous in nature, present little problem of toxicity, and (2) copper porphyrins are very stable to loss of copper ions. Naturally occurring porphyrins complex a variety of metals. Iron porphyrins are present in hemoglobin, myoglobin, and many of the cytochromes. Magnesium porphyrin derivatives are present in the chlorophylls and bacteriochlorophylls. Copper porphyrins are found in the feather pigments of some birds. The nonmetalated porphyrins have found use in tumor photother-

Table 1 ^{67}Cu Nuclear Decay Properties

$T_{1/2}$	Decay mode (%)	Particle energies (%)	Gamma transitions
61.7 hr	β-(100)	182 keV (1)	91 keV (7.8)
		392 keV (56)	93 keV (31.8)
		484 keV (23)	184 keV (48.0)
		576 keV (20)	209 keV (0.1)
			300 keV (0.7)
			309 keV (0.2)

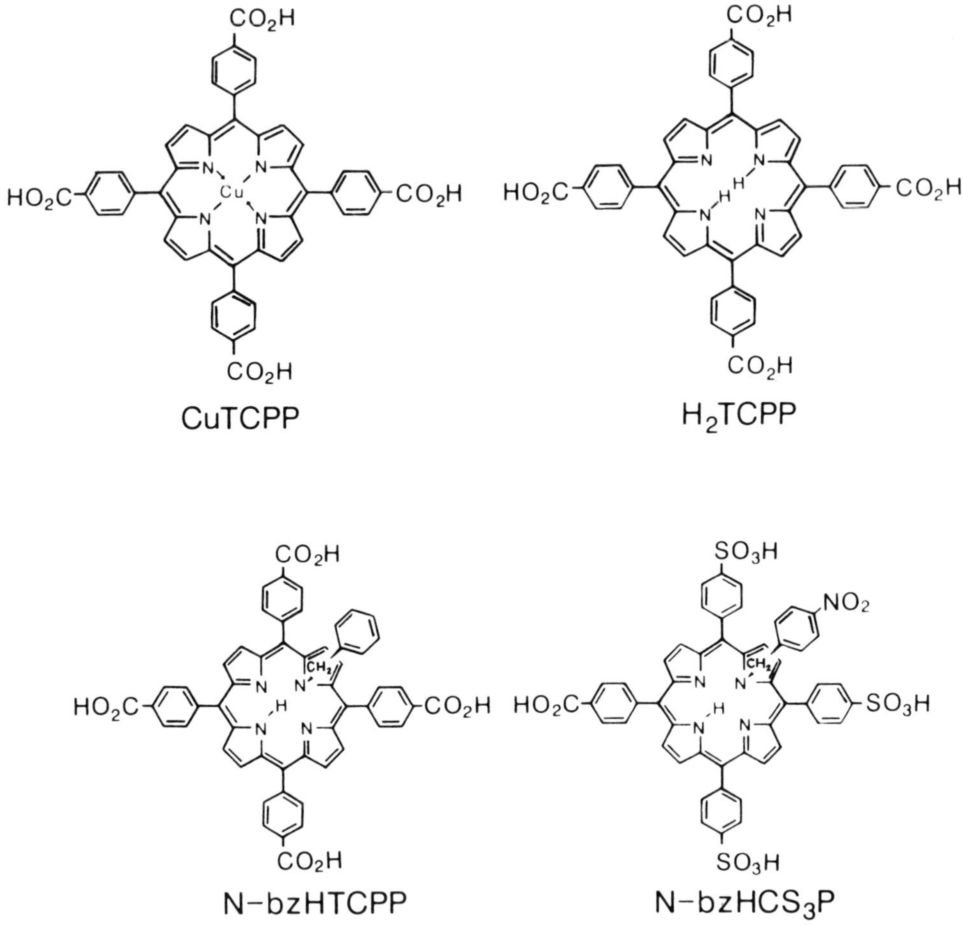

Figure 1 Structure of porphyrins. CuTCPP: 5,10,15,20-tetrakis(4-carboxyphenyl) porphinato copper(II); H_2TCPP: 5,10,15,20-tetrakis(4-carboxyphenyl) porphine; N-bzHTCPP: N-benzyl-5,10,15,20-tetrakis(4-carboxyphenyl) porphine; N-bzHCS_3P: N-4-nitrobenzyl-5-(4-carboxyphenyl)-10,15,20-tris(4-sulfophenyl) porphine.

apy in much larger quantities (9) than would be used for imaging or for radiotherapy. Thus porphyrins should not present a problem of toxicity if they become detached from the antibody in vivo. Copper porphyrins are reported to be extremely stable to loss of the copper dication from the chelate. For example, radiocopper does not exchange with copper porphyrin derivatives during two days in 80% acetone (10), and 100% sulfuric acid is required to remove copper from copper porphyrins (11). Our experiments described herein with copper porphyrins under simulated physiological conditions support these findings. The structures of the porphyrins described in this work are shown in Figure 1.

The objective of our research is to develop "cold kit" methods to attach ^{67}Cu to monoclonal antibodies and antibody fragments by using porphyrins as chelating agents. The "cold kits" would be composed of preformed porphyrin-antibody conjugates that could be radiometalated with ^{67}Cu immediately before use. The ^{67}Cu would be employed to radiolabel porphyrin–antibody conjugates rather than to radiolabel porphyrins that would subsequently be coupled to antibodies. Therefore, loss of the specific activity of ^{67}Cu would be minimized.

In this chapter we report two methods of general utility to form a covalent bond linking N-benzyl-substituted porphyrins to antibodies. The N-benzyl porphyrins are activated for ease of radiometalation with ^{67}Cu; the N-benzyl porphyrin-antibody conjugates can be radiolabeled with $^{67}CuCl_2$ under mild reaction conditions. We also report the stability of the ^{67}Cu porphyrin in human serum under simulated physiological conditions. Our studies of the immunoreactivity of the ^{67}Cu porphyrin–antibody conjugates indicate that little loss of immunoreactivity occurs during the preparation of the radiolabeled conjugates. Thus these studies demonstrate the potential for the development of "cold kits" to prepare ^{67}Cu-labeled antibodies.

II. RESULTS AND DISCUSSION

A. Preparation of Copper-67 Chloride

Copper-67 is produced at LAMPF by a (p,x) spallation reaction on zinc oxide targets. Irradiation of the target in the primary proton beam of 600 to 800 MeV protons at a current of 1 mA produces 2 to 4 Ci of ^{67}Cu after 5 to 7 days of irradiation. The ^{67}Cu is produced in high specific activity, typically 15,000 Ci/g. The spallation reaction produces not only ^{67}Cu: Other spallation reactions also create a variety of isotopes of lighter mass than zinc. The large amount of the target material (70 g) and the presence of isotopes of other elements complicate the purification of ^{67}Cu from the target. In addition, the level of radioactivity is so high that remote handling hot cells must be used to provide adequate shielding during processing of the irradiated targets.

The ^{67}Cu is purified by a series of electrochemical platings that reduce Cu(II) to metallic copper on a platinum working electrode, followed by electrochemical strippings that oxidize the metallic copper deposited on the electrode to Cu(II). This sequence of electrochemical reductions and oxidations serve to isolate ^{67}Cu from zinc in the target material and the other isotopes produced by spallation reactions. The use of an anion exchange column after the electrochemical procedure has been completed further reduces the concentration of entrained zinc. Zinc forms a negatively charged chloride complex, which is retained by the column material, but copper passes through the column. Analysis of the purified ^{67}Cu solution by plasma emission spectroscopy indicates that the final concentration of zinc is in the part per million range, while the concentration of other metals is even lower. Because the 2 M HCl solution of $^{67}CuCl_2$ obtained from the anion exchange column is not suitable for porphyrin metalation, the HCl solution is evaporated to dryness. The $^{67}CuCl_2$ is redissolved in a more suitable solvent (dimethylformamide (DMF) or aqueous buffer) before use.

B. Synthesis and Metalation of N-Benzyl Porphyrins

The remarkable ability of porphyrins to retain bound copper ion and the great stability of synthetic porphyrin ring systems against degradation make them desirable chelators for ^{67}Cu. However, a major drawback to the use of porphyrins has been the slow rates at which the relatively inflexible, planar porphyrins incorporate metal ions. Although copper (II) is one of the most rapidly incorporated metal ions, the metalation rate in aqueous solutions in the pH and temperature range that antibodies are stable is too slow to make the reactions of ^{67}Cu with a protein-linked porphyrin feasible. The only route available for typical porphyrins is the synthesis of the ^{67}Cu complex in refluxing DMF and purification (12), followed by coupling of the radiolabeled porphyrin complex to the antibody. In order to achieve the rapid metal complexation rates that are necessary for a procedure in which a prepurified porphyrin–antibody conjugate could be labeled with ^{67}Cu immediately before use, the porphyrin itself must be synthetically modified.

We have previously shown that N-substitution of synthetic porphyrins of the *meso*-tetraaryl type leads to greatly increased metal complexation rates and that the rate is especially favorable in the case of Cu(II) (13). However, after the Cu(II) ion is bound, the N-substituent must be removed to give a highly stable porphyrin complex because metal ions are readily removed from the N-substituted metalloporphyrins (14). Simple N-substituents, such as a methyl group, are not removed by water as a nucleophile under mild conditions but require such strong nucleophiles as amines (15). The strong nucleophiles necessary to remove the N-methyl substituent require reaction conditions too harsh to be used for porphyrin-antibody conjugates. Recently we have shown that N-

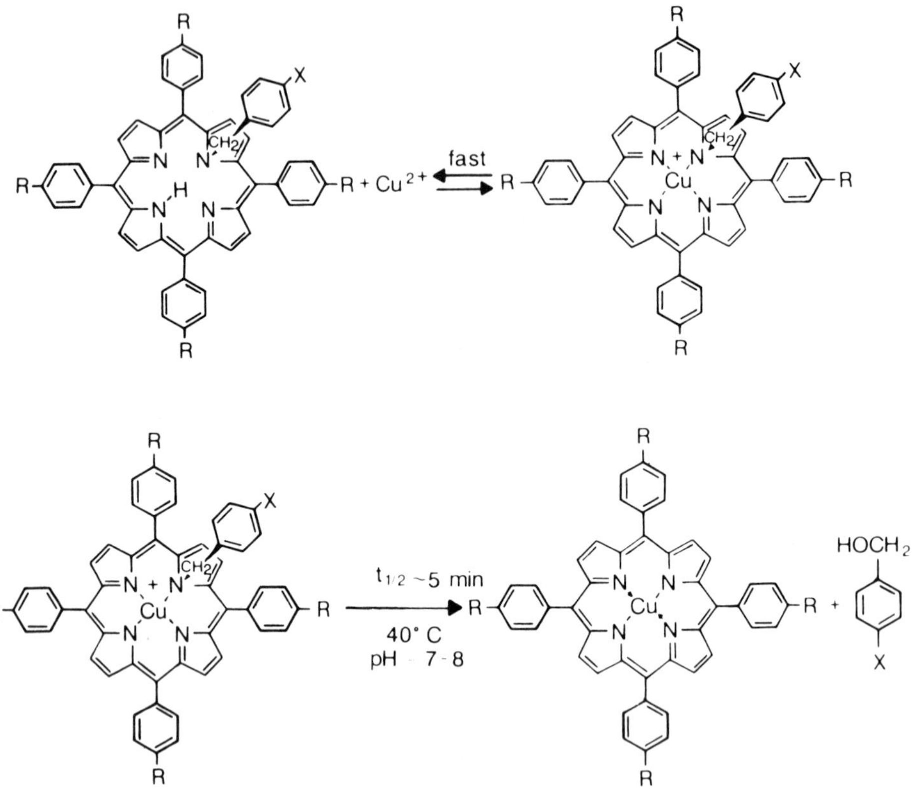

Figure 2 Mechanism of the metalation reaction of N-benzyl porphyrins. N-bzHTCPP: R = CO_2H, X = H; N-bzHCS$_3$P: R = SO_3H, X = NO_2.

benzyl substituents are more easily removed (16). The rate for the overall reaction of metal complexation and N-benzyl group removal in buffered aqueous solution is rapid and independent of Cu(II) concentration (17). The metalation reaction mechanism for the N-benzyl porphyrins is shown in Figure 2.

Thus, the synthetic objective for our study was a water-soluble, N-benzyl-substituted synthetic porphyrin, which could be readily coupled to an antibody. Since the coupling of a carboxylate to an amine site on a protein is a common strategy, the molecule of choice was N-benzyl-5,10,15,20-tetrakis(4-carboxyphenyl) porphine, N-bzHTCPP (Fig. 1). This porphyrin was synthesized in the following stages (shown in Fig. 3): (1) synthesis of benzyldiphenylsulfonium tetrafluoroborate from benzyl alcohol and phenyl sulfide in methanesulfonic acid, followed by reaction with tetrafluoroboric acid; (2) condensation of 4-

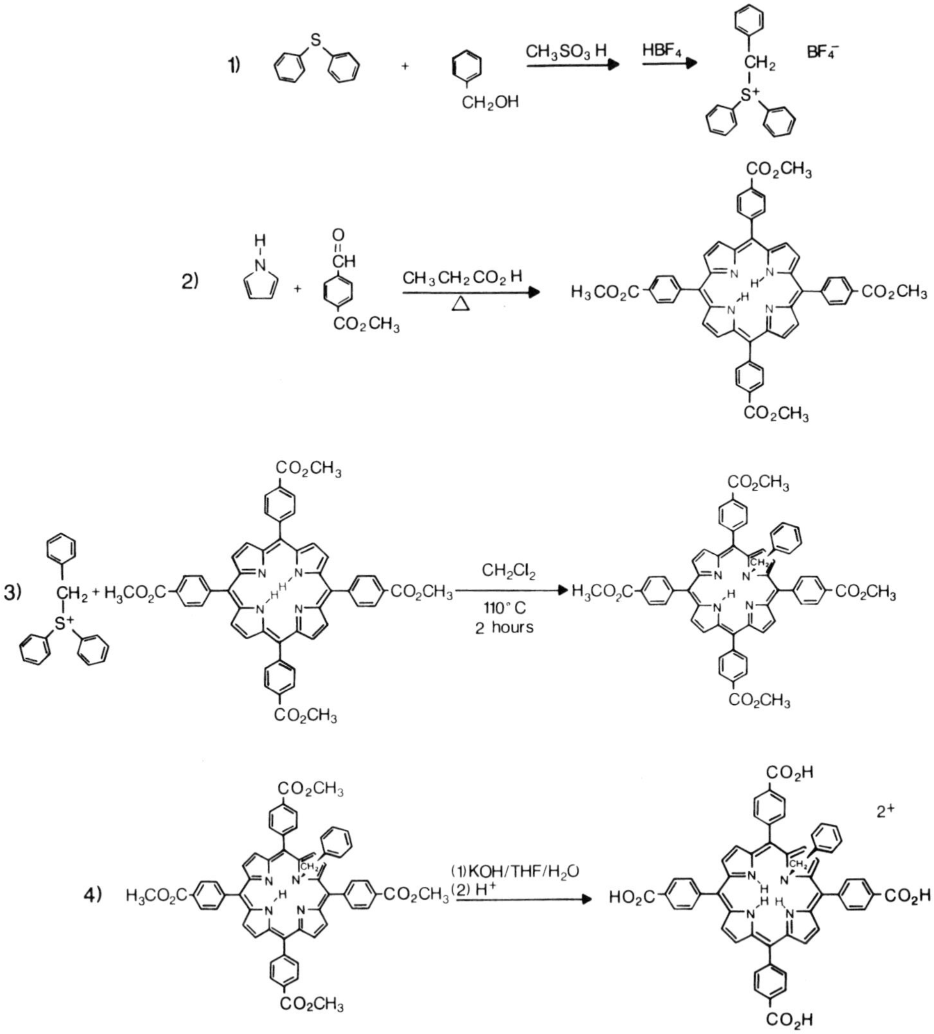

Figure 3 Synthesis of N-bzHTCPP.

Table 2 Electronic Spectral Properties of N-Benzyl Porphyrins

Porphyrin[a]	Absorption maxima (nm)	Log extinction coefficient
N-bzHTCPP	676	3.79
	618 (sh)	–
	578	4.23
	536	4.00
	431	5.18
N-bzHTCPP[b]	695	3.79
	604	4.26
	439	5.22
N-bzH_2TCPP$^+$	669	4.01
	613	4.01
	574	4.02
	433	5.24
N-bzH_3TCPP^{2+}	680	–
	458	–
N-bzHCS_3P	677	3.83
	594	4.16
	544	3.94
	436	4.77
	414	4.72
N-bzH_2CS_3P$^+$	677	4.03
	630	3.94
	441	5.58
	419	5.44
N-bzH_3CS_3P^{2+}	683	4.47
	450	5.25

[a]The spectra were obtained by titration in methanol.
[b]The spectrum was obtained in aqueous 3 M NaOH.

formylmethylbenzoate and pyrrole to form 5,10,15,20-tetrakis(4-methylcarboxyphenyl) porphine; (3) reaction with benzyldiphenylsulfonium tetrafluoroborate to form the N-benzyl derivative; and (4) hydrolysis of the ester in base. The electronic spectral properties of this porphyrin in various degrees of pyrrole nitrogen protonation are presented in Table 2. The degree of protonation affects the ease of metalation of the porphyrin, as well as the optical spectrum. When N-bzH_3TCPP^{2+} is dissolved in acid solution (pH < 4), it retains both of the additional protons, giving a characteristic visible absorption spectrum of a diprotonated N-substituted porphyrin. With both protons present, it is unreactive towards Cu(II). In addition, protonation of all the 4-carboxyphenyl groups at low pH results in low solubility (the spectrum was obtained in acidic methanol). When dissolved in unbuffered water, it retains only one of the additional protons. Since the carboxyl groups are unprotonated, the solubility is increased. In this pH range, the equilibrium of the monoprotonated and free base forms of the porphyrin appears to be sufficient to allow rapid metal ion complexation. (Typically, only the free base form of a porphyrin is capable of binding metal ions (18)). In buffered media with pH greater than 7 and in highly alkaline media (e.g., 0.1 M aqueous NaOH), the same visible absorption spectrum, that of the free base form, is observed.

The four carboxylate groups of the N-bzHTCPP molecule present the potential problem of cross-linking to amine groups on a single antibody or of cross-linking between antibodies. Therefore, we decided to synthesize and study a synthetic N-benzyl porphyrin that would have several peripheral anionic groups to provide water solubility, but only a single carboxylate group that could be used for coupling to the antibody. The reactions to synthesize N-4-nitrobenzyl-5-(4-carboxyphenyl)–10,15,20-tris(4-sulfophenyl) porphine, N-bzHCS_3P (Fig.1), are shown in Figure 4. The first step consists of the formation of 5-(4-methylcarboxyphenyl)-10,15,20,-triphenylporphine by condensation of 4-formylmethylbenzoate, benzaldehyde, and pyrrole in a 1:3:4 ratio. Because the condensation method forms porphyrins with various combinations of unsubstituted phenyl and 4-methylcarboxyphenyl groups, the desired porphyrin (the monoester) was isolated and purified by flash chromatography prior to the remaining synthetic steps. The N-benzylation of the porphyrin by diphenyl-4-nitrobenzylsulfonium tetrafluoroborate can form two different porphyrins, N-4-nitrobenzyl-5-(4-carboxyphenyl)-10,15,20-triphenylporphine and N-4-nitrobenzyl-5-[4-(4-nitrobenzyl)carboxyphenyl] -10,15,20-triphenylporphine, depending upon whether or not the porphyrin monoester from step 1 is hydrolyzed before the initiation of step 2. When 5-(4-methylcarboxyphenyl)-10,15,20-triphenylporphine is the starting material, N-4-nitrobenzyl-5-(4-methylcarboxyphenyl)-10,15,20-triphenylporphine is prepared by substitution of one of the pyrrole protons. (This is shown in the second step in Figure 4). Alternatively, the porphyrin free acid 5-(4-carboxyphenyl)-10,15,20-triphenylporphine (formed by basic hydrolysis of the monoester prepared in step 1), can be employed as the starting material in step 2. In this case, two equivalents of diphenyl-4-nitrobenzylsulfonium tetrafluoroborate must be used because the free acid is converted to the 4-nitrophenyl ester under conditions where N-substitution on the pyrrole occurs. These reactions form N-4-nitrobenzyl-5-[4-(4-nitrobenzyl)carboxyphenyl] -10,15,20-triphenylporphine. In step 3, concentrated sulfuric acid treatment of either of the porphyrins formed in step 2 causes (a) addition of sulfonate groups to the 4-phenyl positions to give water solubility and (b) hydrolysis of the ester to give

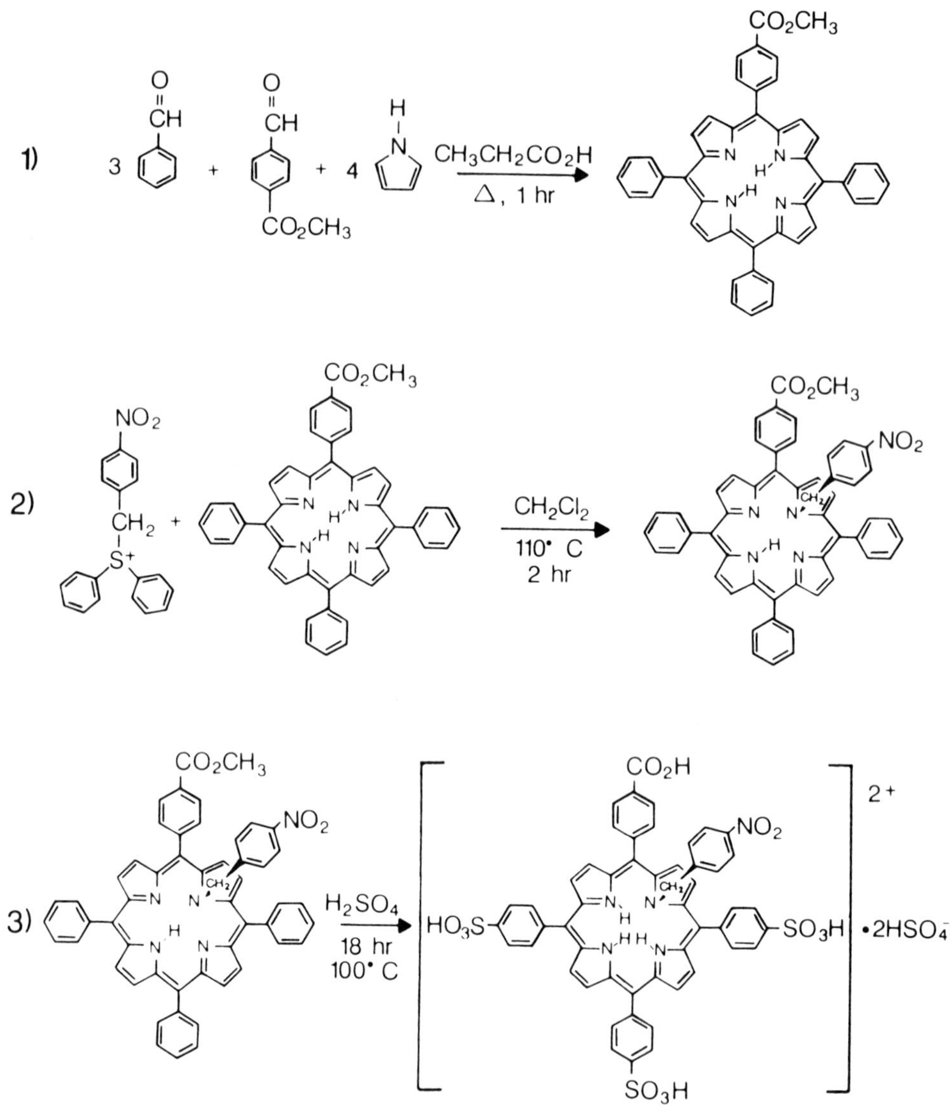

Figure 4 Synthesis of N-bzHCS$_3$P.

the free carboxylate group for conjugation. The sulfuric acid treatment was found to cause elimination of N-substituted benzyl or 4-methylbenzyl groups, but the presence of the 4-nitro group prevents elimination. The porphyrin macrocycle is stable under these reaction conditions. The diprotonated species of the trisulfonated porphyrin, as well as the species of other degrees of protonation, are water-soluble. The electronic spectral characteristics of these species are reported in Table 2.

C. Metalation of N-Benzyl Porphyrins

In borate buffer at pH 8.0, the progress of the reaction of Cu(II) with N-bzHTCPP can be followed spectrophotometrically. With the porphyrin concentration at 10^{-5} to 10^{-3} M and Cu(II) concentrations from 10^{-5} to 10^{-2} M, the half-life for the reaction at 40°C is less than five minutes and is independent of Cu(II) concentration, demonstrating that metal complexion is faster than debenzylation (17). With ^{67}Cu at less than 10^{-6} M (no carrier added) and other conditions as above, ion exchange after separation shows that 95% or more of the ^{67}Cu is incorporated after 10 minutes. The results with cold Cu(II) and free N-bzHTCPP support the results described herein, which indicate rapid binding of ^{67}Cu to N-benzyl porphyrin polyclonal immunoglobulin G (IgG)-antibody conjugates.

D. Serum Stability Studies of CuTCPP

We have developed a method to determine the serum stability of metalloporphyrins and have applied it to 5,10,15,20-tetrakis(4-carboxyphenyl) porphinato copper (II), CuTCPP (Fig. 1). An examination of metalloporphyrin stability in the presence of serum requires special considerations, since porphyrins are known to bind noncovalently to proteins—the "sticky porphyrin" problem. In particular, porphyrins (including CuTCPP) will bind to human serum albumin (19), a protein that binds copper nonspecifically (20). Porphyrins also bind to low density lipoproteins (21). We have observed noncovalent binding of CuTCPP to polyclonal rabbit IgG (RIgG); removal of CuTCPP from IgG by size exclusion high performance liquid chromatography (HPLC) on a TSK Biosil 250 or 400 column is not quantitative. The binding of both copper and porphyrins to albumin would make it impossible to use radiocopper-labeled porphyrins and analyze the proteins binding copper by size exclusion chromatography. This is because these chromatographic methods could not distinguish between loss of copper from the porphyrin with subsequent binding of copper to protein and CuTCPP binding to protein. The fluorescence method which we have developed to determine the stability of metalloporphyrins relies on the fact that copper porphyrins do not fluoresce, whereas nonmetalated porphyrins do fluoresce

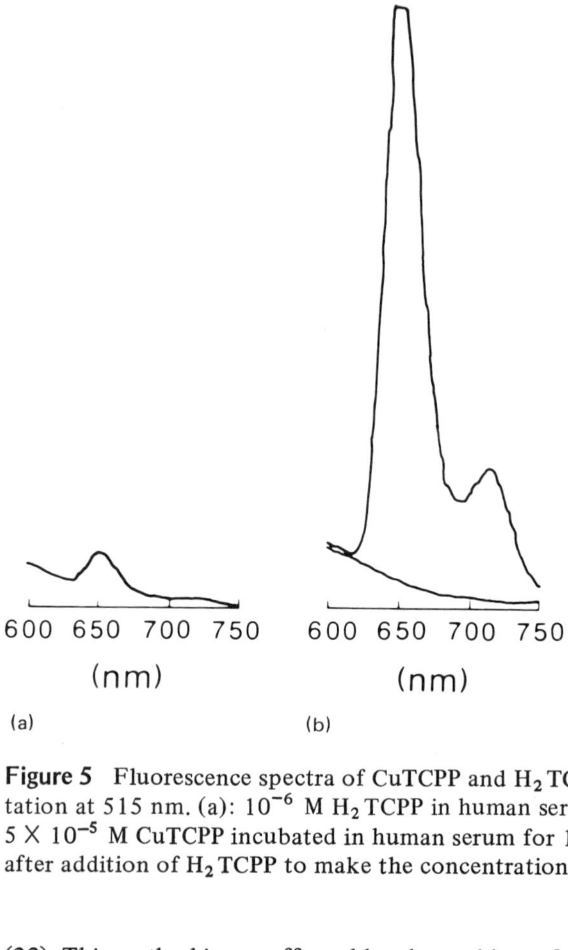

Figure 5 Fluorescence spectra of CuTCPP and H_2TCPP in human serum, excitation at 515 nm. (a): 10^{-6} M H_2TCPP in human serum. (b): bottom spectrum: 5×10^{-5} M CuTCPP incubated in human serum for 12 days. Top spectrum: after addition of H_2TCPP to make the concentration of H_2TCPP 1.4×10^{-5} M.

(22). This method is not affected by the problem of porphyrins binding to proteins and can be used with challengers other than proteins, such as EDTA, since the proteins and simple chelating agents absorb light and fluoresce at shorter wavelengths than do the porphyrins. The fluorescence technique can detect as little as one percent conversion of CuTCPP to the nonmetalated porphyrin, 5,10, 15,20-tetrakis(4-carboxyphenyl) porphine, H_2TCPP (Fig. 1).

We have used the fluorescence technique to determine the stability of CuTCPP in human serum as well as in the presence of human serum albumin, EDTA, and DTPA. CuTCPP was incubated with each of the challengers for 12 days. The fluorescence of each of the CuTCPP challenger solutions was measured. In addition, the UV-visible spectra of the incubated CuTCPP–challenger solutions was compared with freshly prepared solutions to determine whether decomposition of CuTCPP, transcomplexation with other metal ions, or conversion to H_2TCPP had occurred. The fluorescence spectra of H_2TCPP and of CuTCPP in human serum are shown in Figure 5. No loss of copper from the porphyrin could be detected in the presence of any of the challengers, nor did the UV-visible absorption spectrum of CuTCPP show any decomposition of CuTCPP or conversion to H_2TCPP. Thus copper porphyrins are quite stable under simulated physiological conditions in human serum.

E. Conjugation of N-Benzyl Porphyrins to Antibodies

1. Analysis and Purification of N-Benzyl Porphyrin–Antibody Conjugates

The "sticky porphyrin" problem presents special considerations for analytical methods to determine the amount of conjugation of N-benzyl porphyrins to antibodies. Size exclusion HPLC cannot be used, since porphyrins will bind noncovalently to antibodies and thus will be eluted with antibodies, even when conjugation has not occurred. In addition, quantitative measurement of the amount of antibody and porphyrin in a conjugate can be difficult, since the porphyrin electronic absorption bands interfere with many common colorimetric determinations of protein concentration that use dyes. We have found sodium dodecylsulfate polyacrylamide gel electrophoresis (SDS-PAGE) under nonreducing conditions using the Laemmli buffer system (23) to be a useful analytical method to separate noncovalently bound N-benzyl porphyrin from IgG and N-benzyl porphyrin–IgG conjugates. Because we use quartz tubes for SDS-PAGE, the gels can be scanned at 280 nm for the antibody absorbance and at 435 nm for the N-benzyl porphyrin absorbance. The area under the peaks is then integrated to determine the coupling yields based on porphyrin content. The SDS-PAGE method is effective for the determination of coupling yields for N-bzHTCPP- or N-bzHCS$_3$P-antibody conjugates. When the porphyrin–antibody conjugates have been metalated with ^{67}Cu, the gels are removed from the tubes, sliced, and counted for ^{67}Cu activity.

The N-bzHTCPP–antibody conjugates can be purified on a preparative scale by chromatography of the conjugation reaction mixture on Sephadex G25 columns at very slow flow rates. This method removes more than 99% of the uncoupled N-bzHTCPP from the conjugates, as determined by analysis on SDS-PAGE as described above. An average of 89% of the antibody is recovered following this method of purification. However, this chromatographic method is not as effective in removing uncoupled N-bzHCS$_3$P from conjugates; 60 to 75% of the unconjugated N-bzHCS$_3$P was removed by chromatography on Sephadex G25. Other methods of purification (i.e., size exclusion HPLC on TSK Biosil 250 or 400 columns, electrophoretic concentration, and ion exchange chroma-

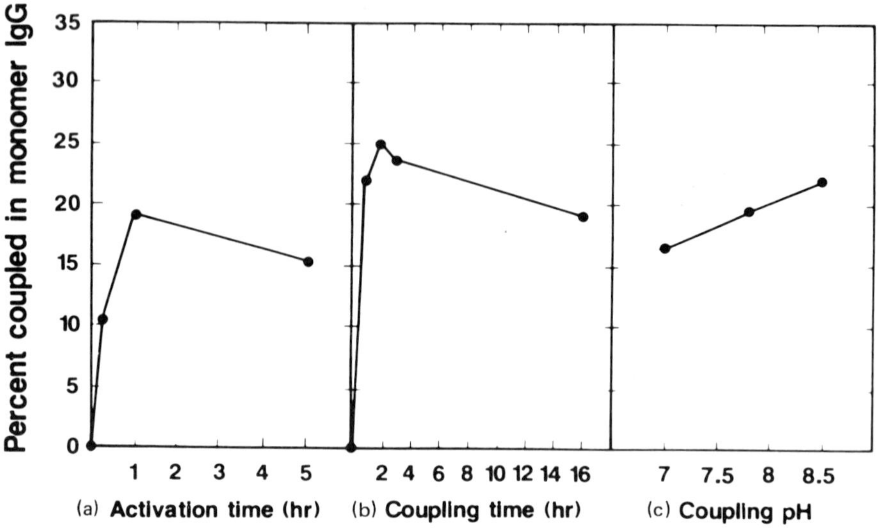

Figure 6 Optimization of the EDAC/NHS coupling method for N-bzHTCPP. (a) Activation time optimization at 16 hours coupling and pH 8.5; (b) coupling time optimization at one hour activation and pH 8.5; (c) pH optimization at one hour activation and one hour coupling. Antibody: N-bzHTCPP:EDAC: NHS molar ratio = 1:10:10:10 for all points. Results are expressed as the average of two determinations.

tography on DEAE sepharose) were less successful in removing free N-bzHTCPP or N-bzHCS$_3$P from the corresponding porphyrin–antibody conjugates.

2. Conjugation Methods

We examined two methods, which are commonly used to form amide bonds between carboxylate groups and the lysine residues of proteins, to attach the carboxylic acid functionality of N-benzyl porphyrins to polyclonal RIgG. (Polyclonal IgG has been used in the developmental phase of this study in order to develop a general method of conjugation and purification of IgG-porphyrin conjugates.) Both conjugation methods involve formation of an activated carboxylate on the N-benzyl porphyrin prior to addition of the antibody. The conjugation methods used were based on modifications of the two-step method of Davis and Preston (24). The two methods studied for the conjugation reaction were the following: (1) formation of an activated carboxylate of the N-benzyl porphyrin by reaction with N-hydroxysuccinimide (NHS) in the presence of 1-ethyl-3-(3′-dimethylaminopropyl) carbodiimide hydrochloride (EDAC), followed by conjugation with IgG (25); and (2) formation of an activated carboxylate of the N-benzyl porphyrin via reaction with 1,1′-carbonyldiimidazole (CDI) prior to conjugation with IgG (26). Both of these methods were optimized for conjugation of N-bzHTCPP to RIgG, then these optimized protocols were applied to conjugation reactions using antibodies derived from a variety of species.

The optimization studies for the EDAC/NHS reaction to couple N-bzHTCPP to antibody are shown in Figure 6. The antibody:N-bzHTCPP:EDAC:NHS molar ratio found to be optimum was 1:10:10:10. The activation step to form the porphyrin succinimidyl ester appeared to be complete after one hour of reaction of porphyrin with EDAC/NHS. Higher concentrations of EDAC/NHS relative to the antibody and N-bzHTCPP did not increase the coupling reaction yield. The coupling yield reached a maximum after one hour of reaction to form the covalent bond linking the porphyrin to the antibody. There was a slight increase in coupling efficiency as the coupling pH increased from pH 7 to 8.5. The optimized coupling protocol for EDAC/NHS with N-bzHTCPP was determined to be one hour activation and one hour coupling time at pH 8.5.

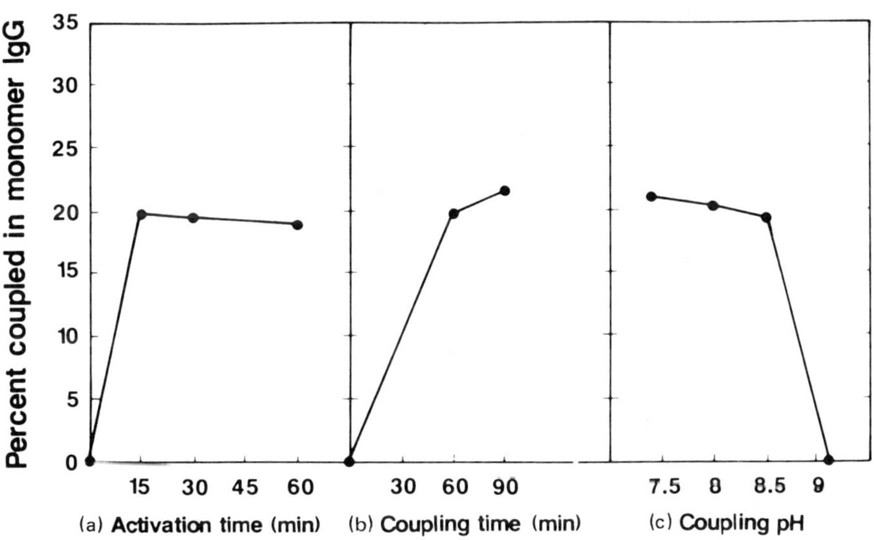

Figure 7 Optimization of the CDI coupling method for N-bzHTCPP. (a) Activatin time optimization at one hour coupling and pH 8.5; (b) coupling time optimization at 30 minutes activation and pH 8.0; (c) pH optimization at 30 minutes activation and 90 minutes coupling. Antibody:N-bzHTCPP:CDI molar ratio = 1:10:10 for all points. Results are expressed as the average of two determinations.

The optimization studies of the CDI coupling method for N-bzHTCPP are shown in Figure 7. The antibody:N-bzHTCPP:CDI molar ratio found to be optimum was 1:10:10. The activation step to form the porphyrin imidazolide by reaction with CDI was faster than the comparable activation step for the EDAC/NHS reaction. The activation step using CDI was essentially complete after 15 minutes of reaction. However, the optimum coupling time to form the amide bond with the antibody was similar to that of the EDAC/NHS method, approximately 60 to 90 minutes. A small increase in coupling efficiency was seen as the pH of the coupling reaction decreased from 8.5 to 7.5. At pH 9, the coupling yield dropped to zero, probably due to immediate hydrolysis of the imidazolide. The protocol found to be optimum for the CDI reaction was a 15-minute activation step, followed by a 90-minute coupling time at pH 7.5 to 8.0.

Cross-linking of the antibody with N-bzHTCPP was observed because this porphyrin has four carboxylate functional groups. Apparently, more than one carboxylate group per porphyrin is activated by either of these coupling methods. Cross-linking was especially evident at a high ratio of CDI to porphyrin and antibody (1:10:100 molar ratio of antibody:N-bzHTCPP:CDI). There was a slight increase in overall conjugation at this molar ratio, but that increase was due to formation of cross-linked antibody. The EDAC/NHS method produced a lower amount of cross-linked material at the higher coupling agent molar ratio (1:10:100:100 molar ratio of antibody:N-bzHTCPP:EDAC:NHS) than did the CDI method. The maximum coupling for both EDAC/NHS and CDI optimized protocols was approximately two porphyrins per IgG monomer, as shown in Table 3.

These two conjugation reactions have similar mechanisms, because an activated carboxylate on the porphyrin is formed as a reactive intermediate prior to the addition of antibody to form the amide bond. In the case of the EDAC/NHS reaction, an activated succinimidyl ester is formed; in the CDI method an activated amide, the imidazolide, is formed. Although some cross-linking occurs for N-bzHTCPP, this cross-linking can be reduced by modification of the reaction conditions to use a small molar ratio of coupling reagent to N-bzHTCPP and antibody (1:10:10 molar ratio of antibody:N-bzHTCPP:coupling reagent). While the two conjugation methods give similar coupling yields under optimized conditions and have approximately the same total reaction time, there is an advantage to the EDAC/NHS method—this method is not moisture-sensitive. The CDI method suffers from the extreme sensitivity of CDI to water. CDI decomposes very rapidly on contact with water; however, the intermediate acylimidazole formed from the reaction with a carboxylate is stable to hydrolysis for short periods of time (26). Therefore, glassware used in the activation step of the CDI method, and the solvent, DMF, must be well dried to prevent decreases in the coupling yields. Thus both of these conjugation methods are useful for coval-

Table 3 Conjugation of N-Benzyl Porphyrins to Antibodies Derived from Various Species

Antibody	Porphyrin	Coupling method[a]	Coupling yield (%)[b]	Porphyrins/ Antibody
Rabbit IgG	N-bzHTCPP	EDAC/NHS	22	2.2
Rabbit IgG	N-bzHCS$_3$P	EDAC/NHS	20	2.0
Rabbit IgG	N-bzHTCPP	CDI	24	2.4
Mouse IgG	N-bzHTCPP	EDAC/NHS	21	2.1
Mouse IgG	N-bzHTCPP	CDI	18	1.8
Goat IgG	N-bzHTCPP	EDAC/NHS	20	2.0
Goat IgG	N-bzHTCPP	CDI	19	1.9
Human IgG	N-bzHTCPP	EDAC/NHS	21	2.1
Human IgG	N-bzHTCPP	CDI	24	2.4
Rat IgG	N-bzHTCPP	EDAC/NHS	18	1.8
Rat IgG	N-bzHTCPP	CDI	18	1.8

[a]Coupling conditions can be found in the Appendix.
[b]Coupling yield is based on starting porphyrin.

ently attaching N-benzyl porphyrins to antibodies, but the EDAC/NHS method is simpler and more reporducible in practice.

3. Conjugation of N-benzyl Porphyrins to Antibodies Derived from a Variety of Species

Our goal is to develop methods which can be used to attach N-benzyl porphyrins to a variety of antibodies. Therefore, we have examined the coupling of N-benzyl porphyrins to antibodies derived from a variety of species. The optimized conjugation conditions developed for RIgG were applied to conjugation reactions using antibodies from other species. The conjugation data are shown in Table 3.

The coupling yields were quite similar for each coupling method regardless of the species of origin of the antibodies. Of special interest are the human and mouse antibody coupling yields, since antibodies of these species are used in hybridoma technology to prepare monoclonal antibodies. In addition, the coupling yields were quite similar for both conjugation methods. The two N-benzyl porphyrins studied, N-bzHTCPP and N-bzHCS$_3$P, gave similar coupling yields for the conjugation to RIgG. These results indicate that both conjugation methods would be generally useful for coupling porphyrins to a wide variety of antibodies.

Table 4 Location of N-bzHTCPP on the Antibody Surface[a]

Coupling method[a]	% N-bzHTCPP Attached			
	Heavy chain	Light chain	$F(ab')_2$	pFc′
EDAC/NHS	64	36	77	23
CDI	66	34	63	37

[a]Experimental details can be found in the Appendix.

4. Location of the Porphyrin on the Antibody

The relative location of attachment of N-bzHTCPP to nonspecific RIgG was determined after two different methods of cleavage of the N-bzHTCPP-RIgG conjugates: (1) pepsin digestion to form $F(ab')_2$ and pFc′ fragments, and (2) treatment with 2-mercaptoethanol to separate the light and heavy chains. The fragments were analyzed by SDS-PAGE to determine where the N-bzHTCPP had been attached. N-bzHTCPP-RIgG conjugates formed by both coupling methods were each examined. The results are shown in Table 4.

The $F(ab')_2$ and pFc′ fragments obtained from the conjugates formed by the two different conjugation methods each showed attachment of N-bzHTCPP. However, the N-bzHTCPP–RIgG conjugates prepared by the EDAC/NHS method had a slightly greater amount of N-bzHTCPP attached to the $F(ab')_2$ fragment than did the N-bzHTCPP–RIgG conjugates formed by the CDI method. N-bzHTCPP attachment was detected on both the heavy and light chains of the antibody. The conjugates prepared by the two different coupling methods showed little difference in the relative amounts of N-bzHTCPP attached to the heavy and light chains of RIgG.

Both of the methods of fragmentation and analysis of N-bzHTCPP–RIgG indicate the random nature of coupling of N-bzHTCPP to antibody; there does not appear to be any site-directed conjugation. While covalent modification remote from the antigen-binding site is considered optimal, the random nature of the conjugation in this study did not greatly affect the antigen-binding capacity of the antibody (see Sec. G).

F. Radiometalation of N-Benzyl Porphyrin–Antibody Conjugates

Radiometalation of the purified N-benzyl porphyrin–antibody conjugates, accompanied by loss of the N-benzyl group to form the ^{67}Cu-labeled porphyrin–antibody conjugate, can be accomplished by treatment with $^{67}CuCl_2$ at 40°C in aqueous buffer. Vacuum dialysis following metalation of the N-bzHTCPP–

Table 5 Protein Recovery

Coupling method	N-bzHTCPP/RIgG	% Yield
A. After Gel Filtration[a]		
CDI	2.3	86
EDAC/NHS	2.5	93
Blank[b]	0	87
B. After Vacuum Dialysis 9- to 10-Fold		
CDI	2.3	49
EDAC/NHS	2.5	48
Blank[b]	0	47
C. After Vacuum Dialysis 2- to 3-Fold		
CDI	2.3	86
EDAC/NHS	2.5	78

[a]Gel filtration conditions are described in the Appendix.
[b]The blank consists of N-bzHTCPP and RIgG mixed together in the absence of coupling reagents.

antibody conjugates removed 98% of the unchelated copper. However, recovery of antibody after concentration by this technique varied with the extent of concentration and was occasionally as low as 48%, as shown in Table 5. Antibody recoveries of 80 to 85% were achieved by careful manipulation and concentration of two- to threefold. Recovery of radioactivity after vacuum dialysis of ^{67}Cu-labeled porphyrin-antibody conjugates routinely averaged 55%.

The ease of radiometalation of the N-benzyl porphyrin-antibody conjugates is a major contribution to the overall success of preparation of these radiolabeled antibody conjugates. In contrast, metalation of the underivatized free base porphyrin, H_2TCPP, requires elevated temperatures and organic solvents (12). The harsh reaction conditions necessary for metalation of H_2TCPP by $^{67}CuCl_2$ would denature antibodies; thus H_2TCPP-antibody conjugates would not be suitable for "cold kit" methods of radiolabeling.

G. Immunoreactivity of Porphyrin-Antibody Conjugates

The results of the studies of the immunoreactivity of porphyrin-rabbit anti-conalbumin (RaCA) conjugates formed by the EDAC/NHS method are shown in Figure 8. A competitive enzyme-linked immunosorbant assay (ELISA) method was used to determine the immunoreactivity of the conjugates in comparison to unmodified RaCA. The immunoreactivity of N-bzHTCPP-RaCA, CuTCPP-RaCA (stable isotope Cu), and ^{67}CuTCPP-RaCA conjugates were examined as a func-

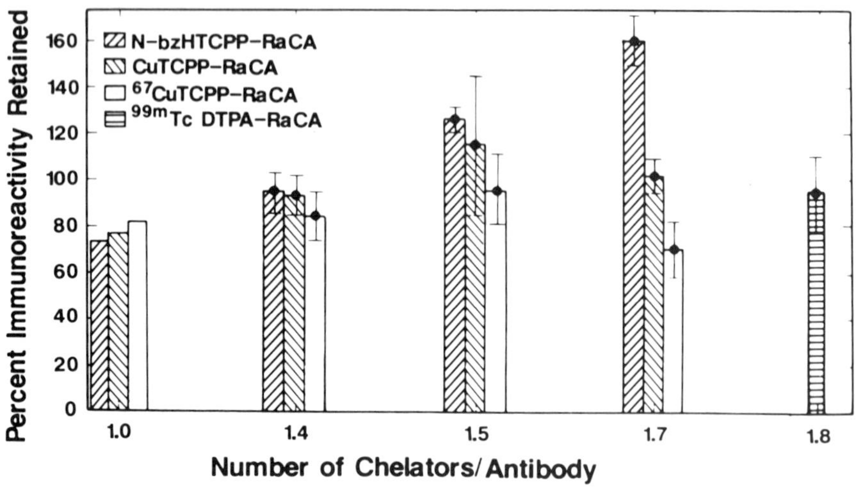

Figure 8 Retention of immunoreactivity of RaCA-^{67}CuTCPP conjugates prepared by the EDAC/NHS method. Details of the competitive ELISA method can be found in the Appendix. Results are expressed as the average ± Standard Deviation for triplicate determinations from three separate ELISA plates. Where no error bars are indicated, n = 2.

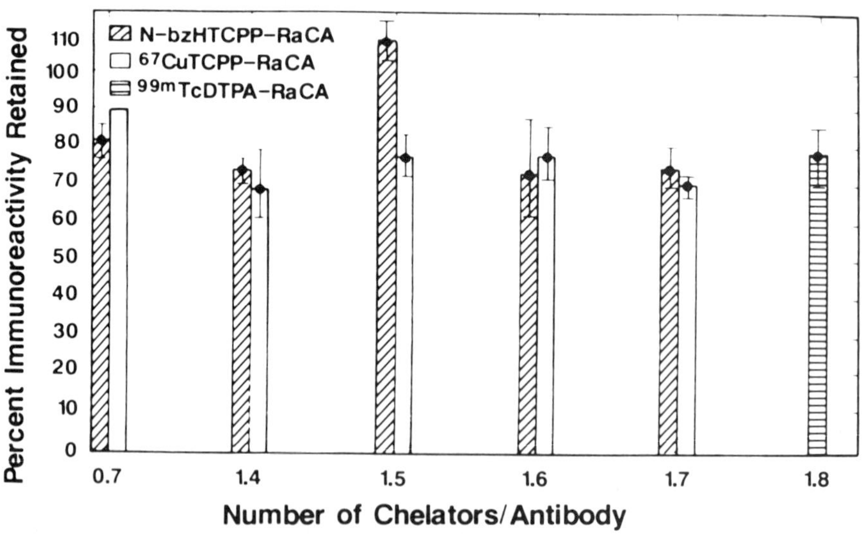

Figure 9 Retention of immunoreactivity of RaCA-^{67}CuTCPP conjugates prepared by the CDI method. Details of the competitive ELISA assay can be found in the Appendix. Results are expressed as the average ± Standard Deviation for triplicate determinations from three separate ELISA plates. Where no error bars are indicated, n = 2.

tion of the number of porphyrins attached per antibody. These experiments illustrate the effect of covalent modification of the antibody, as well as the effect of metalation with stable isotope copper and radiometalation with ^{67}Cu. In most cases there was little difference in the retention of antibody immunoreactivity between metalated and unmetalated porphyrin–RaCA conjugates. In the range examined, the number of porphyrins covalently attached to the antibody appeared to have little effect on the immunoreactivity.

Figure 9 illustrates a similar study of the immunoreactivity of porphyrin–RaCA conjugates which had been formed by the CDI method. Comparable results were obtained that indicated little loss of RaCA immunoreactivity as a function of the number of porphyrins attached per antibody in the range studied. Radiometalation with ^{67}Cu also resulted in little loss of immunoreactivity.

Figures 8 and 9 also show the comparable immunoreactivity of ^{99m}TcDTPA-RaCA conjugates formed by the cyclic anhydride method (27). A comparison of the immunoreactivity of the DTPA conjugates to that reported in the literature indicated that the competitive ELISA was at least as sensitive to loss of immunoreactivity as was the use of antibody binding to affinity columns. Paik and co-workers (27) reported 77.0% active antibody with a range of 64.5 to 85.5% when coupling 1.7 DTPAs per rabbit anti-human serum albumin. This compares favorably with 85% immunoreactivity retained with a range of 57 to 93% for 1.8 DTPAs per RaCA determined with the competitive ELISA. Retention of immunoreactivity greater than 100% appears to be an artifact of the competitive nature of the ELISA method. Negative controls consisting of nonspecific polyclonal RIgG demonstrated no specific binding of the antibody to conalbumin (CA) as a function of antibody concentration.

The good retention of RaCA immunoreactivity as a function of the number of porphyrins attached indicates that both the EDAC/NHS and CDI coupling protocols are feasible methods for preparing N-benzyl porphyrin–antibody conjugates. The similarity of immunoreactivity retained for the N-bzHTCPP–RaCA and ^{67}CuTCPP–RaCA conjugates indicates that radiometalation with ^{67}Cu causes little loss of immunoreactivity of the antibody. Thus these coupling and radiometalation methods show potential for general utility as "cold kit" methods to prepare ^{67}Cu labeled antibodies.

H. Conclusions

Porphyrins fulfill several criteria for use as chelating agents for the preparation of radiolabeled antibodies. Our experiments have shown that copper porphyrins are extremely stable to loss of the copper ion under simulated physiological conditions in human serum, as well as in the presence of chelating agents and a protein which binds copper ions readily. Porphyrins can be synthesized with func-

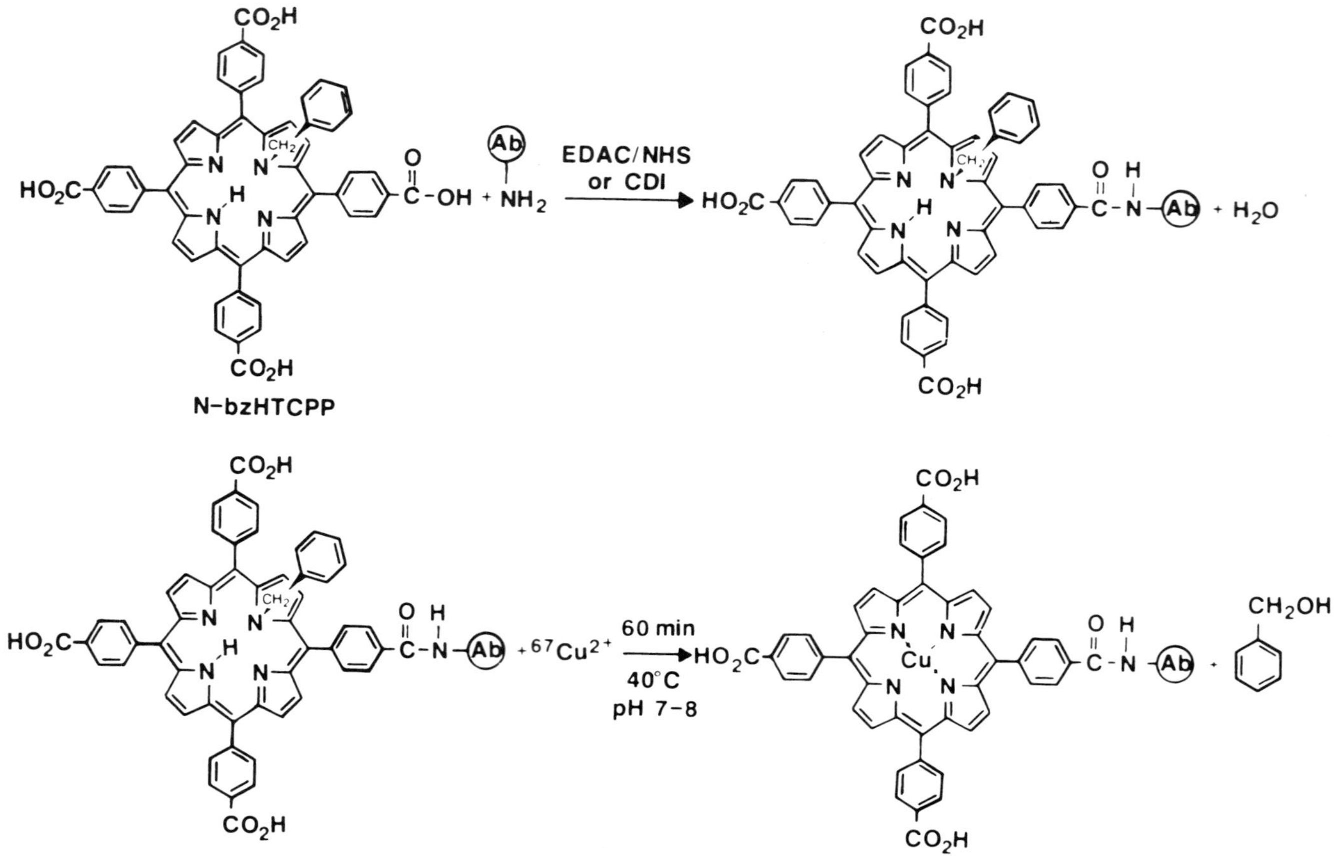

Figure 10 Overall scheme for the preparation of ^{67}Cu antibodies by a "cold kit" method.

tional groups suitable for covalent linkage to antibodies by formation of an amide bond. The N-benzyl porphyrins which have been synthesized can be metalated with $^{67}Cu^{2+}$ readily under conditions which do not denature proteins. All modified antibodies retained a high percentage of the immunoreactivity normally found in the unmodified protein. Thus attachment of N-benzyl porphyrins to antibodies followed by rapid metalation with radiocopper appears to be a very promising method to radiolabel antibodies with ^{67}Cu. The overall reaction scheme is shown in Figure 10. This synthetic strategy is especially pertinent to the "cold kit" type of application.

I. Abbreviations Used

AP, alkaline phosphatase; BBS, borate buffered saline; BSA, bovine serum albumin; CA, conalbumin; CH_2Cl_2, dichloromethane; CH_3CN, acetonitrile; CDI, 1,1′-carbonyldiimidazole; ^{67}Cu, copper-67; CuTCPP, 5,10,15,20-tetrakis-(4-carboxyphenyl) porphinato copper (II); DMF, dimethylformamide; DTPA, diethylenetriaminepentaacetic acid; EDAC, 1-ethyl-3-(3′-dimethylaminopropyl) carbodiimide HCl; EDTA, ethylenediaminetetraacetic acid; ELISA, enzyme-linked immunosorbent assay; HPLC, high performance liquid chromatography; H_2TCPP, 5,10,15,20-tetrakis(4-carboxyphenyl) porphine; IgG, immunoglobulin G; ^{111}In, indium-111; LAMPF, Los Alamos Meson Physics Facility; MW, molecular weight; N-bzHCS$_3$P, N-4-nitrobenzyl-5-(4-carboxyphenyl)-10,15,20-tris(4-sulfophenyl) porphine; N-bzHTCPP, N-benzyl-5,10,15,20-tetrakis (4-carboxyphenyl) porphine; NHS, N-hydroxysuccinimide; PBS, phosphate buffered saline; RaCA, rabbit anit-conalbumin; RIgG, rabbit immunoglobulin G; SDS-PAGE, sodium dodecylsulfate polyacrylamide gel electrophoresis; ^{99m}Tc, technetium-99m; THF, tetrahydrofuran; TLC, thin layer chromatography; tris-HCl, tris(hydroxymethyl)aminomethane-HCl.

J. Acknowledgments

Research carried out at Los Alamos National Laboratory is supported by the U.S. Department of Energy and Office of Health and Environmental Research. The research performed at Hunter College, CUNY is supported by NIH Grant CA25427 and the Center for the Study of Gene Structure and Function, sponsored by the Research Centers at Minority Institutions (NIH). The authors wish to thank Mr. Wayne Taylor, Mr. Richard Staroski, and Dr. Dennis Phillips for preparing the ^{67}Cu; Dr. Timothy Burns, Ms. Sandra Schreyer, and Ms. Suzanne Fehrenbach for excellent technical assistance; Dr. Dean Cole for helpful discussions of the data and experimental methods; and Drs. William Anderson (University of New Mexico) and Sally DeNardo (University of California-Davis) for helpful suggestions.

K. Appendix

1. Biochemicals and Chemicals

All nonspecific polyclonal IgGs were obtained from Sigma and were used without further purification. RaCA was obtained from high-titer, late-course antisera. Rabbits were immunized with 0.5 mg CA (Sigma) emulsified in complete Freund's adjuvant (Sigma) and boosted with incomplete adjuvant. The RaCA was purified sequentially by two different chromatographic methods: (1) protein A chromatography, and (2) affinity chromatography on a 1 cm × 3 cm column of CA covalently attached to Affi-Gel 202 (Biorad) using EDAC (Sigma) following the procedure described in the Biorad Catalog (28). The protein A-purified antibody preparation was applied to the CA affinity column, then the column was washed with 0.02 M sodium phosphate, 0.5 M sodium chloride, pH 7.4. The purified antibody was eluted with the same buffer containing 3.5 M potassium thiocyanate. The potassium thiocyanate was immediately removed either by dilution and dialysis, or by a 1 cm × 12 cm column of Sephadex G25 packed directly under the CA beads. The antibody was concentrated and dialyzed by vacuum dialysis in a negative pressure micro protein dialysis concentrator (Pierce) against two liters of borate-buffered saline (BBS, 0.1 M borate, 0.08 M sodium chloride, pH 8.5).

Pooled normal human serum was obtained from Miles Scientific; Calbiochem was the source of human serum albumin. Immobilized pepsin was purchased from Pierce. Sigma supplied the molecular weight marker proteins, alkaline phosphatase (AP), bovine serum albumin (BSA), cyclic DTPA anhydride, p-nitrophenyl phosphate, NHS, and tris(hydroxymethyl)aminomethane-HCl (tris-HCl) buffer. EDTA was obtained from Mallinckrodt, and DTPA, pyrrole, 4-formylmethylbenzoate, propionic acid, benzaldehyde, phenyl sulfide, benzyl alcohol, and methanesulfonic acid were purchased from Aldrich. Distilled in glass grade DMF was acquired from Burdick and Jackson Laboratories. Linde type 4A molecular sieves were obtained from Union Carbide. Dowex AG1-X8 was purchased from Biorad. Nochromix was supplied by Godax Laboratories. Puratronic grade stable isotope $CuCl_2$ used in the developmental reactions was supplied by Johnson Matthey. The University of New Mexico Radiopharmacy was the source of ^{99m}Tc. The N-benzyl porphyrins (N-bzHTCPP and N-bzHCS$_3$P) were synthesized and metalated with copper by the methods described in the following sections. H_2TCPP was obtained from Porphyrin Products. Thin layer chromatography (TLC) plates (Uniplate XTBO) were obtained from Analtech. Elemental analyses were performed by Analytische Laboratorien Engelskirschen, Federal Republic of Germany.

2. Instrumentation

The negative pressure micro protein dialysis concentrator was supplied by Pierce. Fluorescence was measured with an Aminco-Bowman Model J4-8202 spectrofluorometer (American Instrument). A Hewlett-Packard Model 8450A spectrophotometer was used to measure UV-visible spectra. A Beckman 4420 IR spectrophotometer was used to obtain infrared spectra from KBr pellets. A Biorad Model 250 tube gel electrophoresis cell with an Hoeffer PS 2500 DC power supply were used for the SDS-PAGE. An Isco UA-5 absorbance monitor, model 1310 gel scanner, and type 6 optical unit with filters were used to scan the quartz tube gels. The area under the peaks was integrated with an Hewlett-Packard model 3390A integrator. The flow rates on the Sephadex G25 columns were controlled with a Rabbit peristaltic pump (Rainin). Copper-67 and ^{99m}Tc activity were measured using either (1) an EG&G Ortec and Princeton Gamma-Tech GeLi counter coupled to a Canberra model 8100 multichannel analyzer or (2) a Packard autogamma NaI counter. A Dynatech laboratories Model MR 600 automatic ELISA plate reader was used to measure the absorbance in the ELISA plate wells. Polystyrene ELISA plates were obtained from Flow Laboratories; microtiter plates used in the protein and porphyrin assays were obtained from Becton Dickinson Labware. Lotus 123 (Lotus) and Curve-Fitter-PC (Interactive Labware) were used on an IBM PCXT to analyze the ELISA data. Filter sterilization was accomplished by filtration through a Millex-GV 0.2 μ filter unit (Millipore); a sterile hood (Envirco Enviralab Sterility Module) was used for all filter sterilizations.

3. Preparation of Copper-67 Chloride

The method of producing ^{67}Cu is based on modifications of methods previously described by members of the Medical Radioisotopes Research Program (29,30). Copper-67 is produced at LAMPF by irradiating 70 g of zinc oxide for seven days with 600 to 800 MeV protons. The irradiated target typically had 2 to 4 Ci of activity and a ^{67}Cu specific activity of 15,000 Ci/g. Because the radioactivity of the target is so high, the targets were processed in the remote handling hot cell facilities. The target material was dissolved in 300 ml of 3 M H_2SO_4 and 10 ml of concentrated HNO_3. The ^{67}Cu was removed from the dissolved target material by electrochemical reduction and plating of the copper onto a platinum working electrode at -0.35 volts versus a Ag/AgCl electrode. After an hour of electrochemical plating of ^{67}Cu, the platinum electrode was moved to a different electrochemical cell with fresh electrolyte (0.1 M H_2SO_4). A potential of +0.35 volts was used to strip the ^{67}Cu into solution by oxidizing the copper to the +2 state. The potential was changed to -0.35 volts to replate the copper onto the platinum electrode. The electrochemical stripping and plating process was repeated two times. Then the ^{67}Cu plated onto the platinum electrode was moved to a different electrochemical cell. The ^{67}Cu was stripped, plated onto the electrode, then stripped into a 0.1 M NHO_3 solution. The ^{67}Cu solution was evaporated to dryness on a hot plate and redissolved in 2 M HCl. The resulting ^{67}Cu solution was applied to a Dowex AG1-X8 column and was eluted with 2 M HCl. The $^{67}CuCl_2$ solution was heated on a hot plate and evaporated to dryness under a stream of air. The ^{67}Cu was fumed with HNO_3 to remove any residual anion exchange material; then the ^{67}Cu was heated and evaporated to dryness under a stream of air. The ^{67}Cu was redissolved in appropriate solvent (DMF or aqueous buffer) immediately before use.

4. Synthesis of N-Benzyl-5,10,15,20-Tetrakis(4-Carboxyphenyl) Porphine [N-bzHTCPP]

N-bzHTCPP was synthesized by the following series of steps. The 5,10,15,20-tetrakis(4-methylcarboxyphenyl) porphine precursor was synthesized by modifications of the Adler method (31) of porphyrin synthesis. Pyrrole and 4-formylmethylbenzoate, each 0.35 M in refluxing propionic acid, were used to prepare this porphyrin. After one hour at reflux, the solution was allowed to cool to room temperature. The solution was filtered through a medium porosity glass fritted funnel, giving 15 to 20% yield of fine purple crystals. The crystals were washed with three 25 ml portions of cold methanol, then air-dried. To add the N-benzyl substituent efficiently to the tetrakis(4-methylcarboxyphenyl) porphine, benzyldiphenylsulfonium tetrafluoroborate was employed (17,32,33). The porphyrin and benzyldiphenylsulfonium tetrafluoroborate were combined in equimolar amounts (0.015 M) in dichloromethane (CH_2Cl_2) and either stirred overnight or heated to 110°C for two hours in a pressure bottle. The resulting green solution was neutralized with 1 M aqueous ammonia, extracted with water, and chromatographed on an alumina column with CH_2Cl_2 as the eluent. The purple solution gave a green band on the column (preceded by a small pink band of unreacted porphyrin) which elutes as a purple solution. The solvent was removed by a rotary evaporator. The product can be crystallized from acetonitrile (CH_3CN)/CH_2Cl_2 mixtures. The UV-visible spectrum (logarithm of the molar absorptivities shown in parentheses) of the methyl ester is the following: 437 nm (5.28), 536 nm (3.96), 578 nm (4.12), 618 nm (shoulder), 678 nm (3.66). The ester was converted to the corresponding carboxylate by dissolution in warm tetrahydrofuran (THF), addition of an equal volume of 5 M aqueous KOH, and stirring overnight. In the resulting mixture, the purple aqueous layer contained the porphyrin, and the THF layer was nearly colorless. The aqueous layer was removed, cooled in an ice bath, then carefully neutralized with 1 M HCl to precipitate the green diprotonated porphyrin, N-bzH_3TCPP^{2+}, at approximately pH 4. The precipitate was filtered with a medium porosity fritted glass funnel, washed thoroughly with water, and air-dried. Analyzed for $C_{55}H_{36}N_4O_8 \cdot HCl \cdot 4H_2O$: 66.8% C, 4.54% H, 5.66% N, 3.53% Cl. Found; 67.3% C, 4.20% H, 5.41% N, 2.67% Cl. The electronic spectral properties of the free acid form of this porphyrin in various stages of protonation are given in Table 2.

5. Synthesis of N-4-Nitrobenzyl-5-(4-carboxyphenyl)-10,15,20-tris(4-Sulfophenyl) Porphine [N-bzHCS_3P]

The N-4-nitrobenzyl-5-(4-carboxyphenyl)-10,15,20-tris(4-sulfophenyl) porphine was synthesized by the steps described below.

5-(4-methylcarboxyphenyl)-10,15,20-triphenylporphine The initial species synthesized was 5-(4-methylcarboxyphenyl)-10,15,20-triphenylporphine. Benzaldehyde (20.0 ml, 0.20 mol) and 4-formylmethylbenzoate (10.9 g, 0.066 mol) were mixed and added slowly to a refluxing solution of pyrrole (19.0 ml, 0.27 mol) in propionic acid (1.0 L). Careful addition was necessary to prevent overheating and loss of material. After one hour of refluxing, the solution was allowed to cool to about 60°C, and an equal volume of ethylene glycol was added. The reaction mixture was chilled overnight in an ice bath. Filtration with a medium porosity glass fritted funnel gave 4.5 g (9%) of crude product. After a cold methanol wash, the product was air-dried. In some cases, precipitation did not occur. Then it was necessary to reduce the volume to about 300 ml to obtain a precipitate. After filtration through a medium porosity glass frit, a short alumina column (10 cm high × 7 cm diameter) was used for preliminary purification of 1-g aliquots. CH_2Cl_2 was used as eluent. A rotary flash evaporator was used to remove the solvent. The porphyrin monoester was purified further by flash chromatography on fine mesh silica (15 cm diameter × 20 cm high) at a loading a 2 g of material (34). Good separation was achieved using a column 5 cm in diameter × 38 cm high for a loading of 250 mg of porphyrin. The first band, eluted with CH_2Cl_2, was an undesired porphyrin, 5,10,15,20-tetraphenylporphine, which comprised the bulk of the product. The second band, eluted with CH_2Cl_2 containing 2.5% ethanol, was the mono-4-carboxymethyl porphyrin, (0.5 g, 1% overall yield). Separation of 50-mg portions was also effected on preparative silica gel TLC plates (20 cm × 20 cm, 2 mm silica gel coating) developed in CH_2Cl_2. The UV-visible spectrum in CH_2Cl_2 (with the logarithm of the molar absorptivities in parentheses) is the following: 374 nm (4.30); 414 nm (5.17); 423 nm (5.16); 485 nm (3.54); 515 nm (4.23); 550 nm (3.88); 590 nm (3.71); and 646 nm (3.61). The ester was hydrolyzed in a mixture of equal volumes of 4.0 M NaOH and THF. Analyzed for $C_{45}H_{28}N_4O_2Na{\cdot}H_2O$: 77.28% C, 4.58% H, 8.00% N, 6.86% O. Found: 75.90% C, 4.49% H, 7.81% N, 6.57% O.

N-4-nitrobenzyl-5-(4-methylcarboxyphenyl)-10,15,20-triphenylporphine and N-4-nitrobenzyl-5-[4-(4-nitrobenzyl)carboxyphenyl]-10,15,20-triphenylporphine The 5-(4-methylcarboxyphenyl)-10,15,20-triphenylporphine was converted to N-4-nitrobenzyl-5-(4-methylcarboxyphenyl)-10,15,20-triphenylporphine by the following steps. Diphenyl-4-nitrobenzylsulfonium tetrafluoroborate (17) and 5-(4-methylcarboxyphenyl)-10,15,20-triphenylporphine were combined stoichiometrically in CH_2Cl_2 (typically about 100 mg of the porphyrin to

80 ml of CH_2Cl_2) and heated in a glass and Teflon pressure vessel at 110°C for two hours. (The reaction can also be accomplished at room temperature overnight). The vessel was cooled to room temperature, then the solution was neutralized with 40 ml of 1 M aqueous ammonia and extracted twice with 100-ml portions of water. Chromatography on neutral alumina with CH_2Cl_2 as eluent gave a trace of the starting porphyrin as the first band (pink) and the N-substituted product as the second band (green on the column, eluted as a purple solution). After crystallization from equal volumes of CH_3CN and CH_2Cl_2, yields were 85 to 90%.

Alternatively, the free acid, 5-(4-carboxyphenyl)-10,15,20-triphenylporphine, can be used as the starting material. (This material is easier to purify by flash chromatography than is the methyl ester.) In this case two equivalents of diphenyl-4-nitrobenzylsulfonium tetrafluoroborate were used, because the free acid group is converted to the 4-nitrophenyl ester under the conditions where N-substitution of the pyrrole nitrogen occurs. After using the same procedures described above, N-4-nitrobenzyl-5-[4-(4-nitrobenzyl)carboxyphenyl]-10,15,20-triphenylporphine was isolated in 85 to 90% yield by crystallization from CH_2Cl_2 and CH_3CN. Analyzed for $C_{59}H_{40}N_6O_6$: 76.28% C, 4.34% H, 9.04% N, 10.33% O. Found: 76.35% C, 4.41% H, 8.90% N, 10.47% O.

The UV-visible spectra are nearly identical for the two N-substituted porphyrins, N-4-nitrobenzyl-5-(4-methylcarboxyphenyl)-10,15,20-triphenylporphine and N-4-nitrobenzyl-5-[4-(4-nitrobenzyl)carboxyphenyl]-10,15,20-triphenylporphine (logarithm of the molar absorptivities in parentheses), in CH_2Cl_2: 436 nm (5.29), 531 nm (3.98), 574 nm (4.18), 613 nm (3.70), 677 nm (3.69). The infrared carbonyl stretch for both compounds is in the region typical of esters (1700 cm^{-1} for N-4-nitrobenzyl-5-(4-methylcarboxyphenyl)-10,15,20-triphenylporphine and 1702 cm^{-1} for N-4-nitrobenzyl-5-[4-(4-nitrobenzyl)carboxyphenyl]-10,15,20-triphenylporphine).

N-4-nitrobenzyl-5-(4-carboxyphenyl)-10,15,20-tris(4-sulfophenyl) porphine (hydrogensulfate)hydrate sodium salt Treatment of either N-4-nitrobenzyl-5-(4-methylcarboxyphenyl)-10,15,20-triphenylporphine or N-4-nitrobenzyl-5-[4-(4-nitrobenzyl)carboxyphenyl]-10,15,20-triphenylporphine with concentrated sulfuric acid on a steam bath overnight gave the diprotonated form of N-4-nitrobenzyl-5-(4-carboxyphenyl)-10,15,20-tris(4-sulfophenyl) porphine. The product was isolated by carefully adding water to the H_2SO_4 slurry (5 ml of H_2O to 250 mg of starting porphyrin in 20 ml H_2SO_4), causing precipitation of the dication as the bis(hydrogensulfate) salt. Precipitation was aided by addition of acetone (40 ml). The crude product, the diprotonated porphyrin, was purified by the common procedure for sulfonated porphyrins (35), which consists of dissolution in methanol and reprecipitation with acetone, giving an 87% yield of the monoprotonated porphyrin. (The initial precipitate obtained after treatment with concentrated sulfuric acid is the diprotonated species, N-bzH_3-CS_3P^{2+}; the porphyrin product that results after washing and reprecipitation is the monoprotonated species, N-bz$H_2CS_3P^+$.) The infrared carbonyl stretch for the sodium salt is at 1625 cm^{-1}. Analyzed for $C_{52}H_{31}N_5O_{13}\cdot HSO_4\cdot 4Na\cdot 10$-$H_2O$: 44.65% C, 3.82% H, 5.00% N, 9.17% S. Found: 44.00% C, 2.93% H, 5.10% N, 8.44% S. The electronic spectral characteristics of the porphyrin in varying degrees of protonation are reported in Table 2.

6. Serum Stability Studies of 5,10,15,20-Tetrakis(4-Carboxyphenyl) Porphinato Copper(II) (CuTCPP)

The stability of CuTCPP was determined with each of the following challengers: human serum, human serum albumin, EDTA, and DTPA. A set of 13 tubes was prepared for each challenger; the final concentration of CuTCPP was 5×10^{-5} M. The concentration of the chelating agents, EDTA and DTPA, was 10^{-3} M in pH 7.4 sodium phosphate. The concentration of human serum albumin was 74 mg/ml in pH 7.4 sodium phosphate; filtered (0.2 μ filter) human serum was the fourth challenger. All solutions were filter sterilized (0.2 μ filter) in a sterile hood. The solutions were incubated in a 37°C, 5% carbon dioxide incubator The EDTA and DTPA solutions were not exposed to the carbon dioxide atmosphere in the incubator. CuTCPP was incubated in sterile solution at 37°C with each of the challengers listed above for 12 days. A tube from each set of challengers was removed each day, and the fluorescence from 600 to 750 nm upon excitation at 515 nm was measured. The UV-visible absorbance spectra of freshly prepared solutions of CuTCPP–challenger were compared with those of the 12-day incubations.

7. Determination of Coupling Efficiencies

SDS-PAGE was used as an analytical method to determine the percent of N-benzyl porphyrin covalently attached to protein. The SDS-PAGE method was used under nonreducing conditions using the Laemmli buffer system (23). Aliquots of the conjugation reaction mixture were electrophoresed in tube gels poured in quartz tubes. The running gels consisted of discontinuous polyacrylamide content designed to limit the antibody to the top of the gel, while allowing the uncoupled porphyrin to travel to the bottom of the gel. The lower 6 cm of the running gel was 12% polyacrylamide, on top of which was poured 2 cm of 5% polyacrylamide gel prior to polymerization. The interface of the two gel concentrations was stirred gently to create a slight gradient. This should minimize differences in refractive index resulting from a sharp concentration change that would complicate integration of the absorbance peaks. After electrophoresis was completed, the gels were scanned at 435 nm for N-benzyl porphyrin absorbance and at 280 nm for protein absorbance. The area under the peaks was integrated to determine the coupling yields.

8. Preparative Method of Purification of N-Benzyl Porphyrin–Antibody Conjugates

Purification of the conjugation reaction mixture of N-bzHTCPP–antibody conjugates on a 1 cm × 3 cm Sephadex G25 column at very slow flow rates ($\leq$ 0.05 ml/min) in BBS was used to remove the unconjugated porphyrin from the N-bzHTCPP-RIgG conjugates. Flow rates were controlled with a peristaltic pump. Although greater than 99% of the unconjugated N-bzHTCPP was removed from the conjugates, this method was not as effective in removing unconjugated N-bzHCS$_3$P from the N-bzHCS$_3$P–RIgG conjugates. Approximately 60 to 75% of unconjugated N-bzHCS$_3$P was removed from the conjugates by this chromatographic technique.

9. Optimization of Techniques to Prepare N-Benzyl Porphyrin–Antibody Conjugates

A coupling strategy based on the two-step method of Davis and Preston (24) was used to form the N-benzyl porphyrin–antibody conjugates. The N-benzyl porphyrin was first activated by reaction with the coupling reagent, then the antibody was added. All porphyrin reactions were carried out in the dark or in foil-wrapped vials to prevent porphyrin photooxidation. Nonspecific RIgG was used in the developmental reactions.

Two reagent systems were examined to form a covalent bond linking N-benzyl porphyrins to antibodies: (1) a combination of EDAC and NHS, and (2) CDI. Coupling reactions were optimized as a function of activation time, coupling time, coupling pH, and antibody:N-benzyl porphyrin:coupling agent ratio. The preliminary experiments indicated that the conjugation yield increased as a function of (1) antibody concentration and (2) N-benzyl porphyrin to antibody molar ratio. The N-benzyl porphyrin solubility limited the concentrations used. Therefore, all reactions were carried out at a 10 mg/ml antibody concentration and a 10:1 porphyrin:antibody ratio.

The EDAC/NHS conjugation reaction was based on a combination of the two-step method of Davis and Preston (24) and the method of Anderson and coworkers (25). Because N-bzHTCPP is not soluble at the low pH of the activation reaction, two different methods were used to solubilize the porphyrin: (1) N-bzHTCPP was dissolved in DMF to a concentration which would expose the antibody to less than 20% (v/v) organic solvent, or (2) a small amount of 1 N NaOH was added to the stock porphyrin solutions to solubilize the porphyrin. Ten μl of NaOH in 200 μl of 12.5 mM sodium phosphate, pH 6.0, solubilized the porphyrin. The N-benzyl porphyrin was activated by reaction with EDAC and NHS in aqueous solution, then the antibody was added.

The activation reaction was carried out in neat dry DMF for the CDI method of conjugation. The DMF was purified and dried by modifications of the method of Juillard (36). The DMF was dried over barium oxide for two days, then distilled under vacuum in oven-dried glassware. After the N-benzyl porphyrin had been activated by reaction with CDI, the antibody was added. The maximum concentration of DMF to which antibody was exposed was less than 20% (v/v).

10. Coupling N-Benzyl Porphyrins to Antibodies Derived from a Variety of Species

The optimized conditions used to conjugate N-bzHTCPP which were described in the preceding section were used to attach N-bzHTCPP and N-bzHCS$_3$P to antibodies derived from a variety of species. For the EDAC/NHS reaction, a 1:10:10:10 molar ratio of antibody:porphyrin:EDAC:NHS was used. One hour of activation and one hour to couple to antibody at pH 8.5 were the reaction conditions used in these protocols. The molar ratio of antibody:porphyrin:CDI used was 1:10:10. A 15-minute activation step, followed by 90 minutes of coupling to the antibody at pH 7.5 to 8.0, were the reaction conditions for the CDI coupling.

11. Location of the Site of Attachment of the N-Benzyl Porphyrin to Rabbit IgG

The site of attachment of N-bzHTCPP to nonspecific RIgG was determined by two different methods of cleavage of the antibody, as described below. N-bzHTCPP–RIgG conjugates formed by the EDAC/NHS and CDI methods were each examined.

The site of attachment of N-bzHTCPP to nonspecific RIgG was determined by digesting N-bzHTCPP–RIgG conjugates with immobilized pepsin to create F(ab')$_2$ and pFc' fragments (37) by fivefold assay. The experimental protocol described in the Pierce Catalog (38) was used with the following modifications. A 25-μl sample of immobilized pepsin was washed with 20 mM sodium acetate, pH 4.5, by centrifugation and decantation. The gel was taken up into 25 μl of the same buffer, and 500 μg of N-bzHTCPP-RIgG in BBS was added. Then the mixture was incubated and vibrated at 37°C for two to three days. The supernatant was combined with an equal volume of Laemmli sample buffer (23), excluding 2-mercaptoethanol. The sample was then analyzed by electrophoresis.

The Laemmli method (23) was used to separate the N-bzHTCPP–RIgG antibody heavy and light chains. Triplicate samples of 300 to 400 μg of N-bzHTCPP-RIgG in BBS were combined with an equal volume of the Laemmli sample buffer (23), including 2-mercaptoethanol, and the solutions were immersed in boiling water for two minutes. These solutions were analyzed by electrophoresis.

Molecular weight (MW) marker proteins were combined in 1.0 ml Laemmli sample buffer (23), including 2-mercaptoethanol, and immersed in boiling water for two minutes. The solution contained 0.5 mg α-lactalbumin (MW = 14,200), 1.0 mg trypsin inhibitor (MW = 20,100), 1.0 mg trypsinogen (MW = 24,000),

0.7 mg bovine albumin (MW = 66,000), and 1.0 mg phosphorylase B (MW = 96,700).

All samples were electrophoresed on 10% polyacrylamide gels which were scanned at 435 nm for porphyrin absorbance as described above. The area under the peaks was integrated to give the relative amount of porphyrin attached to each antibody fragment. The molecular weight marker gel was scanned at 280 nm for protein absorbance.

12. Metalation of N-Benzyl Porphyrin–Antibody Conjugates

The N-bzHTCPP–antibody conjugates which had been purified by chromatography on Sephadex G25 were metalated with $CuCl_2$ or $^{67}CuCl_2$ at a 1:1 copper: N-benzyl porphyrin ratio at 40°C for 60 minutes. The metalation reaction was carried out in dim light to prevent photooxidation of the N-benzyl porphyrin; all glassware was acid-washed in Nochromix, then rinsed in copious amounts of deionized water to prevent metalation of the N-benzyl porphyrin by metal ions adsorbed on the surface of the glass. The reaction mixture was vacuum dialyzed against two liters of phosphate buffered saline (PBS, 0.01 M sodium phosphate, 0.15 M sodium chloride, pH 7.4), containing 0.05 M sodium citrate at 4°C to remove unchelated copper and any remaining unconjugated porphyrin. Concentration and dialysis were accomplished simultaneously by vacuum dialysis. Copper-67 was counted using (1) an EG&G Ortec or Princeton Gamma-Tech GeLi counter coupled to a Canberra model 8100 multichannel analyzer, or (2) a Packard autogamma NaI counter.

13. Preparation of Alkaline Phosphatase–Rabbit Anti-Conalbumin Conjugates

AP was covalently attached to RaCA by the method of Avrameas (39). AP in PBS was added to affinity purified RaCA in PBS at final concentrations of 5 mg/ml AP and 1.7 mg/ml RaCA. Glutaraldehyde was added to the solution to make a concentration of 0.05% (v/v). The solution was incubated for one hour at room temperature. An aliquot (typically 0.1 ml per ml of protein solution) of 0.2 M tris-HCl, 2.0 M glycine, pH 7.5, was added to the solution, then the solution was exhaustively dialyzed. First the solution was dialyzed for two days against two changes of 0.1 M tris-HCl, 0.15 M NaCl, 0.1 mM $ZnCl_2$, 0.1 mM $MgCl_2$, pH 7.2. This was followed by three days of dialysis against six changes of PBS containing 0.1 mM $ZnCl_2$ and 0.1 mM $MgCl_2$. The final solution was made 50% (v/v) in glycerol, filter sterilized through a 0.2 μ filter unit, and stored at 4°C.

14. Immunoreactivity Studies (ELISA)

The immunoreactivity of the porphyrin–antibody conjugates was determined by ELISA. Polystyrene ELISA plates were coated overnight at 4°C with CA at 1 μg/

ml CA and 9 μg/ml BSA in BBS. The plates were washed once with deionized water and blocked with 1% BSA (w/v) in BBS to prevent nonspecific adsorption of antibodies to the wells. Wells were typically coated with a volume of 200 μl and blocked with a volume of 300 μl. Samples were assayed in triplicate. In each assay, 100 μl of competing antibody, 100 μl of 1% BSA-BBS, and 100 μl of AP-RaCA conjugate diluted typically 1/2000 were combined and incubated at room temperature for one hour. The plates were washed three times with deionized water. After addition of 300 μl of p-nitrophenyl phosphate at 5 mg/ml in 0.1% (v/v) diethanolamine, 0.02% (w/v) NaN_3, 0.5 mM $MgCl_2$, pH 9.8, the plates were incubated at room temperature until the maximum absorbance at 410 nm reached between 0.7 to 1.0 absorbance units. The absorbances in the wells were read with an automatic ELISA plate reader.

The immunoreactivity of the porphyrin–antibody conjugates was determined by comparing the ability of unmodified RaCA versus porphyrin–RaCA conjugates to inhibit binding of AP–RaCA conjugates to ELISA plate wells coated with the appropriate antigen, CA (40). At the concentrations of conjugates used in the ELISA wells, the porphyrin did not contribute to the absorbance at 410 nm where the product of the substrate-enzyme reaction, p-nitrophenol, is measured. The results were normalized for comparison by plotting percent inhibition versus log μg of competing antibody added per well. The μg of antibody required for 50% inhibition was determined using a curve-fitting computer program on a PC. The percent immunoreactivity (%IR) retained in the conjugate was calculated using the following formula: $\% \text{IR} = (A/C) \times 100$, where C = μg of porphyrin–RaCA conjugate required for 50% inhibition and A = μg of unmodified RaCA required for 50% inhibition. The sensitivity of the ELISA to loss of immunoreactivity was determined by performing the assay on conjugates of RaCA with DTPA. Cyclic DTPA anhydride was coupled to RaCA by the method of Paik et al. (27) and labeled with ^{99m}Tc by the method of Childs and Hnatowich (41) to determine the extent of DTPA coupling. Unbound ^{99m}Tc was removed by vacuum dialysis against the same PBS citrate buffer composition used to remove free copper from the copper porphyrin–antibody conjugates. The immunoreactivity of nonspecific RIgG was assayed as a negative control.

15. Protein and Porphyrin Assays

Protein was assayed by the dye-binding method of Bradford (42). The porphyrin was assayed as copper porphyrin by measuring the absorbance at 410 nm. A standard curve was constructed for the protein-dye and copper porphyrin; the absorbances of each were measured in microtiter plate wells by an automatic ELISA plate reader.

REFERENCES

1. Yelton, Y. E., and Scharff, M. D. (1980) Monoclonal antibodies: a powerful new tool in biology and medicine. *Ann. Rev. Biochem. 50*:657–680.
2. DeNardo, S. J., DeNardo, G. L., Peng, J.-S., and Colcher, D. (1983) Monoclonal antibody radiopharmaceuticals for cancer radioimmunotherapy. In *Radioimmunoimaging and Radioimmunotherapy* (Burchiel, S. W., and Rhodes, B. A., Eds.). Elsevier Scientific, New York, pp. 409–417.
3. Jungerman, J. A., Yu, K.-H. P., and Zanelli, C. I. (1984) Radiation absorbed dose estimates at the cellular level for some electron-emitting radionuclides for radioimmunotherapy. *Int. J. Appl. Radiat. Isot. 35*:883–888.
4. Doherty, P. W., Hnatowich, D. J., Childs, R. L., Kosciuczyk, C., Schwinger, R., Griffin, T., Shealy, D., and Mattis, J. (1984) Behavior of ^{111}In-labeled $F(ab')_2$ fragments (19-9) in patients. *J. Nucl. Med. 25*:P112, Abstract 168.
5. Hnatowich, D. J., Childs, R. L., Lanteigne, D., and Najafi, A. (1983) The preparation of DTPA-coupled antibodies radiolabeled with metallic radionuclides: an improved method. *J. Immuno. Meth. 65*:147–157.
6. Cole, W. C., DeNardo, S. J., Meares, C. F., McCall, M. J., DeNardo, G. L., Epstein, A. L., O'Brien, H. A., and Moi, M. K. (1987) Comparative serum stability of radiochelates for antibody radiopharmaceuticals. *J. Nucl. Med. 28*:83–90.
7. Raman, S., and Pinajian, J. J. (1969). Decay of ^{67}Cu. *Nucl. Phys. A131*: 393–397.
8. Browne, E., Dairiki, J. M., and Doebler, R. E. (1978) *Table of Isotopes* 7th ed. (Lederer, C. M., and Shirley, V. S., Eds.) John Wiley, New York, pp. 211–212.
9. Dougherty, T. J. (1984) An overview of the status of photoradiation therapy. In *Progress in Clinical and Biological Research, Vol. 170, Porphyrin Localization and Treatment of Tumors* (Doiron, D. R., and Gomer, C. J., Eds.). Alan R. Liss, New York, pp. 75–87.
10. Ruben, S., Kamen, M. D., Allen, M. B., and Nahinsky, P. (1942) Some exchange experiments with radioactive tracers. *J. Am. Chem. Soc. 64*:2297–2298.
11. Buchler, J. W. (1975) Static coordination chemistry of metalloporphyrins. In *Porphyrins and Metalloporphyrins* (Smith, K. M., Ed.). Elsevier Scientific, New York, pp. 157–231.
12. Mercer-Smith, J. A., Moody, D. C., O'Brien, H. A., and Taylor, W. A. (1984) Synthesis of copper-67 meso-tetra(4-carboxyphenyl) porphine. American Chemical Society National Meeting, Philadelphia, Abstract NUCL-52.
13. Bain-Ackerman, M. J., and Lavallee, D. K. (1979) Kinetics of metal-ion complexation with N-methyltetraphenylporphyrin: evidence concerning a general mechanism of porphyrin metallation. *Inorg. Chem. 18*:3358–3361.
14. Lavallee, D. K., and Gebala, A. E. (1974) Facile dissociation of a copper porphyrin: chlorocopper (II) N-methyltetraphenyl porphine. *Inorg. Chem. 13*:2004–2008.

15. Kuila, D., and Lavallee, D. K. (1983) Kinetics and mechanisms of reactions of N-alkylporphyrin complexes 3: the effect of porphyrin ring substituents and reaction media. *Inorg. Chem. 22*:1095–1099.
16. Lavallee, D. K., and Kuila, D. (1984) Kinetics of dealkylation reactions of N-alkylporphyrin complexes 4: effect of the N-alkyl and N-aryl subsituents on the dealkylation process. *Inorg. Chem. 23*:3987–3992.
17. Lavallee, D. K., White, A., Diaz, A., Battioni, J. P., and Mansuy, D. (1986) Efficient metalloporphyrin synthesis under mild conditions using N-benzyl porphyrins. *Tet. Lett. 27*:3521–3524.
18. Lavallee, D. K. (1985) Kinetics and mechanisms of metalloporphyrin reactions. *Coord. Chem. Rev. 61*:55–96.
19. Parr, G. R., and Pasternak, R. F. (1977) The interaction of some water-soluble porphyrins and metalloporphyrins with human serum albumin. *Bioinorg. Chem. 7*:277–282.
20. Peters, T. (1977) Serum albumin: recent progress in the understanding of its structure and biosynthesis. *Clin. Chem. 23*:5–12.
21. Reyftmann, J. P., Morliere, P., Goldstein, S., Santus, R., Dubertret, L., and Lagrange, D. (1984) Interaction of human serum low density lipoproteins with porphyrins: a spectroscopic and photochemical study. *Photochem. Photobiol. 40*:721–729.
22. Hopf, F. R., and Whitten, D. G. (1975) Photochemistry of porphyrins and metalloporphyrins. In *Porphyrins and Metalloporphyrins* (Smith, K. M., Ed.). Elsevier Scientific, New York, pp. 667–700.
23. Laemmli, U. K. (1970) Cleavage of structural proteins during the assembly of the head of bacteriophage T4. *Nature 227*:680–685.
24. Davis, M-T. B., and Preston, J. F. (1981) A simple modified carbodiimide method for conjugation of small molecular weight compounds to immunoglobulin G with minimal protein crosslinking. *Anal. Biochem. 116*:402–407.
25. Anderson, G. W., Zimmerman, J. E., and Callahan, F. M. (1964) The use of esters of N-hydroxysuccinimide in peptide synthesis. *J. Am. Chem. Soc. 86*: 1839–1842.
26. Paul, R., and Anderson, G. W. (1960) N,N′-carbonyldiimidazole, a new peptide forming reagent. *J. Am. Chem. Soc. 82*:4596–4600.
27. Paik, C. H., Ebbert, M. A., Murphy, P. R., Lassman, C. R., Reba, R. C., Eckelman, W. C., Pak, K. Y., Powe, J., Steplewski, Z., and Koprowski, H. (1983) Factors influencing DTPA conjugation with antibodies by cyclic DTPA anhydride. *J. Nucl. Med. 24*:1158–1163.
28. *Biorad Catalog* (1986) Biorad, Richmond, CA, p. 56.
29. Bentley, G. E., Steinkruger, F. J., and Wanek, P. M. (1983) Electrochemistry as a basis for radiochemical generator systems. In *Radionuclide Generators: New Systems for Nuclear Medicine Applications* (Knapp, F. F. and Butler, T.A., Eds.). American Chemical Society, Washington, D.C., American Chemical Society Symposium Series No. 241, pp. 169–175.

30. Taylor, W. A., and Bentley, G. E. (1984) Electrolytic isolation of Cu-67 from proton irradiated zinc oxide. 7th Rocky Mountain Regional American Chemical Society Meeting, Albuquerque, NM.
31. Adler, A. D., Longo, F. R., Finarelli, J. D., Goldmacher, J., Assour, J., and Korsakoff, J. (1967) A simplified synthesis of tetraphenylporphyrin. *J. Org. Chem. 32*:476.
32. Badet, B., and Julia, M. (1979) Préparation aisée de sels de sulfonium. *Tetrahedron Lett.* 1101-1104.
33. Badet, B. D. (1980) Synthèses reactivité des sels de sulfonium. Thèse de Doctorat D'Etat, Université Pierre et Marie Curie, Paris.
34. Still, W. C., and Mitra, A. (1978) Rapid chromatographic technique for preparative separation with moderate resolution. *J. Org. Chem. 43*:2923-2925.
35. Lavallee, D. K., McDonough, T., and Cioffi, L. (1982) Fluorometric properties of N-methylporphine and several derivatives: evaluation as standards for the determination of chlorophyll concentrations. *Appl. Spect. 36*: 430–432.
36. Juillard, J. (1982) Dimethylformamide. In *Recommended Methods for Purification of Solvents and Tests for Impurities* (Coetzu, J. F., Ed.). Pergamon Press, New York, pp. 32–37.
37. Tsugikazu, T., Suzuki, T., and Tokunaga, E. (1981) Cleavage of human serum immunoglobulin G by an immobilized pepsin preparation. *Biochim. Biophys. Acta 660*:186–192.
38. *Pierce Handbook & General Catalog* (1986) Pierce Chemical Company, Rockford, IL, p. 20.
39. Avrameas, S. (1969) Coupling of enzymes to proteins with glutaraldehyde: use of the conjugates for the detection of antigens and antibodies. *Immunochem. 6*:43–45.
40. Pijssen, P. (1985) *Laboratory Techniques in Biochemistry and Molecular Biology–Practice and Theory of Enzyme Immunoassays*. Elsevier Science, New York.
41. Childs, R. C., and Hnatowich, D. J. (1985) Optimum conditions for labelling of DTPA-coupled antibodies with technetium-99m. *J. Nucl. Med. 26*: 293–299.
42. Bradford, M. M. (1976) A rapid and sensitive method for the quantitation of microgram quantities of protein utilizing the principle for protein-dye binding. *Anal. Biochem. 72*:248–254.

12

Preparation and Use of DTPA-Coupled Antitumor Antibodies Radiolabeled with Yttrium-90

D. J. HNATOWICH
University of Massachusetts Medical Center, Worcester, Massachusetts

D. SNOOK, G. ROWLINSON, S. STEWART, and A. A. EPENETOS
Hammersmith Hospital, London, England

I. INTRODUCTION

The development of antibodies with specificity for tumor-associated antigens, together with the development of practical methods for their radiolabeling, has led to the use of radiolabeled antibodies in clinical trials in cancer. The majority of these studies have been concerned with tumor detection, although a growing number is concerned with tumor therapy (1–4). In contrast to diagnostic studies where a sizable number of radionuclides with suitable properties are available, in the case of patient therapeutic studies thus far only ^{131}I and ^{90}Y have been employed.

This paucity of choices of therapeutic radionuclides reflects stringent requirements: not only must the radionuclide decay with the emission of high LET (linear energy transfer) radiation, but it should do so with an appropriate physical half-life and without penetrating radiation contributing to unwanted radiation exposure beyond the target. In addition, means must be available to attach the radionuclide to the carrier antibody such that the conjugate is stable at least until localized in tumor. Both ^{131}I and ^{90}Y partially satisfy these requirements but with very different strengths and weaknesses. The 8-day physical half-life of ^{131}I is probably longer than necessary for antibody therapy, where optimal tumor to normal tissue ratios are often reached in 1–2 days (5). In this regard, ^{90}Y with its 64-hour physical half-life is probably superior. The short half-life of ^{90}Y does complicate the logistics of labeling unless the ^{90}Y is obtained from an in-house ^{90}Sr-^{90}Y radionuclide generator (6). The development of generators producing ^{90}Y in a condition suitable for labeling antibodies for human use adds substantially to the attractiveness of ^{90}Y, since this radionuclide then becomes available both inexpensively and on demand.

The absence of radiation other than beta rays in the decay of ^{90}Y is an advantage, in that tissues peripheral to those containing the radioactivity are not exposed. In this sense, the strong gamma-ray emissions of ^{131}I are a drawback. However, the penetrating radiations of ^{131}I may be used to advantage in the quantitation of in vivo radioactivity distribution by external detection in connection with dosimetric calculations.

With regard to the stability of the label, a decided drawback to the use of radioiodinated antibodies is the dehalogenation which occurs in vivo and often results in the rapid release to urine of the greater part of the injected activity (7). It is possible that newer methods of protein radioiodination may limit this instability (8). In the case of ^{90}Y radiolabeled to antibodies via one chelate (DTPA) at least, the label has been shown to be stable in serum, although it appears to redistribute following in vivo catabolism of the antibody (9). It is possible that newer metabolizable chelates may eventually be developed, which will encourage the label to diffuse from normal organs (without similar diffusion from tumor as well) in a chemical form, which is excreted throught the kidneys rather than redistributed with retention (10,11).

A final significant difference between ^{131}I and ^{90}Y is the energy of the beta rays; whereas the maximum range in tissue of the beta rays of ^{131}I is approximately 2 mm, for ^{90}Y this value is 11 mm (12). As a result, the choice between these two isotopes in this regard will depend on the application. With all else equal, ^{90}Y will be the superior therapeutic radionuclide for larger tumors (i.e., 1–2 cm), while ^{131}I may be superior for tumors of smaller size.

It may be obvious from the above that despite the many favorable properties of ^{131}I for therapy, ^{90}Y is in many ways superior (13). This review is concerned, therefore, with ^{90}Y and will describe in useful detail the methods employed in two laboratories for the radiolabeling of antibodies with this radionuclide. In addition, the experiences of these laboratories in animal studies and in recent clinical trials with ^{90}Y-labeled antibodies will also be described.

II. ANIMAL INVESTIGATIONS

Prior to the initiation of clinical trials with ^{90}Y-labeled antitumor antibodies, as much relevant information regarding the in vivo properties of this agent should first be obtained from animal studies. Several animal studies have been reported in which ^{90}Y-labeled antibodies were administered (9,14–16), and some important observations from these are described below.

Although the chemistries of indium and yttrium are similar, and DTPA-coupled antibodies radiolabeled with ^{111}In and ^{90}Y may be expected to behave similarly in vivo, it has been shown that similar biodistributions exist only immediately after administration. Thereafter, significant differences in the distribution of ^{111}In and ^{90}Y become apparent (9). These data suggest that it may not be possible to use existing results with ^{111}In in animals and patients to predict the behavior of ^{90}Y. However, one study has reported similar blood clearances of ^{90}Y and ^{131}I following intraperitoneal administration of the same antibody labeled with these two isotopes (14).

Antibody localization to tumor using an ^{90}Y label has been reported in nude mice bearing a human colon tumor. A more recent work has also reported specific localization in mice of ^{90}Y in tumor, in this case leukemic spleens (16). In addition, these investigators have reported complete remission of this tumor following administration of ^{90}Y labeled to a specific antibody in contrast to the nonspecific control.

The majority of the above animal studies were performed via intravenous administration of intact antibodies. Since ovarian carcinoma is often restricted to the peritoneum, the treatment of this disease with ^{131}I-labeled antibodies has been via intraperitoneal administration (3). Thus a determination of the behavior of ^{90}Y-labeled antibodies in mice following administration by this route is important. Furthermore, since evidence has been presented showing that the $F(ab')_2$ fragments clear the circulation more rapidly than the intact antibodies and may penetrate more deeply into tumor nodules (17–19), it becomes important to evaluate the in vivo behavior of the $F(ab')_2$ fragments versus the intact antibody. Thus, Snook, Rowlinson, and Epenetos at the Hammersmith Hospital have performed a comparison study in mice of ^{90}Y-labeled intact and $F(ab')_2$ antibodies via intraperitoneal administration (20).

The monoclonal antibody HMFG1 (21) and its $F(ab')_2$ fragment were coupled to DTPA using the cyclic anhydride (22). The number of DTPA groups bound per antibody molecule was determined and the immunoreactivity of each conjugate was tested by ELISA using antigen-coated microtiter plates. Labeling of the conjugates was performed in 0.5 M acetate buffer at pH 6.0, and the immunoreactivity of the radiolabeled conjugate was again tested by ELISA and live-cell RIA.

Tumor-free athymic (nude) mice received an intraperitoneal injection of either conjugate. Animals were killed at various times up to 5 days postinjection and dissected. Tissue samples were solubilized and counted on a gamma-counter (see Appendix).

The control animals for this investigation received other chemical forms of ^{90}Y by either intraperitoneal or intravenous injection of (1) free labeled DTPA administered intraperitoneally, (2) colloidal ^{90}Y, intraperitoneally, (3) free ^{90}Y containing 1% human serum albumin in phosphate buffered saline, intraperitoneally, or (4) colloidal ^{90}Y by intravenous administration.

Colloidal ^{90}Y was prepared by adding excess phosphate buffered saline to the ^{90}Y acetate, while labeled free DTPA was produced by the addition of excess free DTPA to ^{90}Y acetate.

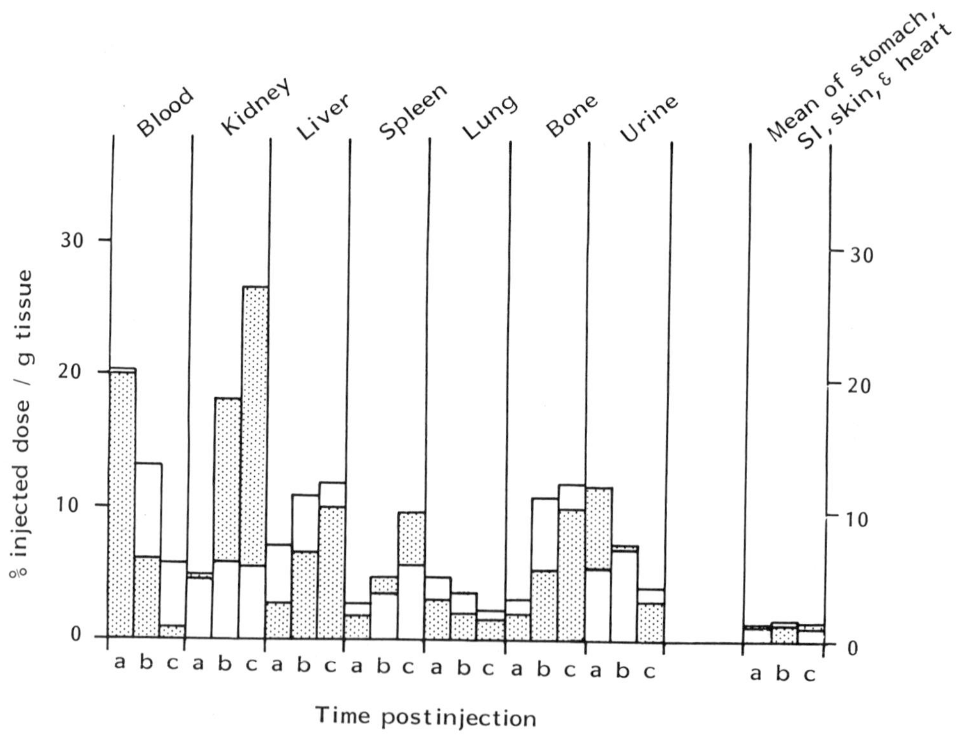

Figure 1 Comparison in nude mice of intraperitoneally administered ^{90}Y-labeled HMFG1 IgG (unshaded) and $F(ab')_2$ fragments (shaded) at (a) 2 hours, (b) 24 hours, (c) 72 hours postinjection.

istration of $F(ab')_2$ fragments radiolabeled with ^{111}In (23,24). Furthermore, the murine model predicts a high systemic radiation dose since blood levels increased rapidly following intraperitoneal administration of intact antibodies with a blood peak at 2 hours in contrast to humans, where a blood peak occurs at two days (25).

One of the important observations of this work was the accumulation of ^{90}Y in bone (rather than bone marrow), regardless of whether the intact antibody or fragments were administered intraperitoneally. The observation of bone uptake of ^{90}Y is in agreement with the work of Hnatowich et al., (26) and is suggested by the work of Epenetos et al. (discussed below), who reported bone marrow toxicity following intraperitoneal administration of ^{90}Y-labeled antibodies.

III. CLINICAL INVESTIGATIONS

A. Pretherapeutic Trials

Since ^{90}Y is a pure beta-ray emitter, the absence of accompanying gamma rays in its decay minimizes radiation exposure to normal tissues. However, it also complicates the evaluation of its biodistribution in patients and thus the estimation of radiation exposure. For pure beta emitters the accumulation of radioactivity in tissues cannot be determined accurately by external imaging. Furthermore, it is unlikely that the biodistribution of ^{111}In-labeled antibodies may be used to estimate the biodistribution of the same DTPA-coupled antibodies labeled with ^{90}Y since these two radiolabels most probably behave differently in vivo (9). It has not yet been shown that the biodistribution of ^{90}Y-labeled antibodies in animals may be used to predict accurately the behavior of this agent in patients.

One approach to the determination of the biodistribution in patients is to administer antibodies to patients scheduled for exploratory surgery so that tissue samples may be obtained by biopsy. This approach was adopted by Hnatowich et al. at the University of Massachusetts Medical Center (26) in a limited pretherapy trial in which the $F(ab')_2$ fragments of the OC-125 antibody were radiolabeled with a tracer dose (1 mCi) of ^{90}Y after conjugating with DTPA. The preparations were administered intraperitoneally to each of five patients who were to receive second-look surgery for ovarian cancer. Several serum and urine samples were obtained prior to surgery and, during surgery, biopsy samples of liver, bone, and bone marrow were obtained along with samples of tumor (if any) and normal peritoneal tissues. The radioactivity content of these samples was then determined and the results used to estimate the biodistribution at the time of surgery. The biodistribution was used in the calculation of radiation-absorbed doses.

Table 1 Mean Biodistribution of ^{90}Y Following Administration of Labeled OC-125 Antibody (as the $F(ab')_2$ Fragment Coupled with DTPA) in Five Patients

	% id	SD
Urinary excretion	6	(4)
Serum	8	(4)
Liver	10	(5)
Bone marrow	7	(4)
Bone	19	(19)

Results expressed as the mean percentage of the injected dose (corrected for decay) in total urinary excretion, in total serum, and whole organ, standard deviation in parentheses (NET).

Patients underwent surgery between 16 and 47 hours postadministration. The mean biodistribution at surgery is listed in Table 1 in percent of the administered dose per total organ, total urine excretion, or total blood volume. It will be apparent from the large standard deviations listed that the distributions varied considerably from patient to patient. One example of this variability is obvious from the values for bone radioactivity; it has been estimated that in patient 2 accumulation in bone at surgery was approximately 49% of the injected ^{90}Y, while in two others (patients 1 and 5) this value was between 2-4%. A second important variability observed in this study concerned the retention of activity in the peritoneum. Although retention was not directly determined, it was possible to estimate this value for each patient by examination of the radioactivity excreted in urine, present in circulation, and accounted for in liver, bone, and bone marrow. By this consideration, patient 1 retained a significant fraction of the administered dose within the peritoneum; not only were serum levels at surgery much lower than that of the other patients in this study, but only about 20% of the dose is accounted for by the above analysis. That this patient also presented with ascites may indicate blockage of the lymphatics and may offer an explanation for low levels of diffusion. However, patient 5 showed similarly poor diffusion without evidence of ascites. In this case circulating activity was also low at surgery and only about 35% of the dose was accounted for. The highest serum levels were observed in the case of patients, 2, 3, and 4, while the radioactivity accounted for in these patients was approximately 80, 50, and 70% respectively. An important conclusion from these findings is that the degree of bone uptake may be related to degree of diffusion from the peritoneum.

The accumulation of radioactivity in tumor also varied from patient to patient. Activity in tissues free of tumor cells by histopathological examination averaged 0.003% id/g with a modest standard deviation. Tumor was not present in tissues obtained from patients 4 and 5, while the radioactivity accumulated in tumor tissues from patients 1, 2, and 3 was 0.05% (0.035 SD, $n = 6$); 0.020%, (0.004 SD, $n = 6$), and 0.009% (0.005 SD, $n = 10$) of the injected dose per gram, respectively. The tumor/normal tissue ratios were therefore 25, 7, and 3, respectively.

On the basis of these results, it was possible to estimate the radiation dose to tumor and to normal tissue resulting from this procedure. However, it was necessary to adopt certain assumptions to arrive at these estimates. First, since tissue activity levels were determined at only one time point (at surgery) it was assumed that the observed levels were reached immediately upon antibody administration and that the label remained in these tissues at that level until completely decayed. Second, it was assumed that the activity levels determined in the biopsy sample for liver, bone, and bone marrow were representative of the entire organ. The assumption of uniform distribution in bone is particularly important in the estimate of bone marrow dose. Since bone marrow is found primarily in trabecular bone, which constitutes only 20% of bone mass, dose estimates to bone marrow will be considerably increased on the assumption of uniform bone distribution as opposed to the assumption of higher accumulation in cortical bone. A final assumption applies to tissues within the peritoneum and concerns their irradiation from radioactivity in the peritoneal fluid or on the surfaces of the peritoneum. It was calculated in the case of organs the size of the liver that this additional dose is negligible, while for tumor and thin-walled organs the added dose may be more significant and will depend on the surface-to-volume ratio of the tissues in question.

Under these assumptions it was estimated that 1 mCi of ^{90}Y-labeled antibody administered interperitoneally will deliver approximately 50 rads to tumor and between 5 and 9 rads to normal tissues. As such, bone marrow is likely to be the dose-limiting organ with radiation exposure of about 8 rads/mCi. The radiation dose to tumor is marginal considering the need to limit exposure to other organs, such as bone marrow, especially since a tumor dose of 1500 rads may be required for therapy (1). However, it was pointed out that tumor dose will depend on tumor geometry, and the estimates presented are subject to large uncertainties.

The authors concluded that under the conditions of their study, it may be possible to treat ovarian cancer with ^{90}Y-labeled antibodies, although it will be necessary to proceed with caution. The use of intraperitoneal rather than intravenous administration may be important to this application, since it apparently offers a means of reducing radiation exposure to bone marrow, the critical organ, without reducing exposure to tumor within the peritoneum.

B. Clinical Trials

Although clinical trials of ^{90}Y-labeled antibodies for cancer therapy are under consideration at a number of centers, this work is at present underway in only a few laboratories. The earliest investigation, and one which continues, is the use of ^{90}Y-labeled antiferritin antibody by Order et al. for the treatment of liver carcinoma (27). The antibody is administered intravenously, and preliminary reports have been encouraging, although significant bone marrow toxicity has apparently been observed.

Over the past three years, Epenetos et al. at the Hammersmith Hospital in London have been conducting clinical therapy trials with labeled monoclonal antibodies for the treatment of malignant effusions and chemoresistant ovarian cancer (3,12). Whereas initially ^{131}I was the label used in this study, it has been recently replaced with ^{90}Y. These investigators were the first to consider intraperitoneal administration for therapy and have continued to employ this route (2). This approach is possible in the case of ovarian cancer since the disease is often restricted to the peritoneum. Administration by this route may limit the uptake of label in normal tissues by limiting access of the label to the circulation, while permitting access of the antibody to tumor associated antigen by diffusion throughout the mass of small tumors.

In a small pilot study in ten patients preliminary to the treatment of ovarian cancer, pleural and pericardial effusions were controlled by intracavitary administration of up to 60 mCi of ^{131}I-labeled intact antibodies (12). Most of these effusions had failed previous treatment but were controlled by the antibody administration until the patients died of metastatic disease. It has been previously shown that tumoricidal quantities of ^{131}I-labeled antibodies will bind to cells suspended in malignant effusions (28), and it has therefore been assumed that this was the mechanism of palliation in these patients.

A more ambitious trial of ^{131}I-labeled intact antibodies was then conducted for the treatment of chemoresistant ovarian cancer by intraperitoneal administration. Twenty-nine patients received up to 30 mg of an antibody selected from a panel of four: HMFG1, HMFG2, AUA1, and H17E2 (21,29). The relevant antibody was labeled with escalating dose of ^{131}I from 20 to 157 mCi in a phase I/II trial. Patient responses were divided into groups according to the amount of disease prior to treatment. None of the eight patients with bulky disease (individual tumor nodules greater than 2 cm) achieved an objective response as assessed clinically. Of the 15 patients with nodules less than 2 cm in size, two patients with minute nodules (several millimeters in size) responded, one completely and the other with a greater than 50% reduction in size. One of the surprising results of this investigation was the rapid transport of the intact antibody from the peritoneum to the circulation, such that up to 30% of the administered label was found in blood after 48 hours. This rapid egress was also noted in the trial by Hnatowich et al. in three of the five patients studied, however only about 8% of the ^{90}Y-labeled F(ab′)$_2$ antibody was found in circulation in this study. It may be assumed that the lymphatics are responsible for this transport, since in both investigations patients with ascites showed lower blood levels. Using MIRD formulism (30) and the integrated blood levels, the Hammersmith group have estimated that 150 mCi of ^{131}I-labeled antibody delivers 300–400 rads to bone marrow as a result of this transport. Iodine-131 doses above 120 mCi were associated with marrow toxicity resulting in neutropenia and thrombocytopenia at three to six weeks after therapy. Thrombocytopenia was marked in four of the six patients receiving 150 mCi ^{131}I-labeled antibody, and in one case platelet transfusions were required until marrow recovery.

It appears from this pilot study that ^{131}I-labeled antibody may destroy single cancer cells, either in effusions or as microscopic residual disease. However, there is little evidence that, even with regional administration, tumoricidal doses are delivered to macroscopic disease by this therapy. Therefore, in the past six months Epenetos et al. at Hammersmith have initiated a new phase I clinical trial using ^{90}Y as the label in place of ^{131}I. Thus far, ten patients have been treated with ^{90}Y-labeled HMFG1. Only patients with confirmed or suspected disease persistent to adjuvant therapy have been accepted into the trial, and only if their tumors have been shown by immunoperoxidase staining to be positive for the HMFG1 antibody.

All patients were assessed at laparoscopy prior to therapy and a peritoneal dialysis catheter inserted. At the same time, a second catheter, about 38 cm in length, was also inserted containing 40 lithium fluoride thermoluminescence rods, each about 1 × 6 mm in dimension. Lithium fluoride is of a similar atomic number to tissue with respect to radiation and absorbs radiation in a similar manner. As such, these thermoluminescence dosimeters may be used to estimate the radiation dose delivered to the peritoneal cavity from ^{90}Y. In this way, the radiation dose to the pelvis, paracolic gutters, and subdiaphragm was estimated. The catheter was left in situ in the peritoneal cavity for five days following administration. Between 10 and 20 mg of the antibody was administered along with increasing doses of ^{90}Y, at present up to 20 mCi. The antibody was infused over 20 minutes along with 1.5 liters of normal saline. Blood samples were taken twice daily and total urine was collected for five days postadministration. Thereafter, blood samples were obtained weekly for the determination of cell counts.

As shown in Table 2, only five of the ten patients have thus far been assessed for response. There have been two partial responses with greater than 50% reduction in tumor size. Three patients have developed progressive disease, although one of these had complete palliation of ascites until her death eight weeks after treatment. Two patients have received adjuvant therapy and are therefore not

Table 2 Response and Toxicity Data in Patients Receiving Intraperitoneal ^{90}Y-labeled Monoclonal Antibodies

Pt. no.	Tumor size	Dose	Response	Platelet nadir (10^9/L)	WBC nadir (10^6/L)
1	>2 cm, ascites	14 mCi	PD	279 (38)	4.3 (30)
2	<2 cm	5 mCi	PR	151 (28)	3.9 (30)
3	Not assessed	6 mCi	Not assessable	286 (36)	5.4 (44)
4	"Adjuvant"	16 mCi	Not assessable	141 (36)	3.1 (42)
5	<2 cm	12 mCi	PR	107 (44)	3.5 (51)
6	<2 cm	15 mCi	PD	69 (38)	2.8 (52)
7	<2 cm	15 mCi	Not yet available	115 (24)	2.9 (24)
8	"Adjuvant"	15 mCi	Not assessable	83 (37)	2.6 (58)
9	<2 cm	15 mCi	Not yet available	62 (49)	3.6 (15)
10	>2 cm	20 mCi	PD	23 (43)	2.3 (49)

PD = progressive disease; PR = partial response.
The times (days) of the platelet and WBC nadirs are listed in parentheses.

assessable for response. Figure 3 shows that, like ^{131}I-labeled antibodies, the ^{90}Y-labeled antibody is also transported into circulation. However, unlike ^{131}I, where 70% of the administered dose appeared in urine in five days, in the case of ^{90}Y this value is less than 15%, in fair agreement with Hnatowich et al., who reported 8% over 2 days.

Even though blood levels are lower with ^{90}Y, bone marrow toxicity is still apparent. All patients receiving more than 15 mCi of ^{90}Y developed thrombocytopenia or leukopenia. Marrow suppression was only evident after three weeks, with mean platelet and WBC nadirs at 37 and 40 days, respectively. Patient 10, who received 20 mCi, required a platelet transfusion for spontaneous hematomas. This patient therefore responded similarly to the one patient, described earlier, who received 150 mCi of ^{131}I-labeled antibody. However, the bone marrow dose estimated by integrating the blood activity is quite low for ^{90}Y and is less than about 100 rads for the 20 mCi administration. Undoubtedly the observed bone marrow toxicity is more a result of bone uptake of ^{90}Y, such as that observed both by Hnatowich et al. (26) and Snook, Rowlinson, and Epenetos (20) and is presumably the result of antibody catabolism.

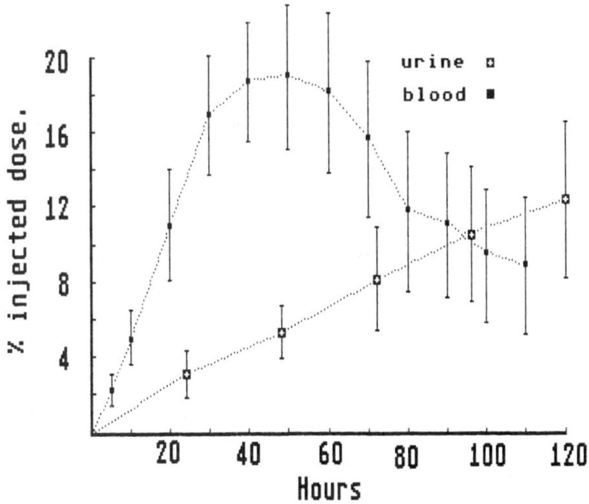

Figure 3 Blood ^{90}Y levels and cumulative urine excretion in ten patients treated with intraperitoneal ^{90}Y-labeled HMFG1. All values are decay-corrected (bars represent 2 SEM).

The radiation dose to tissues due to ^{90}Y within the peritoneum was estimated by use of the thermoluminescence dosimeters to be between 200 and 600 rads, with at least a twofold difference apparent along the length of the catheter. These values are similar to those observed earlier in the case of patients receiving ^{131}I-labeled antibody and are clearly insufficient to explain the observed tumor responses. It is possible, therefore, that the radiation dose to tumor within the peritoneum is much greater than that estimated for normal tissues and due to specific antibody-associated localization of label at tumor sites.

Epenetos et al. (25) have concluded from these therapy trials that one of the advantages of ^{90}Y over that of ^{131}I therapy is the decreased radiation exposure to staff due to the absence of gamma radiation in the decay of ^{90}Y. Furthermore, since ^{90}Y is not excreted in urine to the same extent as ^{131}I, patients may be nursed on general wards. Their results also suggest that in the absence of bone marrow transplantation, a 20 mCi dose of ^{90}Y administered intraperitoneally may be close to the tolerable limit, although the favorable responses seen at this and even lower levels of ^{90}Y suggest that a therapeutic response is possible.

IV. FUTURE PROSPECTS

One significant and universal observation regarding the use of radiolabeled antibodies for tumor localization studies is the tiny percentage of the administered dose that ultimately localizes in tumor, regardless of the label employed (31). In many cases the observed uptake must be considered marginal for diagnostic imaging purposes and may be even more questionable for therapeutic purposes. Unfortunately so little is known of the pharmacokinetics of the activity distribution in tumor and normal tissue, and on the radiosensitivity of these tissues toward radioactivities at these levels, that it is impossible to predict with certainty the success of present attempts at antibody-mediated radiotherapy of tumor. However, evidence of efficacy has already been provided in the work of Order et al. (27), in which ^{90}Y antibodies were administered intravenously and, as described herein, in the work of Epenetos et al. and Hnatowich et al. with intraperitoneal administrations. Several additional studies employing ^{131}I-labeled antibodies have also reported successful therapies (32). Nevertheless, it is obvious that improved tumor localization and improved target/nontarget ratios would be desirable. These improvements may result from the introduction of superior antitumor antibodies, possibly human or chimeric. However, the anticipated benefits from similar improvement in the past, such as the introduction of monoclonal to replace polyclonal antibodies, never materialized and the tumor localization reported at present is not much improved over that reported by Pressman et al. in their pioneer work (33). The message from these observations is that poor target/nontarget radioactivity ratios may be expected if tumor tissues are normally exposed to only a small fraction of the injected antibodies due to their limited blood flow (31). Furthermore, since blood flow to normal organs is not similarly limited, and if antibodies are extracted from circulation and catabolized in normal organs, such as the liver (34), background radioactivity will normally reach high levels. If so, the desired improvements in targeting must result from new approaches.

In the case of antibodies radiolabeled by the bifunctional chelate approach, the use of alternative chelators to DTPA may be useful. One observation common to the animal and patient studies conducted by the Hammersmith Group and the study of Hnatowich et al. is that DTPA, the chelator most often used in diagnostic and therapeutic studies, may not be ideal for use with ^{90}Y due to accumulation of this label in bone following administration of ^{90}Y labeled to DTPA-coupled antibodies. If the unwanted accumulation of label in bone is due to free ^{90}Y released during catabolism of the antibody, then stronger chelators may restrict this but possibly with resulting increased accumulation of label in liver and other sites of catabolism. Chelators covalently attached to antibody via metabolizable linkages may have an advantage if the radioactivity is released, not as the free ion, but as the free chelate, which is more likely than the free ion to be cleared through the kidneys and excreted (10,11).

An alternative approach, which may be useful in improving targeting, exploits the strong affinity of avidin for biotin (35). It may be possible to obtain more favorable results by administering the antitumor antibody labeled, not with radioactivity, but with biotin. If sufficient time is allowed for the clearance of antibody from circulation and from normal tissues before the administration of the radiolabeled avidin, it is possible that the tumor/normal tissue ratio will be improved by this approach, if not the absolute tumor uptake.

The results obtained using ^{90}Y-labeled antibodies for tumor therapy described within this chapter, point to the success that may be anticipated in the use of this approach, at least in the treatment of ovarian cancer. However, the same results also illustrate the potential difficulties of the treatment as it is now practiced, namely the dose-limiting bone marrow toxicities resulting from the accumulation of label in bone. It is possible that widespread use of ^{90}Y-labeled antibodies for therapy may await improved techniques for the delivery of radiation dose specifically to the tumor tissue. Fortunately, as described, a number of approaches are now under active investigation to achieve this goal.

V. APPENDIX: RADIOLABELING ANTIBODIES WITH YTTRIUM-90

Like most metals, yttrium does not form stable covalent bonds, and as such ^{90}Y cannot be attached to proteins via processes that can be successful for nonmetals, such as iodine. The solution to this (the bifunctional chelate approach) was described originally for ^{111}In (36) and has now been applied to ^{90}Y in a similar manner (9). A chelating agent is first covalently attached to the protein to serve as a site for the subsequent stable binding of the radionuclide. The chelating agent most often selected for this purpose is DTPA, since it forms stable chelates with a variety of metallic radionuclides, and a simple method for its conjugation to proteins employing its cyclic anhydride has been described (22). Methods in use in most laboratories for the conjugation of antibodies with DTPA via the cyclic anhydride and for their subsequent radiolabeling with ^{90}Y will be described in this section. First, however, past experiences in one laboratory's use of a ^{90}Sr-^{90}Y radionuclide generator to provide the ^{90}Y will be described.

A. ^{90}Y-Radionuclide Generators

Yttrium-90 is one of only two therapeutic radionuclides at present that may be obtained as generator products, the other being ^{186}Re. The considerable advantages in terms of cost and convenience resulting from the use of an in-house generator should be exploited. Fortunately, ^{90}Sr-^{90}Y generator systems have been developed that provide ^{90}Y in good yield with minimal ^{90}Sr breakthrough, with levels of trace metal contamination that do not interfere with radiolabeling at reasonable specific activities.

The one generator system that has thus far been adapted for in vivo therapeutic use with antibodies has recently been described (6). Up to 25 mCi of ^{90}Sr has been loaded on a cation exchange resin without evidence of radiation degradation over more than one year. The generator is eluted with a small volume (5 ml) of 0.003 M EDTA solution at pH 4.6, and under these conditions about 98% of the ^{90}Y is extracted. The breakthrough of ^{90}Sr was found to be 0.003% of the ^{90}Y, and thus 20 mCi of ^{90}Y contains less than 1 μCi of ^{90}Sr.

One unfortunate property of all ^{90}Sr-^{90}Y generators results from the need for high concentrations of complexing agents to extract ^{90}Y. In the above case, ^{90}Y in the eluant is chelated to EDTA and is consequently largely unavailable for protein labeling. An additional step must therefore be added to destroy the EDTA and to convert the radioactivity into some weak complex. The conversion process is not simple, but it may be performed semiremotely and may be completed in less than one hour (6). Concentrated HNO_3/H_2SO_4 has been used to destroy the EDTA during evaporation of the generator eluant so that the radioactivity could be dissolved in a minimal volume (usually 0.5 ml) of 0.5 M acetate buffer, pH 6.0. In this form it is suitable for protein labeling.

B. Protein Conjugation with DTPA via the Cyclic Anhydride

The use of the cyclic anhydride of DTPA for covalently attaching this chelator to proteins has been described in detail elsewhere (22) and will be discussed here only briefly. Because of the documented adverse effects of overconjugation of proteins with DTPA, as well as other groups (16), most investigators attached an average of no more than 1-2 groups per protein molecule. This may usually be achieved by adding the cyclic anhydride at an anhydride:protein molar ratio of 2:1 and at a protein concentration of 10-20 mg/ml. Since the quantity of antibody to be conjugated is usually small, the weight of anhydride required under the above conditions is normally too small to be weighed directly with accuracy. Therefore, the anhydride is either suspended, for example in dry chloroform, or dissolved in dry dimethylsulphoxide (DMSO) so that an accurate aliquot may be removed. The protein in 0.05 M bicarbonate buffer, pH 8.0, is added to the anhydride either as the solid (after evaporation of the chloroform) or as the solution in DMSO. The mixture is agitated for 1-5 minutes at room temperature to permit conjugation to proceed to completion. Free DTPA can be purified from the conjugated antibody by Sephadex G50 gel filtration using a suitable elution buffer (e.g., 0.1 M acetate, pH 6.0, or 0.05 M bicarbonate, pH 8.0). Absorbance at 280 nm is measured and the protein fractions pooled and sterilized by 0.22 μm millipore filtration. The immunoreactivity of the conjugate should be tested by an ELISA (enzyme-linked immunosorbent assay). This conjugate may be stored for several months, either at 4 or -70°C, depending on the antibody.

It is important, following each conjugation, to determine the average number of DTPA groups attached to each protein molecule. This may conveniently be accomplished using an aliquot of reaction mixture from the coupling reaction. In addition to the coupled antibody, this sample contains free DTPA and unmodified antibody. When reacted with a trace amount of ^{111}In, the isotope will distribute itself between the protein-bound DTPA and free DTPA in proportion to their relative concentrations, since the binding affinity of DTPA for indium is uncompromised by attachment to a protein (21). Subsequent separation by gel filtration or other separation techniques may be used to determine the percentage of added ^{111}In bound to the protein. Since the antibody to DTPA molar ratio is known, the number of DTPA groups per antibody can be estimated (percent radioactivity bound × molar ratio/100).

C. Radiolabeling DTPA-conjugated Antibodies with ^{90}Y

One of the fortunate features of radiolabeling by the bifunctional chelate approach is that the labeling procedure is generally simple and involves merely adding the coupled antibodies to the radioactivity, usually solubilized as a weak complex. Using ^{90}Y obtained from a generator, radiochromatographic purities of 95% or better have been routinely achieved with antibodies coupled with about one DTPA group per molecule, provided that the specific activity does not exceed approximately 1-3 mCi/mg of antibody (6). The activity is added in 0.5 M acetate buffer, pH 6.0, to the antibody conjugate to a final pH of 5.5. The mixture is agitated and then allowed to stand for a minimum of 30 minutes. Postlabeling purification can be carried out on a small Sephadex G50 column using phosphate buffered saline, pH 7.4, (PBS) as elution buffer. Human serum albumin (HSA) may be added to this buffer when a radioprotecting molecule is required, for example, during the preparation of large activities of ^{90}Y-labeled conjugates for patient administration. The protein-containing fractions are pooled and sterilized by 0.22 μm millipore filtration. The absolute activity may be measured in an ^{90}Y calibrated ionization chamber or by liquid scintillation counting. The immunoreactivity of the ^{90}Y-labeled antibody can be tested by a radioimmunoassay (RIA) using antigen-positive cells in solution (see below).

As in any labeling, it is important to determine the radiochemical purity of the labeled antibody preparation prior to its use. This is most conveniently accomplished by size exclusion HPLC (or FPLC) analysis in which good labeling efficiency will be evident in part by a radiochromatographic profile showing most of the radioactivity present in a single peak co-eluting with the protein. However, it is important also to determine the recovery of radioactivity during this analysis. Unbound and colloidal radioactivity may be retained by the columns used in these analyses such that these species do not appear in the radiochromatograms. Thus the radiochemical purity of a labeled antibody preparation may be seriously overestimated in the absence of information on recovery. This is especially important in the case of ^{90}Y, as there are indications that the trapped radioactivity is in a chemical form, which may localize in bone following administration (6).

When low anhydride-to-protein molar ratios are used for antibody conjugation, the investigator may choose between purification of the coupled protein from free DTPA (generated by hydrolysis of the anhydride during coupling) prior to radiolabeling or doing the purification after radiolabeling. The latter approach is more likely to result in an acceptable preparation, since any free activity (possibly present due to trace metal contamination) will be removed along with the free DTPA. The former approach occasionally results in a poor label with considerable free activity (poor labeling efficiency), especially if an attempt is made to radiolabel at too high a specific activity. However, when successful, labeling in this case is by "kit" methods since postlabeling purification is not performed, and is therefore particularly attractive for patient preparations. In any case, purification may be achieved simply on a small gel filtration column of Sephadex G50 eluted with normal saline or some suitable buffer.

D. Immunoreactivity Assays

1. ELISA

The antibody to be tested in an enzyme-linked immunosorbent assay (ELISA) is applied (in serial dilution) to a microtiter plate previously coated with either antigen-positive cells or purified antigen (human milk fat globule in the case of HMFG1). Unmodified antibody is used as a standard. The plate is incubated at 37°C for 1 hour and then washed using PBS containing 0.05% Tween 20 (PBS/Tween). A rabbit antimouse antibody conjugated to peroxidase is then added and the plate incubated for 1 hour at 37°C. The plate is washed in PBS/Tween. ABTS (2,2′-azino di-[3-ethylbenzthiazoline sulphonate]), the substrate for peroxidase, is then added and the plate developed for 30 minutes at room temperature. The absorbance is then measured at 405 nm. A plot of absorbance against μg of antibody should be superimposable for the standard and the derivatized antibody.

2. Radioimmunoassay

A live-cell radioimmunoassay (RIA) can be carried out on both antigen-positive and antigen-negative cells. The radiolabeled antibody is added in serial dilution to a standard number of cells (e.g., 10^6/ml) in tissue culture medium (RPMI) containing 0.08% azide. Incubation for 1 hour at 37°C is followed by three RPMI washes. The cells are resuspended in the original volume and samples take for counting by liquid scintillation. A plot of counts bound/counts added against antibody concentration is then made and compared to that for the antibody labeled in a conventional manner (e.g., with ^{111}In or ^{125}I). No significant binding should be seen on the antigen-negative cells.

E. Animal Biodistribution

The animals used in this study were 2-month-old female beige nude mice. The mice were specific pathogen–free and housed in sterile filter-top cages with sterile bedding and maintained on irradiated diet and acidified water (pH 2.8) throughout the experiment.

The monoclonal antibody HMFG1 was raised against delipidated human milk fat globule: It is an IgG_1 class antibody directed against a large mucinlike molecule normally produced by the lactating human mammary epithelial cell. It has been found to react with both ovarian and breast carcinomas (21).

Mice were injected intraperitoneally with 14 μg of either HMFG1 or its $F(ab')_2$ fragment in 100 μl of PBS containing 1% HSA. These conjugates were labeled with ^{90}Y to specific activity of between 0.8 and 1.3 μCi/μg. At times varying from 1 hour to 5 days after antibody administration, groups of 5 mice were killed by partial exsanguination via cardiac puncture, and immediately dissected. Samples of kidney, liver, spleen, lung, femur, stomach (empty), small intestine (empty), skin, and heart were washed twice in PBS containing 250 units of heparin/100 ml, blotted dry, and weighed. Samples were never greater than 250 mg in weight. Blood and urine samples were also taken and weighed. Tissues were solubilized in 1 ml Soluene-350 (Packard) at 37°C overnight. The radioactivity was measured using a gamma-counter. This method is both accurate and simpler than liquid scintillation counting. The counting efficiency of the gamma-counter method was found to be approximately 8% by measuring a colorless ^{90}Y standard by both liquid scintillation and gamma counting. The linearity was determined by counting the activity of different weighted samples from the same liver before and after solubilization. The counts from nonsolubilized samples became nonlinear with weight after 150 mg, whereas the linearity of the solubilized samples was maintained up to weights greater than 250 mg, the largest tissue weight used in this study. Tissue activity was expressed as percentage of the injected dose per gram of wet tissue.

ACKNOWLEDGMENTS

The authors wish to express their appreciation to Ruth Parks for her cheerful cooperation throughout the preparation of this chapter and especially during its completion. We also wish to thank the Imperial Cancer Research Fund of London for financial assistance. One of us (DJH) also thanks the U.S. National Cancer Institute for financial assistance (CA 33029).

REFERENCES

1. Larson, S. M., Carrasquillo, J. A., and Reynolds, J. C. (1984) Radioimmunodetection and radioimmunotherapy. *Cancer Invest. 2*:363–381.
2. Epenetos, A. A., Courtenay-Luck, N. S., Halnan, K. E., et al. (1984) Antibody guided irradiation of malignant lesions: Three cases illustrating a new method of treatment. *Lancet 1*:1441–1443.
3. Epenetos, A. A., and 16 others. (1987) Antibody-guided irradiation of advanced ovarian cancer with intraperitoneally administered radiolabeled monoclonal antibodies. *J. Clin. Oncol. 5*:1890–1899.
4. Epenetos, A. A., Pickering, D., Hooker, G., Courtenay-Luck, N. S., Durbin, H., and McKenzie, C. G. (1985) Antibody guided irradiation of brain glioma by arterial infusion of radioactive monoclonal antibody against epidermal growth factor receptor and blood group A antigen. *British Medical Journal 290(6480)*:1463–1466.
5. Mach, J. P., Buchegger, F., Forni, M., et al. (1981) Use of radiolabeled monoclonal anti-CEA antibodies for the detection of human carcinomas by external photoscanning and tomoscintigraphy. *Immunol. Today 2*:239–249.
6. Chinol, M., and Hnatowich, D. J. (1987) Generator-produced yttrium-90 for radioimmunotherapy. *J. Nucl. Med. 28*:1465–1470.
7. Sullivan, D. C., Silva, J. S., Cox, C. E., et al. (1982) Localization of I-131-labeled goat and primate anti-carcinoembryonic antigen (CEA) antibodies in patients with cancer. *Invest. Radiol. 17*:350–355.
8. Wilbur, D. S., Jones, D. S., Fritzberg, A. R., et al. (1986) Radioiodination of monoclonal antibodies. Labeling with para-iodophenyl (PIP) derivatives for in vivo stability of the radioiodine label. *J. Nucl. Med. 27*:959 (abstract).
9. Hnatowich, D. J., Virzi, F., and Doherty, P. W. (1985) DTPA-coupled antibodies labeled with yttrium-90. *J. Nucl. Med. 26*:503–509.
10. Quadri, S. M., Paik, C. H., and Yokoyama, K. (1986) Biodistribution of an In-111 labeled antibody DTPA conjugate containing ester bonds. *J. Nucl. Med. 27*:959.
11. Haseman, M. K., et al. (1986) Metabolizable 111-Indium chelate conjugated anti-idiotype monoclonal antibody for radioimmunodetection of lymphoma in mice. *Eur. J. Nucl. Med. 12*:455–460.
12. Austegen, M., Schlimner, P., Wilhelm, P., Wilhelm, H., Trendelenburg, F., et al. (1984). Palliative therapy of tumor induced pleural effusions with *90*yttrium silicate. *Eur. J. Resp. Dis. 65*:64–67.
13. Wessels, B. W., and Rogus, R. D. (1984). Radionuclide selection and model absorbed dose calculations for radiolabeled tumor associated antibodies. *Med. Phys. 11*:638–645.
14. Vaughn, A. T. M., Keeling, A., and Yankuba, S. C. S. (1985) The production and biological distribution of yttrium-90 labeled antibodies. *Int. J. Appl. Radiat. Isot. 36*:803–806.
15. Washburn, L. C., Hwasun, T. T., Crook, J. E., et al. (1986) ^{90}Y-labeled monoclonal antibodies for cancer therapy. *Nucl. Med. Biol. 13*:453–456.

16. Anderson-Berg, W. E., Squire, R. A., and Strand, M. (1987) Specific radioimmunotherapy using ^{90}Y-labeled monoclonal antibody in erythroleukemic mice. *Cancer Res. 47*:1905–1912.
17. Covell, D. G., Barbet, J., Holton, O. D., et al. (1986) Pharmacokinetics of monoclonal immunoglobulin G1, $F(ab')_2$, and Fab′ in mice. *Cancer Res. 46*:3969–3978.
18. Sutherland, R., Buchegger, F., Schreyer, M., et al. (1987) Preparation and binding of radiolabeled anti-carcinoembryonic antigen binding fragments in human colon multicellular tumour spheroids. *Cancer Res. 47*:1627–1633.
19. Buchegger, F., Halpern, S. E., Sutherland, R. M., et al. (1986) In vitro and in vivo tumor models for studies of distribution of radiolabeled monoclonal antibodies and fragments. *Nucl. Med. 25*:207–209.
20. Snook, D., Rowlinson, G., and Epenetos, A. A. (1987) Preparation and in vivo study of yttrium-90 labeled immunoconjugates. *Nucl. Med. Comm. 8*: 257 (Abstract).
21. Taylor-Papadimitriou, J., Peterson, J. A., Arklie, J., et al. (1981) Monoclonal antibodies to epithelium-specific components of the human milk fat globule membrane: Production and reaction with cells in culture. *Int. J. Cancer 28*:17–21.
22. Hnatowich, D. J., Childs, R. L., Lanteigne, D., et al. (1985) The preparation of DTPA-coupled antibodies radiolabeled with metallic radionuclides: an improved method. *J. Imm. Method 65*:147–157.
23. Hnatowich, D. J., Griffin, T. W., and Kosciuczyk, C. (1985) Pharmacokinetics of an indium-111 labeled monoclonal antibody in cancer patients. *J. Nucl. Med. 26*:849–858.
24. Hnatowich, D. J., Gionet, M., Ruschowski, M., et al. (1988) Pharmacokinetics of indium-111 labeled OC-125 antibody in cancer patients—a comparison with the 19-9 antibody. *Can. Res.* (in press).
25. Stewart, S. (1987) Private communication.
26. Hnatowich, D. J., Chinol, M., Siebecker, D. A., et al. (1988) Biodistribution of intraperitoneal-administered antibody radio-labeled with yttrium-90. *J. Nucl. Med.*, (in press).
27. Order, S. E., Klein, J. L., Leichner, P. K., et al. (1986) Yttrium-90 antiferritin—a new therapeutic radiolabeled antibody. *Int. J. Radiation Oncology Biol. Phys. 12*:277–281.
28. Ward, B. G., Mather, S. J., et al. (1986) Prospects for antibody-targeted radiotherapy of cancer. *Lancet 1*:1441–1443.
29. Ward, B. G., Lowe, D. G., and Shepherd, J. H. (1987) Patterns of expression of a tumor associated antigen, defined by the monoclonal antibody HMFG2, in human epithelial ovarian carcinoma. Comparison with expression of HMFG1, AUA1 and F36/22 antigens. *Cancer 60*:787–793.
30. Snyder, W. S., Ford, M. R., Warner, G. G., and Watson, S. B. (1975) "S" absorbed dose per unit cumulated activity for selected radionuclides and organs. *MIRD pamphlet No 11*, New York, Published by the Society of Nuclear Medicine, Inc.

31. Epenetos, A. A., Snook, D. E., Durbin, H., et al. (1986) Limitations of radiolabeled monoclonal antibodies for localisation of human neoplasms. *Cancer Res. 46*:3183-3191.
32. Larson, S. M., Carrasquillo, J. A., McGuffin, R., et al. (1985) Use of I-131 labeled, murine Fab against a high molecular weight antigen of human melanoma: preliminary experience. *Radiology 155*:487–492.
33. Pressman, D. (1980) The development and use of radiolabeled antitumor antibodies. *Can. Res. 40*:2960-2964.
34. Sands, H., and Gallagher, B. M. Physiological, pharmacological and immunological aspects of antibody targeting. In *Antibodies in Radiodiagnosis and Therapy* (Zulatsky, M. R., Ed.). Baton Rouge, LA, CRC Press, in press.
35. Hnatowich, D. J., Virzi, F., and Ruskowski, M. (1987) Investigations of avidin and biotin for imaging applications. *J. Nucl. Med. 28*:1294-1302.
36. Sundberg, M. W., Meares, C. F., Goodwin, D. A., et al. (1974). Selective binding of metal ions to macromolecules using bifunctional analogs of EDTA. *J. Med. Chem. 17*:1304-1307.

Index